I0622989

SEASONAL AFFECTIVE DISORDER AND BEYOND

Light Treatment for SAD and Non-SAD Conditions

NATIONAL UNIVERSITY
LIBRARY   SAN DIEGO

SEASONAL AFFECTIVE DISORDER AND BEYOND

Light Treatment for SAD and Non-SAD Conditions

Edited by

RAYMOND W. LAM, M.D.

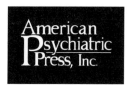

Washington, DC
London, England

Note: The authors have worked to ensure that all information in this book concerning drug dosages, schedules, and routes of administration is accurate as of the time of publication and consistent with standards set by the U.S. Food and Drug Administration and the general medical community. As medical research and practice advance, however, therapeutic standards may change. For this reason and because human and mechanical errors sometimes occur, we recommend that readers follow the advice of a physician who is directly involved in their care or the care of a member of their family.

Books published by the American Psychiatric Press, Inc., represent the views and opinions of the individual authors and do not necessarily represent the policies and opinions of the Press or the American Psychiatric Association.

Copyright © 1998 American Psychiatric Press, Inc.
ALL RIGHTS RESERVED
Manufactured in the United States of America on acid-free paper
01   00   99   98   4   3   2   1

First Edition
American Psychiatric Press, Inc.
1400 K Street, N.W., Washington, DC   20005
www.appi.org

Library of Congress Cataloging-in-Publication Data

Seasonal affective disorder and beyond : light treatment for SAD and
    non-SAD conditions / edited by Raymond W. Lam.
        p.   cm.
    Includes bibliographical references and index.
    ISBN 0-88048-867-0 (alk. paper)
    1. Seasonal affective disorder–Phototherapy.   2. Neuroses–
Phototherapy.   I. Lam, Raymond W., 1956–   .
    [DNLM: 1. Seasonal Affective Disorder–therapy.   2. Phototherapy–
methods.   3. Depressive Disorder–therapy.   4. Bulimia–therapy.
5. Sleep Disorders–therapy.   6. Circadian Rhythm.   WM 171 S4385
1988]
RC545.S42   1998
616.85'27–dc21
DNLM/DLC
for Library of Congress   97-47208
                                                                CIP

British Library Cataloguing in Publication Data
A CIP record is available from the British Library.

CONTENTS

LIST OF CONTRIBUTORS

David H. Avery, M.D.
Associate Professor, Department of Psychiatry and Behavioral Sciences, University of Washington School of Medicine, Seattle, WA, U.S.A.

George C. Brainard, Ph.D.
Professor of Neurology and Professor of Biochemistry and Molecular Pharmacology, Jefferson Medical College, Philadelphia, PA, U.S.A.

Ziad Boulos, Ph.D.
Senior Scienetist, Institute for Circadian Physiology, Cambridge, MA, U.S.A.

Scott S. Campbell, Ph.D.
Department of Psychiatry, Laboratory of Human Chronobiology, Cornell University Medical College, White Plains, NY, U.S.A.

Elliot M. Goldner, M.D.
Assistant Professor of Psychiatry, University of British Columbia; St. Paul's Hospital, Vancouver, BC, Canada

Rod J. Hughes, Ph.D.
Director, Chronobiology and Sleep Laboratory, Air Force Research Laboratory-HEPM, Brooks AFB, TX, U.S.A.

Daniel F. Kripke, M.D.
Professor of Psychiatry, Department of Psychiatry, University of California, San Diego; Sam and Rose Stein Institute for Research on Aging, La Jolla, CA, U.S.A.

Raymond W. Lam, M.D.
Associate Professor of Psychiatry and Head, Division of Mood Disorders, University of British Columbia; Vancouver Hospital & Health Sciences Centre, Vancouver, BC, Canada

Anthony J. Levitt, M.D.
Associate Professor, Department of Psychiatry and Department of Nutritional Sciences, University of Toronto; Sunnybrook Hospital, Toronto, ON, Canada

Alfred J. Lewy, M.D., Ph.D.
Professor, Departments of Psychiatry, Pharmacology, and Ophthalmology; Sleep and Mood Disorders Laboratory, Oregon Health Sciences University, Portland, OR, U.S.A.

Michael J. Norden, M.D.
Clinical Associate Professor , Department of Psychiatry and Behavioral
Sciences, University of Washington School of Medicine, Seattle, WA,
U.S.A.

Barbara L. Parry, M.D.
Associate Professor of Psychiatry, Department of Psychiatry, University of
California, San Diego, La Jolla, CA, U.S.A.

Edwin M. Tam, M.D.
Clinical Assistant Professor of Psychiatry, Division of Mood Disorders,
University of British Columbia; Vancouver Hospital and Health Sciences
Centre, Vancouver, BC, Canada

Michael Terman, Ph.D.
Professor, Department of Psychiatry, Columbia University; New York State
Psychiatric Institute, and Center for Environmental Therapeutics, New
York, NY, U.S.A.

Virginia A. Wesson, M.D.
Research Associate, Department of Psychiatry, McMaster University;
Hamilton Psychiatric Hospital, Hamilton, ON, Canada

Lakshmi N. Yatham, M.D.
Assistant Professor of Psychiatry, Division of Mood Disorders, University
of British Columbia; Vancouver Hospital and Health Sciences Centre,
Vancouver, BC, Canada

Athanasios P. Zis, M.D.
Professor of Psychiatry and Head, Department of Psychiatry, University of
British Columbia; Vancouver Hospital & Health Sciences Centre,
Vancouver, BC, Canada

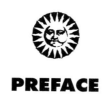

PREFACE

Raymond W. Lam, M.D.

In 1994, when organizing a symposium on light therapy for the Annual Meeting of the American Psychiatric Association, I realized that a decade had passed since the publication of the article on seasonal affective disorder (SAD) and light therapy by Dr. Norman Rosenthal and colleagues (Rosenthal et al. 1984). Their 1984 paper first sparked my interest in the biologic and therapeutic effects of light in mood disorders. Obviously I was not alone—several hundred research articles on SAD and light therapy have since been published. A number of other developments also signaled the emergence of this new research field. The Society for Light Treatment and Biological Rhythms, a nonprofit organization dedicated to the promotion of research and clinical application of light and chronobiology, was established in 1987. In 1988, *Current Contents* (a bibliography and citation service) identified SAD, light treatment, and chronobiology as some of the most rapidly expanding areas of biomedical research (Garfield 1988). By 1991, Seasonal Affective Disorder was added as a Medical Subject Heading to the Medline computer database in recognition of the many publications on winter depression and light therapy. Finally, in 1993, the Rosenthal article was designated a "Citation Classic" by *Current Contents* by virtue of more than 385 citations in other publications, indicating its stature as a seminal research paper (Rosenthal 1993).

Although SAD was the initial clinical focus for light therapy, the therapeutic use of light has expanded well beyond treatment of seasonal depression. The clinical interest in light has extended along research lines based on the identification of other seasonal syndromes (e.g., bulimia nervosa) and on the effects of light on human circadian rhythms (e.g., sleep disorders, jet lag and shift work disorders, premenstrual disorders). However, the biologic effects of light are numerous, and there is also increasing interest in using light to treat nonseasonal, noncircadian disorders (e.g., nonseasonal depression).

This book addresses the expanded clinical interest in therapeutic effects of light. The contributing authors are respected clinical researchers who are actively studying light treatment. The chapters provide both a summary of the literature—what is known and not known—and details of new findings. Thus, this book should prove useful to clinicians (those who are using light therapy, and those who would like to add light therapy to their treatment repertoire) and to researchers in the field. Basic scientists in the area of biological rhythm and light research will be very interested in the "end result" of their research, and clinical scientists will benefit from the critical appraisals of methodology used in studies. Finally, our students and knowledgeable consumers will also be interested in this succinct volume which summarizes current opinion on the scientific aspects of light treatment.

We begin with Dr. Brainard's chapter on biological and physical properties of light. He reminds us that although light is omnipresent, there are numerous methods for measuring and quantifying the effects of light. What is most easily measured and understood (e.g., lux, the measurement of illumination used in most light studies) may not necessarily be most relevant for understanding the biological or therapeutic mechanisms of light.

The next five chapters discuss the use of light therapy for seasonal and nonseasonal depressive disorders. Drs. Wesson and Levitt summarize the light therapy studies in SAD, with an emphasis on the controversial topics of placebo response and critical parameters of light therapy. Despite some conflicting data, the evidence for efficacy of light in SAD is certainly greater than for many interventions that are in wide clinical use in psychiatry (and other medical disciplines, for that matter). Dr. Terman then tackles new ways of thinking about the therapeutic effects of light on seasonal symptoms. He also suggests important future research directions for light treatment.

The initial interest in light therapy arose from photoperiodic models for depression. However, Dr. Tam and colleagues remind us that the therapeutic effects of light on SAD may involve biological effects other than through circadian mechanisms. They review psychobiological studies of light effects in SAD, with a particular emphasis on the serotonergic effects of bright light. These findings may be most important for understanding the use of light in the treatment of psychiatric disorders in which serotonin dysregulation is implicated (including nonseasonal depression, bulimia nervosa, and premenstrual depression).

Drs. Avery and Norden go on to present a dimensional approach to seasonality by discussing subsyndromal SAD, with studies suggesting that light therapy is also effective in this seasonal group. Because subsyndromal SAD is likely more prevalent than SAD in the general population (affecting up to 15% of the population in more northerly latitudes), the public health implications for treating subsyndromal SAD are potentially very important. Dr. Kripke follows with a provocative chapter exploring the evidence for light treatment of nonseasonal depression. He argues that light therapy should be more widely used as adjunctive or alternative treatment for patients with nonseasonal mood disorders.

Following are two chapters about light treatment for other psychiatric syndromes. Dr. Parry summarizes studies on light therapy for premenstrual depression, with a focus on chronobiological mechanisms. Dr. Goldner and I review the growing literature on seasonality of eating disorders and our studies of light therapy for bulimia nervosa.

A joint Task Force of the Society for Light Treatment and Biological Rhythms and the American Sleep Disorders Association, chaired by Dr. Michael Terman, recently published their report on the use of light for treating sleep disorders as a special issue in the *Journal of Biological Rhythms* (1995). Members of the Task Force highlight the chronobiological effects of light in the next chapters of this book. Drs. Hughes and Lewy include a comprehensive summary of the use of light and melatonin to treat sleep disorders involving disturbances of circadian phase. Dr. Boulos then reviews studies of light treatment for jet lag and shift work disorders, followed by Dr. Campbell describing his studies of light treatment for insomnia in the elderly. The final chapter includes some of my comments on the important clinical issues raised by the chapter contributors.

I also want to acknowledge and thank those people who were important to me in the preparation of this book: Dr. Ronald A. Remick for igniting my clinical interest in mood disorders, Dr. J. Christian Gillin and Dr. Daniel F. Kripke for their research mentorship and career support, my colleagues for contributing chapters for this book, and, finally, to my wife and partner, Tracy A. Defoe, for her patience and encouragement throughout this project.

References

Garfield E: Chronobiology: An internal clock for all seasons. Part 2. Current research on seasonal affective disorder and phototherapy. Current Contents 2:3–9, January 11, 1988

Journal of Biological Rhythms (Special Issue): Task Force Report on Light Treatment for Sleep Disorders. J Biol Rhythms 10:99–176, 1995

Rosenthal NE: This week's citation classic: a decade of SAD and light therapy. Current Contents 10:8, March 8, 1993

Rosenthal NE, Sack DA, Gillin JC, et al: Seasonal affective disorder: a description of the syndrome and preliminary findings with light therapy. Arch Gen Psychiatry 41:72–80, 1984

ONE

The Healing Light:
Interface of Physics and Biology

George C. Brainard, Ph.D.

For the rest of my life I will reflect on what light is.
—*Albert Einstein, 1917*

All the fifty years of conscious brooding have brought me no closer
to answer the question, "What are light quanta?" Of course today
every rascal thinks he knows the answer, but he is deluding himself.
—*Albert Einstein, 1951*

Light is nothing short of miraculous. Light makes our world luminous, dazzles our senses, and quietly controls the chemical tides in

The author appreciates the generous assistance of Robert Levin, Ph.D, (Table 1–3) and
Sharon Miller (Figure 1–4) for supplying some of the radiometric details and editorial com-
ments; Raymond W. Lam, M.D., Gerald Grunwald, Ph.D., David Sliney, Ph.D., Robert Landry,
Michael Baumholtz, and Arthur Zajonc, Ph.D., for scientific review; and John Hanifin and Laine
Brainard for manuscript preparation and editorial review. The author extends special thanks to
Robert L. Fucci Jr. for his substantive input on the form and content of the manuscript. This re-
search was supported in part by FDA Grant #785346, NIMH Grant #MH-44890, NASA
Grant #NAGW1196, the National Electrical Manufacturer's Association (#LRI 89:DR:1), the
Lighting Research Institute (#LRI 88:SP:LREF:6), USUHS Grant # R07049, Jefferson's
Dean's Overage Research Program, and the Philadelphia Chapter of the Illuminating Engineer-
ing Society. Finally, none of this work would have been possible without the inspired guidance
of William Lederer and Christopher Bird.

our bodies. Humans are predominantly visual creatures—from moment to moment our waking consciousness is filled with the sense of vision. Little wonder, then, that exploring the behavior of light and color has been a passion for philosophers and scientists for two millennia or more. The finest minds from Plato to Goethe and from Newton to Einstein have puzzled over the mystery of light and its interaction with the human eye (Zajonc 1993).

In contrast to the sense of vision, nonvisual responses to light are less obvious to humans and tend not to enter everyday awareness. Our physiological and hormonal rhythms can be powerfully controlled by light, but these events remain subtle to the conscious mind, which is often preoccupied with the myriad sensations of the external world. Perhaps because it is less immediately obvious, the scientific study of the internal, biological effects of light is much more recent—spanning only a small handful of decades—compared to centuries of study on the physics of light and the physiology of vision. Despite its relative youth, this field of study is an important frontier of science in which light may increasingly be harnessed as a therapeutic force (Wetterberg 1993).

The ancient Egyptians, Romans, and Greeks, among other distant cultures, revered the healing power of light. Throughout recorded history, many different methods have been developed for treating disease, trauma, and human dysfunction with different qualities of light (Birren 1961; Kaiser 1984; Lieberman 1991; Ott 1973). At times, these practices were in the domain of mysticism, sometimes being connected to religious or spiritual beliefs. Traditionally, the scientific community has been ambivalent or skeptical about the various claims made for the healing potency of light and color. What, then, is different about the use of light for therapeutic purposes today? A major compelling difference is the application of controlled empirical methods for testing the efficacy of light treatment. Increasingly, the data from careful experimentation are yielding a clear result: light can heal specific physical and mental dysfunctions and restore human health. Thus, the community of scientists working on this frontier appears to be confirming what philosophers and mystics have proposed over the centuries. The chapters of this book explore the growing data that indicate that light may be used to alleviate the depressed mind, resolve

TABLE 1–1

Therapeutic applications of radiant energy in humans

Therapeutic applications	Ultraviolet (200–400 nm)	Visible light (380–760 nm)	Infrared (760–3,000 nm)
Phototherapy	Psoriasis	Bilirubinemia	Radiant heating
	Photodynamic therapy	Photodynamic therapy	
	Herpes simplex	Seasonal depression	
	Vitiligo	Nonseasonal depression	
	Dentistry	Circadian disruptions (e.g.) Shift work Jet lag	
		Sleep disorders	
		Menstrual cycle disturbances	
		Low-level laser (?) Wound healing Pain	Low-level laser (?) Wound healing Pain
		Chromotherapy (?)	
Photosurgery[1]		Laser surgery (e.g.) Retinal detachment Glaucoma Tattoo removal[1]	Laser surgery (e.g.) Retinal detachment Glaucoma Tattoo removal[1]

[1] These therapeutic applications of radiant energy are not based on classical photobiological mechanisms, because they occur at higher than normal physiological temperatures. Therapies that remain controversial are indicated by a question mark.

sleep disruption, normalize eating problems, quiet mood swings, ameliorate menstrual dysfunctions, and stabilize the disrupted rhythms of shift workers and jet travelers.

Currently, light is used as a therapeutic tool for many medical applications. Table 1–1 summarizes the range of how light can be used to heal human disease. In some cases, light is employed as a medical tool to destroy tissues. Examples of this include laser surgery, cauterization of bleeding vessels, and destruction of tumors. In these examples, the energy of light is sufficiently intense to sever, burn, or eradicate living tissue (Sliney and Wolbarsht 1980). In contrast, other medical uses of light rely on nonthermal, photobiological mechanisms for healing diseased tissues or organisms.

As research determines the efficacy and utility of the newer forms of light therapy, it becomes increasingly important to clarify the underlying biological mechanisms that mediate the therapeutic benefits of light. Presumably, for each of the maladies discussed in the following chapters, light works as a healing agent via nonthermal, photobiological principles. Indeed, as light is found to have a specific therapeutic value for a given disorder, there is a fundamental underlying event that triggers the healing response. *Specifically, for any photobiologically driven healing to occur, the first cause is the singular event of a photon being absorbed by an organic molecule that initiates a cascade of biological events that ultimately results in restoration of physiological homeostasis and biological/psychological health.* Thus, photobiologically driven healing relies on the interface between the physical nature of light and human biochemistry. It follows, then, that those interested in these therapies must consider the fundamentals of light energy as well as the fundamentals of how living tissues respond to light.

Quantifying Light

Photobiology is based on the interaction between optical radiation and living organisms. Specifically, the science of photobiology involves the study of how the infrared, visible, and ultraviolet (UV) portions of the electromagnetic spectrum influence biological processes (Horspool and Song 1994; Smith 1989). Light can be considered from different viewpoints, as Table 1–2 illustrates. Light can be understood in experiential terms of color and appearance, or in more physical terms of wavelengths and photons.

Most individuals prefer to think about and discuss light from an experiential perspective—its apparent color and brightness. This way of describing light is serviceable for purposes of general communication, but it is less useful as a descriptor in photobiology. It is important, however, to recognize that the specific photopigments and photoreceptor mechanisms for transducing light stimuli for therapeutic purposes have yet to be identified (Brainard et al. 1993). Until the

TABLE 1-2

Photobiologically active portion of the electromagnetic spectrum: spectral bandwidths, wavelengths, and photon energies

Spectral band width (color appearance)	Wavelength range	Photon energy (eV)
Far-infrared (IR-C)	1,000–3 μm	0.001–0.413
Middle-infrared (IR-B)	3–1.4 μm	0.413–0.886
Near-infrared (IR-A)	1.4–0.76 μm	0.886–1.63
Visible range	760–380 nm	1.63–3.26
Red	760–610 nm	1.63–2.03
Orange	610–585 nm	2.03–2.12
Yellow	585–575 nm	2.12–2.16
Yellow–green	575–530 nm	2.16–2.34
Green	530–495 nm	2.34–2.50
Blue–green	495–485 nm	2.50–2.56
Blue	485–465 nm	2.56–2.67
Violet (indigo)	465–380 nm (460–440 nm)	2.67–3.26 (2.70–2.82)
Near-ultraviolet (UV-A)	400–315 nm	3.10–3.94
Middle-ultraviolet (UV-B)	315–280 nm	3.94–4.43
Far-ultraviolet (UV-C)	280–100 nm	4.43–12.4

Note. The infrared bandwidths, visible range, and ultraviolet bandwidths are defined by the Commission Internationale de l'Eclairage (1987). The specific color limits in this table are approximate (Kelly 1943). Many authors no longer include the color appearance of indigo as separate from violet, but its wavelength range and photon energy are included in parentheses.

specific underlying photoreceptor system(s) for light therapy is determined, the optimum technique for specifying and measuring the light used in therapy will be somewhat arbitrary.

There are two broad categories of light measurement techniques: radiometric and photometric (Illuminating Engineering Society 1993). Each measurement technique has its merits and drawbacks relative to light therapy. Radiometry is based exclusively on the physical properties of light—its energy and wavelength. A radiometer measures the radiant power of a light source over a defined range of wavelengths. Figure 1–1 illustrates an example of a radiometer detector response that measures radiant power from the middle UV spectrum (290 nm) into the near-infrared spectrum (770 nm). Radiometers can

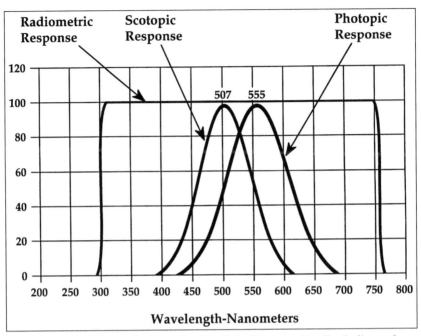

FIGURE 1–1. Response functions for three light detectors. One line indicates the characteristic response of a radiometer that has a flat sensitivity from 310 nm to 750 nm. The two other curves represent photometric responses for photopic lux and scotopic lux, based on the Commission Internationale de l'Eclairage standard observer (Commission Internationale de l'Eclairage 1987).

be configured to measure different bandwidths across the electromagnetic spectrum. The wavelengths within the designated bandwidth can be detected equally, as shown in Figure 1–1, or they can be filtered for differential sensitivity across the various wavelengths. Instead of detecting the total radiant energy emitted across a defined waveband, spectroradiometers are used to characterize the energies of specific wavelengths emitted by lamps and light sources. In terms of light therapy, spectroradiometers provide a spectral power distribution (SPD), or the radiant power per unit wavelength emitted by the therapeutic device. This information can be useful in comparing various light therapy devices that emit different combinations of wavelengths.

Radiometric quantification of stimuli is particularly important for research as opposed to clinical purposes in light therapy. Comparisons between data on treatment efficacy obtained with different therapeutic light devices can be facilitated when radiometric values of the stimulus along with the wavelength characterization of the stimulus are reported. Increased availability of radiometric data also will ultimately help clarify comparisons of treatment efficacy and the photoreceptive process that mediates light therapy. When using a radiometer to quantify the energy from a light therapy device, however, it is important to understand that a radiometer measures all wavelengths within its sensitivity range whether or not those wavelengths have any therapeutic potency.

In contrast to radiometry, photometry is based on the selective responsiveness of the human visual system (Commission Internationale de l'Eclairage 1987; Illuminating Engineering Society 1993). A photometer is a radiometer that has filters added to the detector that "shape" the detector sensitivity to resemble the luminance (brightness) response of the human visual system. Thus, photometry is a special branch of radiometry. Figure 1–1 illustrates the well-characterized visual responses: photopic (or day vision) and scotopic (or night vision). Between individual humans, there are substantial differences in visual responses. The curves shown in Figure 1–1 represent sketches of the average response curves for the "standard observer" as determined by the Commission Internationale de l'Eclairage (1987). The photopic and scotopic visual functions are defined with reference to the adaptive state of the rod and cone photoreceptors in the human retina. Radiometers can be filtered to detect only those relative proportions of wavelengths that compose the photopic or scotopic visual response. Such photometers will detect photopic lux or scotopic lux, respectively. Specifically defined, lux is a measure of illuminance—the amount of light, or luminous flux, falling on a surface. One photopic lux is one lumen per square meter (lm/m^2).

Most investigators have operated from the assumption that light therapy is mediated via a photoreceptive mechanism in the human eye as opposed to a photoreceptive mechanism in the skin or some other part of the body. Indeed, in terms of light therapy for seasonal affective disorder (SAD) (Wehr et al. 1987), and in terms of light stimulation of the circadian and neuroendocrine systems of mammals and humans (Aschoff 1981; Binkley 1990; Klein et al. 1991;

Wetterberg 1993), there is experimental data supporting this assumption. What remains unproved is whether the photoreceptive mechanism that mediates light therapy is similar or identical to the photoreceptive system that mediates the sensory capacity of vision.

In 1996 an intriguing theory proposed that blood-borne elements in the eye might be responsible for transducing photic stimuli for circadian and neuroendocrine regulation (Oren 1996). Two landmark studies have drawn considerable attention to this theory. First, it was deomonstrated that there are multiple, independent photoreceptive circadian clocks distributed throughout the bodies of fruit flies (*Drosophila*) (plautz et al. 1997). Subsequently, it was reported that a single 3-hour briht light pulse of 13,000 lux delivered to the backs of the knees of healthy human subjects systematically reset circadian rhythms of body temperature and melatonin (Campbell and Murphy 1998). Thus photoreception for circadian regulation in humans may not employ visual photoreceptors, and the eye may not be the exclusive site for circadian photoreception.

Over the past 15 years, scientists and clinicians working with light therapy have predominantly used a photometric description and measurement system—specifically photopic photometry. Thus, test subjects or patients are given light treatment at a specified illuminance (photopic lux) for a specific length of time. Consequently, the elements of photopic lux and exposure time are the principal ingredients in formulating the intended "dose" of light. Similarly, the various light therapy devices are characterized as providing illuminances at a given distance or on a given surface. Light therapy devices have also been characterized photometrically as emitting a level of luminous intensity (candelas), luminous flux (lumens), or luminance (candelas per square meter). It is useful to distinguish between the illuminance provided by a light therapy device versus the device's luminance. Currently, illuminance measures (lux) are the standard in the field of light therapy and are taken with a standard photometer at the level of the human cornea. In contrast, luminance is related to the perceived "brightness" of the light source and is measured with a more sophisticated device, a telephotometer, which has optics for imaging the light-emitting surface. Two light sources with two very different luminances can produce an equal illuminance at the level of the human cornea. For example, a small, bright lamp can provide the same corneal illuminance as a large white reflecting wall that appears considerably less bright. The radiometric terms for irradiance and radiance are parallel to the photometric terms of illuminance and luminance, with the key difference being that the radiometric quantities are measured without the bias of the sensitivity characteristics of the human eye.

Although most light therapy scientists adhere to the International System of Units (SI), which specifies lux, candelas, and lumens as the preferred terminology for photometric measurement, some authors have described light therapy in terms of the older photometric terminology that includes footcandles for illuminance and footlamberts for luminance. It is easy to convert the older photometric measures to the preferred SI photometric units. If light therapy is described in terms of footcandles, multiply the footcandle number by 10.76 to obtain the lux value. If there is need to change a lux value to footcandles for comparative purposes, multiply the number of lux by 0.093 to obtain the footcandle value.

The photopic photometric system provides a serviceable nomenclature and measurement technique for describing light therapy, but its use implies that the community of professionals involved with light therapy accepts that the human visual system, and specifically the daylight-sensitive or photopic visual system, is responsible for mediating light therapy. As will be discussed later, not only is this acceptance unproved, but data have emerged that make the assumption questionable. Although it remains reasonable to *hypothesize* that the daytime, or photopic, visual system mediates the effects of light therapy, the traditional use of photopic measurement values should not be misconstrued as general acceptance that this hypothesis has been proved. Just as a radiometer may measure the energy of wavelengths that are not relevant to the efficacy of light therapy, photometers may not detect wavelengths that are relevant to the therapeutic response. Similarly, photometers may detect wavelengths relevant to therapy but measure their energies in the wrong proportion.

For example, what would be the consequences of the discovery that a single cone—for the sake of argument, the blue cone—was responsible for mediating all the therapeutic effects of light? Such a discovery would mean that all previous publications based solely on lux values would be misrepresenting the dosage of light applied to patients or test subjects. Specifically, in this scenario, the lux readings would have significantly underrepresented energies in the blue, indigo, and violet portions of the spectrum, overrepresented the green and yellow portions of the spectrum, and incorporated energies in the red portion of the spectrum that are irrelevant to the efficacy of therapy. This example is *not* meant to suggest that there is better evidence for a single cone versus a photopic or three-cone mechanism mediating light therapy. The sole purpose of this example is to illustrate the potential measurement problems the professionals in the light therapy community may have. Such difficulties in measurement will be resolved only when the photobiological physiology that mediates light therapy is clarified.

If photometric descriptors and measures are not the best system for light therapy, what is? Because there is no clear answer to that question, it remains reasonable to continue using photometric terminology and measurements for light therapy. It is important to remember, however, that the use of the photometric standard is arbitrary, and when the underlying photoreceptive mechanism is determined, this nomenclature and measuring system may need to be revised. Meanwhile, whenever possible, investigators may consider providing some radiometric detail along with their standard photometric values. This added information will enable investigators to trace back to the electromagnetic energies that were applied clinically and experimentally. Specifically, it is optimum to provide the spectral power distribution along with irradiance or photon density emitted by the light therapy device. Lamps can vary quite significantly in their radiance and spectral output because of factors such as lamp aging, operating temperature, manufacturing changes, and the like (Illuminating Engineering Society 1993). Thus, direct measures on the specific therapeutic equipment used in a given study are always preferable to referencing previously published values from manufacturers or other laboratories. If it is not feasible to make direct measurements because of a lack of available radiometric equipment, then, minimally, the therapeutic lamp type along with its operating system should be identified. Rough conversions of photometric values into radiometric values are also possible, as indicated in Table 1–3. These conversions, however, will only approximate the real radiometric values for the light sources indicated.

TABLE 1-3

Factors for converting photometric to radiometric values for selected light sources

multiply lux of → to obtain ↓ by ↗	Average daylight sun & sky 5,500 K CRI 100	Incandescent 3,000 K CRI 100	Cool white fluorescent 4,200 K CRI 65	Daylight fluorescent 6,300 K CRI 75	"Full-spectrum" fluorescent 5,500 K CRI 91	Tri-phosphor fluorescent 4,100 K CRI 75
Irradiance (μW/cm^2)	0.50	0.60	0.30	0.33	0.38	0.30
Quantum density (photons/sec/cm^2)	1.4×10^{12}	1.9×10^{12}	8.1×10^{11}	8.9×10^{11}	1.1×10^{12}	8.2×10^{11}

Note. The radiometric measures in this table are for a 290–770 nm bandwidth. CRI indicates the Color Rendering Index, while K indicates the Corrected Color Temperature. Although conversions made using this table will yield reasonable estimates of radiometric and photometric values, direct measurements are preferable.

Source. Portions of the data in this table were provided by Robert Levin, Ph.D. (personal communication), and the Durotest Corporation (Form 955-7711U, 1977).

Photobiological Principles
Relevant to Light Therapy

Light therapy is based on the interface between the physical energy of the electromagnetic spectrum and the biochemistry of the human eye. In general, a relatively restricted portion of the electromagnetic spectrum—the middle and near-ultraviolet, the visible and the near-infrared wavebands—mediates all photobiological responses. Certainly, other portions of the electromagnetic spectrum can induce changes in living organisms. For example, wavelengths shorter than 200 nm can ionize cellular molecules, whereas wavelengths longer than 1.4 μm can heat or burn tissues. Those processes induce biological change that ultimately may lead to the destruction of the living organism. Nearly all of the species inhabiting the earth have evolved specific photobiological physiology that allow them to survive by using UV, visible, or infrared solar energies. Single-celled organisms and higher-order plants capture light energy to produce food. In contrast, fish, birds, and mammals do not use sunlight to generate nutrients directly. Instead, these creatures use light to mediate visual sensation and to regulate daily and seasonal rhythms.

Despite a wide diversity of processes by which living organisms use visible and near-visible electromagnetic energy for survival, nearly all living species share a common feature in their ability to respond to light stimuli. All photobiological responses are mediated by specific organic molecules that absorb photons and then undergo physiochemical changes that ultimately lead to an overall physiological change in the organism (Horspool and Song 1994; Smith 1989). Organic molecules that absorb light energy and initiate photobiological responses are called *chromophores,* or *photopigments.* This basic photobiological process is called *phototransduction.* The example shown in Figure 1–2 is based on the photopigment rhodopsin, which is responsible for initiating a cascade of biochemical changes within rod cells of the retina that ultimately leads to the sensory capacity of night, or scotopic, vision. Rhodopsin is composed of a protein portion called *opsin* that combines with an organic compound formed from vitamin A called *retinal*. The retinal is actually the light-absorbing part of the rhodopsin complex. Figure 1–2 provides a diagrammatic sketch of phototransduction, which is the fundamental photobiological event of a chromophore molecule absorbing a photon and undergoing a conformational modification. In general, different chromophores, or photopigments, do not absorb energy equally across the electromagnetic spectrum. Each chromophore molecule has a characteristic absorption spectrum that depends on that molecule's atomic structure. For example, in the case of the human rhodopsin photopigment, there are three peaks of electromagnetic energy absorbance. The rhodopsin absorption spectrum has a large, broad peak at 498 nm (α peak), in the visible portion of the spectrum; a smaller, broad peak at 340 nm (β peak), in the near-ultraviolet range; and a strong, sharp peak at 278 nm (γ peak), in the far-ultraviolet range (Wald 1955).

In considering light therapy from the photobiological viewpoint, it is important to understand the principle of an action spectrum. Strictly defined, an action spectrum is the relative response of an organism to different wavelengths. The concept of action spectra was first introduced in the nineteenth century when plant biologists observed that plant growth depends on the spectrum of light to which the plant is exposed. In more recent times, photobiologists have evolved a refined set of acceptable practices and guidelines to determine action spectra that are applicable to all organisms from simple plants to complex animals such as humans (Coohill 1991; Horspool and Song 1994; Smith 1989). Although it is not a trivial task to develop a complete action spectrum, there are both pragmatic and scientific benefits to determining the action spectrum for light therapy.

Generally, an action spectrum is determined by establishing a set of dose-response curves (fluence-response curves) at different monochromatic wavelengths for a specific biological response. The action spectrum is then formed by plotting the reciprocal of incident photons required to produce the biological response versus wavelength. Despite the potential difficulty of developing action spectra, this fundamental photobiological technique has high utility. In the case of light therapy, an action spectrum will determine the best combination of wavelengths that should be emitted from light therapy equipment to optimize treatment efficacy. Additionally, determining an action spectrum for light therapy will help to identify the underlying photoreceptor physiology that mediates the therapeutic benefits of light.

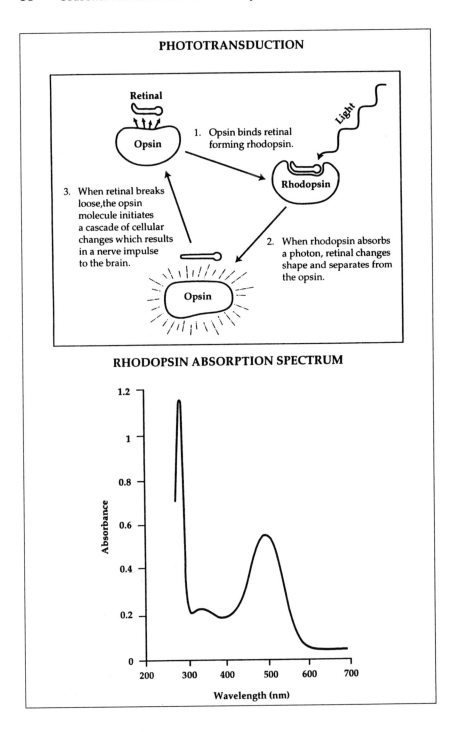

PHOTOTRANSDUCTION

Retinal

Opsin

Light

1. Opsin binds retinal forming rhodopsin.

Rhodopsin

3. When retinal breaks loose, the opsin molecule initiates a cascade of cellular changes which results in a nerve impulse to the brain.

2. When rhodopsin absorbs a photon, retinal changes shape and separates from the opsin.

Opsin

RHODOPSIN ABSORPTION SPECTRUM

Absorbance

Wavelength (nm)

It is important to recognize that all the different types of light therapy discussed in this book may not share a single photoreceptor mechanism. Thus, the photopigment(s) that mediates the therapeutic benefits of light therapy for winter depression may not be the same photopigment(s) that mediates light-induced phase shifting of shift workers' circadian rhythms. In a parallel example, the human visual system has at least three separate action spectra for visual responses at different levels of light adaptation. The action spectra for scotopic (night) vision and photopic (day) vision are quite similar to the photometric response curves illustrated in Figure 1–1. Not shown in that figure is a distinct set of action spectra for mesopic vision, or vision in twilight levels of illumination. Scotopic vision appears to be mediated by a single chromophore (rhodopsin) in a single photoreceptor cell type (rods), as illustrated in Figure 1–2. There is a close match between the action spectrum for scotopic vision and the absorption spectrum of rhodopsin in the visible portion of the spectrum. The scotopic action spectrum is not completely identical to the rhodopsin absorption spectrum because of how light is modified as it is transmitted through ocular media and retinal cells. In contrast, photopic vision is mediated by three different chromophores (cyanolabe, chlorolabe, and erythrolabe) in three different cone cells (the short wavelength–sensitive, or blue, cone; the middle wavelength–sensitive, or green, cone; and the long wavelength–sensitive, or red, cone, respectively). The action spectrum for photopic vision does not match the absorption spectrum of any one of the cone photopigments. Instead, the three cone mechanisms work together with the entire visual system pathway to produce the action spectrum for day vision, which

FIGURE **1–2.** *(opposite)* The efficacy of light as a therapeutic agent for humans ultimately depends on the activation of a photobiological process. This sketch illustrates a simplified example of the physicochemical change that a chromophore molecule goes through as it absorbs a photon—an event that is fundamental to all photobiological responses. This specific example is of the photopigment rhodopsin, which undergoes a conformational change as it absorbs a photon. This photochemical event initiates a cascade of biochemical changes within rod cells of the retina that ultimately leads to the sensory capacity of scotopic or night vision. The graph to the right illustrates the absorption spectrum for rhodopsin and is adapted from Wald 1955.

is essentially represented in Figure 1–1 by the photopic response curve. From these examples in the visual system, it should be clear that one or more chromophores may mediate a given photobiological response. Thus, if only a single photopigment mediates a given type of light therapy, then it is reasonable to predict that the action spectrum for that therapy will resemble the absorption spectrum of the underlying chromophore. Alternatively, if two or more photopigments mediate the benefits of light therapy, the action may not resemble a single chromophore absorption spectrum.

From Photons and Molecules to Human Health

One of the beauties of light is its capacity to restore human health. Until recently, psychologists and psychiatrists had little reason to be concerned with the physics of light, the principals of radiometry, and the organic chemistry of chromophores. In 1982, however, a case study was published that has ultimately created an upheaval in the community of clinicians who treat patients with various mood and affective disorders. It was found that a patient who experienced depression annually during the fall and winter months seemed to improve from daily treatment with bright light exposure (Kern and Lewy 1990; Lewy et al. 1982). That single observation opened the door for defining the SAD syndrome and extensive testing of the efficacy of bright light therapy (American Psychiatric Association 1994; Rosenthal et al. 1984). Since that time, considerable research has been directed toward determining the specific lighting parameters and exposure techniques for light treatment of winter depression (Rosenthal and Blehar 1989; Rosenthal et al. 1988; Terman and Terman 1992; Terman et al. 1989a; Wesson and Levitt, this volume). Although there are continuing disputes over the optimum method for light treatment of this affective disorder, there is a general consensus that this therapy is effective for many patients who are afflicted with SAD (Society for Light Treatment and Biological Rhythms 1991; Rosenthal 1993).

During the past 15 years, the majority of studies on light therapy have been concerned with treating winter depression. Other research, however, has sought to extend the applications of light therapy. Investigators have had some success in treating nonseasonal depression with light therapy (Kripke, this volume; Kripke et al. 1989). In addition, light therapy may benefit individuals with specific sleep disorders (Campbell, this volume; Rosenthal et al. 1990; Terman et al., this volume), difficulties associated with the menstrual cycle (Kripke 1993; Parry, this volume), or eating disorders (Lam and Goldner, this volume; Lam et al. 1994). Beyond these specific clinical disorders, light therapy is being evaluated for its capacity to resolve health and performance problems resulting from the desynchronization of biological rhythms associated with shift work and long-distance jet travel (Boulos, this volume; Czeisler et al. 1986, 1990; Daan and Lewy 1984; Eastman 1990a, 1992; Lewy et al. 1987; U.S. Congress 1991). Much more work needs to be done to determine the utility of light for treating both clinical and nonclinical disorders. It is clear, however, that we are entering a medical frontier in which the human biological response to light is being harnessed for improving health and well-being.

The most commonly used light for treating SAD is white-appearing light. These "white" light sources include at least five different fluorescent lamp types and three different incandescent lamp types. Thus, the wavelength emissions from these devices will vary tremendously, making comparisons between different intensities less valid. The color temperature, expressed as kelvins (K), varies from approximately 2,900 K to 6,300 K for these eight white light sources—a range that indicates how very different these white light sources are from one another in spectral balance (Illuminating Engineering Society 1993). Studies that employed these eight different white light sources all showed that they could effectively reduce SAD symptoms. It is critical to note that these findings *do not* support the notion that these eight white light sources are therapeutically equivalent, or that white-appearing light represents the optimum therapy for winter depression. It is also important to understand that there are numerous wavelength compositions that appear white to human observers. For example, two narrow bandwidth wavelengths at 440 nm (indigo-violet-appearing monochromatic light) and 560 nm (yellowish-green-appearing light) can be mixed to produce a light that appears white to an observer. In contrast, whole sets of visible wavelengths can be mixed together to produce white-appearing light. Thus, the possible combinations of wavelengths that can produce white light are nearly infinite. In general, the white light sources that have been employed for treating SAD are broad bandwidths of polychromatic light with a great amount of variability in the different wavelengths that are emitted across the spectrum.

Researchers have debated the role of UV in light treatment, based on the early studies on light therapy for winter depression that successfully utilized white light fluorescent lamps that emitted a portion of the UV wavelengths (Lewy et al. 1982; Rosenthal et al. 1984; Terman et al. 1989a). The early results supported the idea that "full-spectrum" light, or light that includes a balance of both visible and UV wavelengths, is necessary for successful therapy. Indeed, one study demonstrated that white light stimuli with UV wavelengths produced better therapeutic responses than white light without UV wavelengths (Lam et al. 1991). Later studies, however, found no significant difference in therapeutic response to white light treatment with or without UV wavelengths (Bielski et al. 1992; Lam et al. 1992). Numerous other studies have indicated that SAD symptoms can be reduced by lamps that emit little or no UV (Avery et al. 1993; Oren et al. 1991; Stewart et al. 1990; Terman et al. 1990). Thus, UV wavelengths do not seem *necessary* for eliciting beneficial effects when using light to treat winter depression. Does this rule out UV having any role in light therapy? Many species including insects, fish, and birds have specific UV photoreceptors in their eyes (Vision Research 1994). In addition, some mammalian species appear to have UV photoreceptors (Jacobs 1992; Jacobs and Deegan 1994), and in some animals UV-A or UV-B radiation can regulate circadian rhythms, seasonal reproduction, and melatonin production (Brainard et al. 1986a, 1986b, 1992, 1994a). Furthermore, in young, normal, healthy humans from age 6 up to at least 25 years, near-ultraviolet radiation (UV-A) can be visually detected (Brainard et al. 1992, 1993; Sanford et al. 1996; Tan 1971). In older adults, the lens of the eye develops a pigmentation that ultimately prevents UV wavelengths from reaching the retina. Thus, though the latest studies show positive therapeutic responses when UV is excluded in SAD treatment, they do not demonstrate that UV is necessarily non-contributory. Whether UV wavelengths contribute to the optimum balance of wavelengths for SAD therapy remains unanswered.

It must be recalled that overexposure to infrared, visible, or UV can be a hazard to both skin and eye tissues (Illuminating Engineering Society 1993; Lerman 1980; Waxler and Hitchens 1986). Fortunately, at typical therapeutic illuminances and durations, the lamp types currently used in light therapy are not known to emit harmful levels of infrared, visible, or UV wavelengths (American Conference of Governmental Industrial Hygienists 1989; Illuminating Engineering Society 1993, 1996a, 1996b). It is prudent, however, for patients with eye disease, photosensitive skin, or those taking photosensitizing drugs to consult their ophthalmologist or dermatologist before undergoing light therapy (Terman et al. 1990). It is ultimately important to discern between wavelengths and doses of light that are effective therapeutically yet are safe in terms of potential tissue damage. This is best accomplished by developing the action spectrum for light therapy.

Given the growing use of light as a therapeutic agent, it becomes increasingly important to identify the photobiological processes that mediate the therapeutic effects of light in humans. What is our current understanding of how the eye transduces light for use in healing? More specifically, what are the photopigments that transduce light for therapy? Where are they located in the eye? What are their operating range and adaptational capacities? What conditions optimize the therapeutic benefits of light treatment? Unfortunately, this scientific field is still at a very rudimentary stage. For example, in terms of light therapy for SAD, no dose-response curve for light therapy with a single light source has ever been established. Indeed, there have been direct comparisons of two different light intensities or two different durations of light therapy, which suggest that light treatment of SAD follows a dose-response function. Similarly, researchers who analyzed light therapy data from several different laboratories also concluded that light therapy appears to exhibit dose-response characteristics (Terman and Terman 1992). A complete dose-response function that identifies the threshold, the 50% response (ED50), and the saturation intensities for a single light therapy device will require either a substantial multicenter effort or the commitment of a single laboratory over a series of winters.

The issue of dosage is complicated by the diversity in the configuration of light therapy devices now available to patients and researchers. Originally, it was thought that a light panel must provide an illuminance of 2,500 lux or more to patients' eyes to be therapeutically effective. However, recent work with dawn simulators and light visors suggests that substantially lower illuminances may provide equivalent therapeutic benefit (Avery and Norden, this volume; Avery et al. 1993; Joffe et al. 1993; Rosenthal et al. 1993; Stewart et al. 1990; Terman et al. 1989b). Do such devices work at lower illuminances because they stimulate the photoreceptive mechanism for light therapy more effectively than do light panels? Alternatively, does the novelty of these devices produce strong therapeutic benefits because such devices elicit a greater placebo response in patients than do light panels or workstations? Such questions will remain unanswered for all light therapy equipment until the photoreceptor physiology for light therapy has been elucidated and the general degree of placebo response in light therapy has been further clarified. It is doubtful that there will ever be a generic dosage of illuminance or intensity that is recommended for light treatment of SAD. The optimum dosage used in light therapy will always depend on the configuration of the therapeutic device, its time and method of use, the duration of use, and the type of light source within it.

Just as there has been no elucidation of a dose-response function, there also has been no elucidation of an action spectrum for light therapy. The feasibility of determining an action spectrum for light treatment of SAD has been demonstrated by a set of three experiments that compared different portions of the spectrum for clinical efficacy. In the first study, patients were treated with an equal photon dose (2.3×10^{15} photons/cm^2/sec) of white-, blue-, or red-appearing light for 1 week. (This photon density was selected because it is equivalent to a dosage of white light known to be therapeutically effective [Rosenthal et al. 1988; Terman et al. 1989a]). The photon density emitted from the white light source elicited a significantly stronger clinical response compared to the response obtained from an equal photon density from the blue and red light (Brainard et al. 1990). That result implied that light sources for SAD light therapy could not be improved by substituting narrower bandwidths of blue or red light in place of broadband white light.

A second study was done to compare restricted bandwidths of green light to those of red light at 2.3×10^{15} photons/cm^2/sec for treating winter depression. Data from this study is illustrated to provide an example of the techniques and therapeutic results characteristic of the three wavelength studies. Figure 1–3 illustrates the spectral power distribution, photometric values, and radiometric values of the red and green light sources used in the second study. As is also shown in Figure 1–3, 1 week of light treatment with either green or red light sources produced an improvement in depression symptoms in the groups of patients tested. The percent reduction in mean Hamilton Rating Scale for Depression (HAM-D) scores (Hamilton 1967) was 51% and 30% for the green and red light sources, respectively. The reduction in HAM-D scores was statistically significant for the green light treatment ($P < .005$) but not for the red light treatment ($P > .10$). Hence, at this photon density, green light was significantly stronger than the red light for treating winter depression (Oren et al. 1991).

Considered alongside the results from the study comparing red, white, and blue light therapy at the same photon density, the results of the study with red and green light therapy suggest that broad-spectrum white light and narrower band green light are equivalent in their capacity to reduce symptoms of SAD. Between the two studies, white and green light treatments were associated with statistically significant reductions in mean HAM-D scores of 48% and 53%, respectively. Comparisons of group responses between different studies, however, are not conclusive.

The final study in this series compared the efficacy of green versus white light at a lowered equal photon density (1.23×10^{15} photons/cm^2/sec). The results suggested that at this lower photon density, white light may have a narrow superiority to green light for treating SAD (Stewart et al. 1991).

Together, the results from these three wavelength studies form the basis for determining an action spectrum for light therapy for winter depression. The traditional approach to defining a complete action spectrum, however, requires testing with narrower bandwidth light stimuli and more tightly controlled light exposures than are feasible in outpatient clinical trials (Brainard et al. 1993; Coohill 1991; Smith 1989). A serious complication for the majority of studies on SAD involves the fact that they are performed on an outpatient basis. Thus, patient compliance on treatment timing, frequency, and duration can-

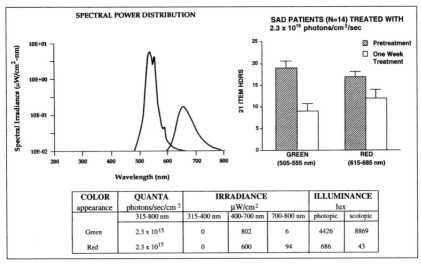

FIGURE 1–3. The graph on the left illustrates the wavelength emissions of the red and green light sources used in this study. The chart under this graph shows both radiometric and photometric information for these sources. The graph on the right indicates mean (± SEM) HAM-D values for patients before treatment (hatched bars) and after 1 week of treatment with equal photon densities of green or red light (open bars). The reduction in HAM-D scores was statistically significant for the green light treatment ($P < .005$) but not for the red light treatment ($P > .10$). Numbers in parentheses indicate the half-peak bandwidth of the light source (Oren et al. 1991).

Source. Reprinted from Brainard GC, Gaddy JR, Bartker FM, et al.: "Mechanisms in the Eye That Mediate the Biological and Therapeutic Effects of Light in Humans," in *Light and Biological Rhythms in Man.* Edited by Wetterberg L. Stockholm, Pergamon, 1993, pp. 29–53. Used by permission of Elsevier Science, Ltd.

not be closely controlled even with the most cooperative subjects. Did patients have different gaze behaviors or different patterns of light usage with the different wavelength light sources? As will be discussed below, very small changes in gaze direction and patient position relative to the light source can cause great variability in the amount of light transmitted to the patients' eyes. The optimum method of comparing different wavelengths—or any other photic parameter—for SAD therapy is to work with more carefully controlled exposures.

In conclusion, this nascent field of research has not yet evolved some of the key data—dose-response curves and action spectra—

necessary for understanding the physiology of how the eye mediates the healing power of light. Two significant impediments confront those who would elucidate the ocular mechanisms that mediate the beneficial effects of light. First, considerable experimental "noise" needs to be eliminated by improving patient compliance and standardizing gaze behavior during the therapeutic period. Tighter experimental control and thus lower exposure variability can be achieved with inpatient studies, but such studies require significantly greater time and expense. Secondly, the inability to accurately separate nonspecific or placebo responses from genuine clinical responses produces another element of noise in phototherapy data, which seriously hinders the accurate discrimination of the underlying neurobiology that mediates light therapy. The experimental confound of placebo responses is not unique to the field of psychological and psychiatric research in general (Eastman 1990b; Ross and Olsen 1981), and, specifically with light therapy, placebo issues have been discussed most insightfully by Eastman (Eastman 1990b; Eastman et al. 1993). Despite such impediments, progress can still be made toward identifying how the eye processes light as a nonvisual stimulus by examining light regulation of the pineal gland.

Ocular Physiology That Mediates the Biological Effects of Light

Throughout history there has been an intriguing array of ideas about the human pineal gland ranging from the well-known contention by Rene Descartes (1596–1650) that the pineal is the seat of the human soul, to the ancient Eastern wisdom that the pineal is an inner eye that serves spiritual enlightenment. Through the development of modern science, such concepts were largely ignored, and as recently as 1950 the pineal gland was still considered to be a vestigial, nonfunctioning organ. Since that time, however, four decades of studies on various animal species have clearly demonstrated that the pineal gland is an actively functioning neuroendocrine transducer that secretes melatonin, is strongly regulated by light stimuli, and functions as an important component of the circadian timing system (Binkley 1988; Klein et al.

1991; Reiter 1991). As the basic physiology was revealed through animal experimentation, it was soon discovered that the human pineal gland is also active in neuroendocrine and circadian physiology.

A landmark finding was published in 1980 by Lewy and colleagues who showed that exposing the eyes of healthy volunteers to 2,500 lux of white light during the night produced a strong suppression of plasma melatonin. In that same study, these investigators also showed that the nocturnal rhythm of melatonin was not disturbed by exposing the eyes to 500 lux of white light, which is an illuminance typical of home and office lighting (Lewy et al. 1980). Prior attempts to influence human biological rhythms and pineal physiology with illuminances ranging from 100 to 800 lux failed to produce similar biological responses, which had already been documented in other animal species (Akerstedt et al. 1979; Jimerson et al. 1977; Lynch et al. 1978; Vaughan et al. 1976, 1979; Wetterberg 1978). Lewy and his collaborators succeeded in their experiment because they used a substantially stronger light stimulus to suppress human melatonin synthesis. This seminal finding opened the door to numerous studies that probed for the clinical utility of exposing humans to light at an illuminance of 2,500 lux. The subsequent success of employing light to treat depression and other disorders has generated both scientific and public enthusiasm for light therapy.

As researchers and clinicians demonstrated that "bright" light illuminances of 2,500 lux or more were effective for inducing nonvisual biological and behavioral effects, a prevailing idea emerged that light *must* be bright to be biologically and behaviorally effective. This concept is, in part, incorrect. For example, under proper conditions, illuminances 25–100 times *lower* than 2,500 lux can suppress melatonin. Specifically, a study was done to determine more precisely the dosages of light needed to suppress melatonin in normal, healthy humans. In that study, subjects were exposed to five different intensities of monochromatic green light (509 nm) for 1 hour during the night between 2:00 A.M. and 3:00 A.M. During the light exposure, the volunteers' pupils were fully dilated and their heads were held steady relative to the light source, which produced a constant and uniform illumination over the whole retina. As indicated in Table 1–4, data from this experiment demonstrated that light affects human mela-

TABLE 1–4

Dose-response curve for melatonin suppression by monochromatic light at 509 nm

Quanta (photons/sec/cm^2)	Irradiance (μW/cm^2)	Illuminance (lux)		Melatonin suppression (%)
		Photopic	Scotopic	
9.2×10^{13}	0.01	0.03	0.17	−9.67
2.8×10^{15}	0.30	1.03	5.25	1.83
1.5×10^{16}	1.60	5.50	27.98	37.33
4.6×10^{16}	5.00	17.18	85.90	51.67
1.2×10^{17}	13.00	44.66	227.37	60.67

Source. Based on data from Brainard et al. 1988.

tonin in a dose-response fashion, as is typical of other photobiologically mediated responses (Brainard et al. 1988).

The volunteers and the experimenters reported seeing each stimulus as appearing green, therefore all stimuli used in that study activated the photopic visual system. However, the low-stimulus intensities did not suppress melatonin, whereas the higher intensities induced a 60%–80% decrease in this hormone. Thus, for both animals and humans, much more light is needed for circadian control and melatonin regulation than for vision. (Brainard et al. 1983, 1988; Czeisler et al. 1986; Lewy et al. 1980; Minors et al. 1991; Nelson and Takahashi 1991).

The human melatonin dose-response data shown in Table 1–4 also confirm that very bright light is not necessarily needed for melatonin suppression. Only 5–17 lux was needed to significantly suppress melatonin in normal volunteers—an illuminance equal to civil twilight and well below typical indoor light. Thus, when conditions are carefully controlled, 25–100 times less light can suppress melatonin than originally believed (Brainard et al. 1988; Lewy et al. 1980). Furthermore, low illuminances do not necessarily need to be composed of a monochromatic green wavelength to have a strong impact on melatonin regulation. Other recent studies have shown that illuminances from 100 to 630 lux of white light can suppress plasma melatonin levels in humans when exposure conditions are more carefully controlled (Bojkowski et al. 1987; Brainard et al. 1994b; Brainard et al. 1997; Gaddy et al. 1992; 1993; McIntyre et al. 1989). Some of those data will be reviewed later to demonstrate the physiological components that are involved in melatonin regulation and perhaps other circadian and therapeutic effects of light.

The demonstration that relatively dim illuminances can suppress melatonin in normal humans created an apparent paradox. Why did the earlier attempts to suppress melatonin in humans fail when illuminances from 100 to 800 lux were tested? This paradox can be resolved by examining the ocular physiology involved in transducing light stimuli to the circadian system and pineal gland (Brainard et al. 1993, 1994b, 1997). Figure 1–4 illustrates a simplified version of the physical and anatomical elements involved in photic regulation of the melatonin generating system. This model system comprises two general categories of elements: 1) components for physical/biological stimulus processing and 2) structures involved in sensory/neural signal processing. To resolve the paradox of why dim light can suppress melatonin in one circumstance but not in another, it is important to consider the physical nature of the light stimulus, the geometrical relationship of the light stimulus to the eyes, gaze direction, status of the ocular media, pupillary dilation, retinal field exposure, photoreceptor sensitivity, the capacity of the system to integrate photic stimuli over time and space, and the adaptational state of the system. Each of these factors is likely to contribute to the effectiveness of a photic stimulus in regulating melatonin. Clarification of this physiology will ultimately help to explain how light is processed by the broader circadian system and may open the door to a better understanding of the potency of light as a therapeutic force.

The magic of light—its capacity to regulate melatonin or to provide therapeutic benefit—is not just in the light source itself, but in the *relationship* of the light source to the human eye. It is critically important to recognize that light emitted from a natural or artificial source may have very different physical characteristics from the light that is ultimately received at the photoreceptor surface. A given lamp may emit a specific balance of wavelengths, but that specific balance does not necessarily reach the retina. Similarly, a lamp may provide an illuminance or irradiance that is detected by the appropriate meter,

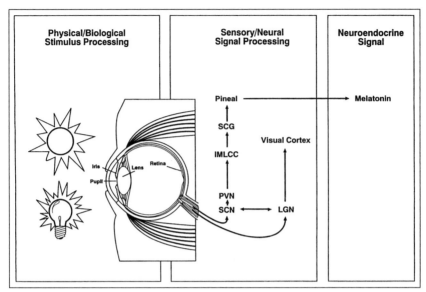

FIGURE 1–4. A simplified version of the physical and anatomical elements involved in light regulation of the melatonin-generating system. Clarification of this physiology may open the door to a better understanding the potency of light as a therapeutic force. SCN: suprachiasmatic nuclei; LGN: lateral geniculate nuclei; PVN: paraventricular nuclei; IMLCC: intermediolateral cell column; SCG: superior cervical ganglion (Brainard et al. 1994b).

Source.   Reprinted from Brainard GC, Gaddy JR, Ruberg FL, et al.: "Ocular Mechanisms That Regualte the Human Pineal Gland," in Advances in Pineal REsearch, Vol. 8 Edited by Møller M, Pévet P. London, John Libbey, 1994, pp. 415–432. Used by permission of John Libbey and Co., Ltd.

but that quantity of light may not reach the retina. Three factors can greatly modify the quantity and quality of light reaching the photoreceptive surface in the eye: 1) gaze behavior relative to a light source, 2) the condition of the clear ocular media, and 3) pupillary dilation.

The behavior of the human eye is dynamic; our head and eyes are in constant motion relative to light sources. In contrast, when used properly, photometers and radiometers are static relative to light sources. In most of the early human studies that failed to demonstrate light-induced melatonin suppression with illuminances of 100 to 800 lux, the behavior of the volunteers relative to the experimental light source was not rigorously controlled. Often, the experimental light stimulus was the overhead light provided with the experimental room, and illuminance was measured by placing a light meter on the desktop, aimed directly at the overhead lights. This measurement technique, although standard for characterizing architectural lighting (Illuminating Engineering Society 1993), may have over- or underestimated the actual corneal illuminance experienced by the subjects.

Studies have shown that when subjects are free to alter their gaze and/or distance from a light source, they can lose 80%–99% of their putative corneal irradiance (Dawson and Campbell 1990). Furthermore, the loss of corneal illuminance is compounded by the eye's optics, which focus an image of the light source on the retina rather than diffuse the light across it (Gaddy 1990). Thus, in almost any given room with a typical illumination level of 500 lux, the occupants may be able to see 500 lux when they look directly toward the light fixtures, but if they look at the floor or walls, the illuminance reaching their eyes may drop to 50 or even 5 lux. Light entering the eyes can be further reduced if the volunteers close their eyes, squint, or gaze into shadowy areas. Such gaze aversion not only reduces general corneal illuminance, it also reduces the total area of the retinal image produced by a discrete light source.

Also, the iris of the eye can modify the illuminance or intensity of light that reaches the retina by adjusting pupillary diameter from 2 mm to 9 mm relative to the brightness of the light. Pupil dilation increases retinal light exposure whereas pupil constriction decreases retinal illumination. Although it is well known that the iris enhances vision, provides visual comfort, and protects the retina (Lowenstein and Lowenfeld 1962; Sliney and Wolbarsht 1980), little work has been done to assess the role of the iris and pupil in modulating the therapeutic or biological effects of light.

To test how pupillary dilation affects melatonin regulation, groups of healthy subjects were studied on three separate nights with at least 1 week between each night of study (Gaddy et al. 1993). On test nights, subjects were exposed to 1) darkness only, 2) a 100-lux spatially uniform white light stimulus that filled the visual field while their pupils were pharmacologically dilated, or 3) the 100-lux stimulus while their pupils were free to constrict. During the light exposures, the pharmacologically dilated pupils were significantly larger ($P < .001$) than pupils that were free to constrict (means 7.3 and 3.3 mm, respectively). As shown in Figure 1–5, light exposure in both the dilated and free pupil conditions suppressed melatonin blood levels over the 90-minute period ($P < .002$), with a significantly greater drop in the dilated pupil condition than in the free ($P < .04$). These data confirm that when the pupil is dilated, melatonin suppression increases significantly (Gaddy et al. 1993). In addition, these results suggest that the iris may modify the illuminance that reaches the retina from a light therapy device.

Like the iris, the ocular media of the eye may modify the characteristics of light emitted from a lamp before it reaches the photoreceptors. It is well known that the cornea, aqueous humor, and vitreous humor of the healthy human eye are clear tissues that transmit nearly 100% of visible and UV wavelengths (down to 300 nm) to the retina; there is little change in the transmission characteristics of these tissues with age (Boettner and Wolter 1962; Lerman 1987). In contrast, the crystalline lens yellows with age and acts as a filter that greatly attenuates the total transmission of radiant energy to the retina, particularly in the shorter wavelength portion of the spectrum (Brainard et al. 1993; Lerman 1987). Thus, the lens has a role in de-

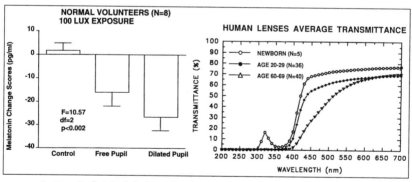

FIGURE 1–5. Left, Modulation of melatonin light regulation by pupillary dilation. The data illustrate mean ($\pm$ SEM) percent change scores from baseline plasma melatonin levels (2:00 A.M.) to final melatonin levels (3:30 A.M.) in eight subjects studied on three separate nights. There was a significantly greater melatonin suppression ($P < .04$) when pupils were dilated compared to when they were free to constrict (Gaddy et al. 1993). Right, mean transmittance of visible and ultraviolet wavelengths of postmortem human lenses from 5 newborn donors, 36 donors aged 20–29 years, and 40 donors aged 60–69 years (Brainard et al. 1994b).

termining both the quantity and quality of photic stimuli that can reach photoreceptors for the circadian and neuroendocrine systems.

To quantify the lenticular transmission of UV, visible, and infrared wavelengths, postmortem lenses (n = 288) were collected from human donors ranging from prenatal to 92 years of age. Figure 1–5 shows the mean percent transmittance data from three age groups: 0–2, 20–29, and 60–69 years old. Those data demonstrate how greatly lenticular transmission can vary over the human life span. This study indicated that longer visible and infrared wavelength transmission is not substantially different between age groups. However, significant, gradually occurring differences do exist between age groups for the shorter wavelength and visible ranges. For example, it was observed that a set of 36 lenses from humans between 20 and 29 years of age transmitted significantly more blue (440 nm) and green (540 nm) light than a set of 40 lenses from humans aged 50–59 years (P < .0001 and P < .03, respectively) (Brainard et al. 1993, 1994b). These results show that the age of the human lens significantly modulates the total quantity of light and the balance of wavelengths that reach the retina. Thus, measures of corneal illumination are not necessarily equivalent to measures of retinal illumination. For any broad-spectrum light source applied as a biological or therapeutic stimulus, there will be a progressive decrease in energy reaching the retina from the UV, violet, indigo, blue, and green portions of the spectrum as patients age.

Beyond the modification of light stimuli by ocular tissues and behavior, there is the physiology of sensory and neural signal processing. Specifically, the capacity of the system to integrate photic stimuli over time and space, the adaptational capacity of the system, and the photoreceptor spectral sensitivity are likely to contribute to determining the effectiveness of a photic stimulus in regulating melatonin. Compared to what is known about how light stimuli are processed for visual sensation, the sensory and neural processing of light stimuli for light therapy is virtually unexplored.

In the psychophysics of the visual system, it is well known that the retina exhibits spatial summation of photic stimuli. Specifically, the area of retinal stimulation determines the minimum intensity necessary for light perception (Riggs 1965). A recent study demonstrated that the stimulation of a larger portion of the bilateral visual field resulted in greater melatonin suppression in healthy human subjects (Gaddy et al. 1992). With the indication that photic stimuli were spatially summated within the retinas, the following experiment tested the possibility of spatial summation between the two retinas (Gaddy et al. 1993). Following a protocol similar to that already described for pupillary studies, light-induced melatonin suppression was examined in healthy volunteers on three different nights separated by 1-week intervals. On different nights, subjects were exposed to 1) darkness only, 2) a monocular corneal illuminance of 630 lux of white light (the nondominant eye was patched), or 3) a binocular exposure to 630 lux of white light. The results illustrated in Figure 1–5 show that on both light exposure nights, plasma melatonin levels demonstrated a significantly greater suppression in the binocular condition than in the monocular condition ($P < .03$). These results demonstrate the additive effect of the two retinal inputs to the suprachiasmatic nuclei (SCN) for melatonin control. Thus, retinal spatial summation appears to include cross-retina as well as within-retina summation for neuroendocrine regulation.

With pineal regulation, there appears to be a physiology for spatial summation at the level of the retina—the more retinal area that is exposed to light, the greater the suppression of melatonin. Neuroanatomical evidence from rodents, sheep, and nonhuman primates lends support to this concept. Morphological studies indicate that retinal ganglion cells projecting to the SCN are distributed across the entire retina (Tessonneaud et al. 1994; Moore et al. 1995; Pickard 1982). This suggests that photoreceptors from the entire retinal field may contribute to stimulation of the SCN. Further support for this principle comes from a study that examined melatonin suppression in healthy humans with two different exposures to 1,000 lux of white light: one exposure illuminated the central visual field 5° from the center of gaze whereas the other exposure was directed to the peripheral visual field 60° lateral to the direction of gaze. The results suggested that melatonin suppression can be effected by either central or peripheral illumination (Adler et al. 1992). Many questions remain unanswered about how the retina processes photic stimuli for melatonin regulation. What are the receptive field characteristics of the ganglion cells that project to the SCN from the retina? Do certain areas of the retina send stronger signals to the SCN than others? Does the superior retinal field have a greater role than the inferior retinal field? The anatomical spread of ganglion cells in the retina does not guarantee a homogeneity of physiological function. Further studies are needed to determine more precisely how the physical location of photoreceptors in the retina mediates nonvisual responses to light.

While the initial research indicates that for melatonin regulation, light is summated over the area of the retinas that it reaches, it is unclear if photic stimuli are also summated over time. Are constant light stimuli equivalent to intermittent stimuli in their influence on the pineal gland? For example, it is known from animal studies that light pulses or "skeleton" photoperiods can entrain circadian rhythms and modulate seasonal reproduction as do full cycles of light and darkness (Evered and Clark 1985; Pittendrigh and Daan 1976).

In light therapy for SAD, a standard instruction to patients is to "engage in such activities as reading, writing or eating" while concentrating the eyes "on the surfaces illuminated by the lights and not the lights themselves" (Society for Light Treatment and Biological Rhythms 1994). Though clinically effective, this exposure method can introduce a wide variability in the actual dose of photons that reaches patients' retinas; the dose depends on how often and how long the patients' eyes receive the therapeutic light stimuli. Do the retinas and associated neural structures integrate variable photic stimuli over the treatment period? A series of experiments have been designed to test questions about the effects of light on circadian regulation. In the initial study, pulses of light were compared to continuous light exposure for their capacity to suppress nocturnal melatonin (Brainard et al. 1994c). On three separate nights with at least 1 week between each study, nine healthy subjects were exposed for 90 minutes to 1) darkness only; 2) continuous, full-field 200-lux white light; or 3) pulsed full-field 200-lux white light (lights on and off in 10-minute intervals). As shown in Figure 1–6, both continuous and pulsed light exposures at 200 lux suppressed plasma melatonin. Continuous light exposure caused a significantly greater suppression of melatonin compared to the pulsed exposure ($P < .03$). Thus, over a 90-minute exposure period, a set of 10-minute light pulses is not as

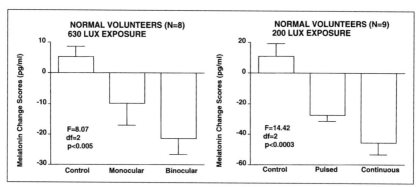

FIGURE 1–6. Mean (± SEM) change scores from baseline plasma melatonin levels (2:00 A.M.) to final melatonin levels (3:30 A.M.) in sets of subjects studied on three separate nights (Gaddy et al. 1993; Brainard et al. 1994b). The graph on the left shows that exposure of both eyes to 630 lux produces a stronger melatonin suppression than the exposure of a single eye (*P* < .03). The graph on the right shows that continuous light exposure caused a significantly greater suppression of melatonin (*P* < .03) compared to light exposure in 10-minute pulses (Brainard et al. 1994c).

Source.   Reprinted from Brainard GC, Gaddy JR, Ruberg FL, et al.: "Ocular Mechanisms That Regualte the Human Pineal Gland," in Advances in Pineal REsearch, Vol. 8 Edited by Møller M, Pévet P. London, John Libbey, 1994, pp. 415–432. Used by permission of John Libbey and Co., Ltd.

effective as a continuous exposure for suppressing melatonin. Additional testing is needed to determine the limits of the melatonin system in summating photic stimuli over time and if similar responses are shared for other circadian or therapeutic effects of light.

It is not known what photoreceptors and photopigments transduce light stimuli and provide the nonvisual biological and therapeutic effects in humans. Nearly all researchers acknowledge that the peak sensitivity of the circadian and neuroendocrine system is in the blue-green portion of the visible spectrum. Some investigators have discussed the hypothesis that rhodopsin or a rhodopsin-based molecule is the primary receptor for circadian and neuroendocrine regulation (Brainard et al. 1984, 1988; Bronstein et al. 1987; Cardinali et al. 1972; Podolin et al. 1987; Takahashi et al. 1984; Thiele and Meissl 1987). It has also been hypothesized that one or more of the known cone photopigments may be involved in these regulatory effects (Brainard et al. 1984, 1986a; Foster et al. 1993; Holtz et al. 1990; Milette et al. 1987; Podolin et al. 1987; Thiele and Meissl 1987). Recent data raise the possibility that neither the rods nor the cones used for vision participate in regulating the circadian and neuroendocrine systems. The retinally degenerate mouse (rd/rd) exhibits normal circadian responses to 515-nm light pulses despite a nearly total loss of classical visual photoreceptors (Foster et al. 1991). This concept is further supported by the finding that rats with total or near-total destruction of retinal photoreceptors caused by prolonged constant light exposure still exhibit acute light-induced suppression of nocturnal melatonin and entrain their melatonin rhythms normally to the ambient light-dark cycle (Webb et al. 1985). Similarly, it has been shown that in some humans with complete visual blindness, melatonin suppression can be induced by exposing the eyes to white light at 6,000 lux (Czeisler et al. 1995). In that study, the neuroendocrine sensitivity to light remained despite a loss of pupillary reflex, outer retinal functioning as determined by electroretinographic testing, or conscious perception of the light stimulus. Such data suggest that for the circadian and neuroendocrine systems, light detection may not rely on the rods or cones used for vision.

One approach to determining the nature of the photoreceptors involved in melatonin regulation is to study whether a retinal deficiency in the color perceptual system could affect light-mediated melatonin suppression. In one study, volunteers were screened for color vision defects using the Ishihara, Farnsworth-Munsell, and Nagel anomaloscope tests (Ruberg et al. 1996). Fourteen volunteers with color vision deficiencies were compared to seven volunteers with normal color vision in the melatonin suppression protocol similar to that described earlier. Subjects with color vision deficiencies were diagnosed as follows: five subjects had protanopia (functionally lacking the red cone pigment), six subjects had deuteranopia (functionally lacking the green cone pigment), one subject had an unspecified dichromism (with an unknown cone deficiency), and three subjects had anamolous trichromism. All subjects were studied on two nights separated by at least 1 week: 1) a control night during which they were exposed only to darkness, and 2) a night during which they were exposed to 200 lux of white light in a full visual field with their pupils dilated from 2:00 A.M. to 3:30 A.M. The data from this study revealed that melatonin was suppressed after light exposure both in subjects with normal color vision and subjects with color vision deficiencies ($P < .001$), with no significant difference in the degree of suppression between the two groups. These findings suggest that a normal trichromatic photopic system is not necessary for light regulation of the pineal gland. A second study done on subjects with color vision deficiencies further reinforced the conclusion that a normal trichromatic visual system is not necessary for light-induced suppression of melatonin or for regulating acute circadian characteristics of the melatonin rhythm (Ruberg et al. 1996).

What are the implications of determining that a normal trichromatic visual system is not necessary for melatonin regulation and perhaps other circadian and therapeutic effects of light? At the beginning of this manuscript, the physics of light and the principles of light measurement were reviewed briefly. Specifically, Figure 1–1 illustrates the photometer response for daytime vision based on the standard observer (Commision Internationale de l'Eclairage 1987). Predominantly, scientists and clinicians working with light therapy have used photopic nomenclature and measurement techniques for specifying light dosages for patients and characterizing light therapy equipment. This is all based on a standard, normal, three-cone visual system adapted to daytime light levels. If the normal, three-cone visual system does not mediate the effects of light on the neuroendocrine system, as has been suggested by the recent studies discussed here (Czeisler et al. 1995; Ruberg et al. 1996), then the use of "lux" or other photopic measures becomes questionable. At this time, the photopic system is still serviceable for describing light therapy, but the community of professionals involved with light therapy should be cautious in being too attached to this nomenclature and measurement technique.

Conclusion

Light can be a potent force for healing and biological change. There is now extensive empirical evidence that human well-being can be powerfully influenced by light that enters the eyes. Despite 15 years of vigorous research examining the efficacy of light therapy for the improvement of various biological, behavioral, and mood problems, surprisingly little is known about the underlying physiology through which light produces its beneficial effects. Are there separate photo-biological processes for the different applications of light therapy? Are the eyes the exclusive mediator of light's beneficial effects? How do the nervous and endocrine systems process photic signals to eventually produce health benefits? These and many other questions remain largely unanswered.

Humankind has had a long and enthusiastic love affair with light—a history spanning more than two millennia. The research reviewed here represents one of the newer chapters in this passionate relationship. By clarifying the salient details—the physics of light, the techniques for its measure, and the underlying photobiological physiology—clinicians and researchers are bound to make further advances for improving human health and well-being. However, will elucidating the underlying ocular and neurophysiology sufficiently explain how light interacts with biology to ultimately alter human consciousness?

Much of modern biology is based on a relentless pursuit of finer and finer grades of physiological detail in an effort to understand the complexity of life. While scientists possess an incredible ability to measure things—photons with spectroradiometers and hormone molecules with radioimmunoassays, such a tight focus on submicro-scopic measures may obscure our grasp of the bigger picture. Perhaps there is a synergism at work in our neurobiological processes that escapes the reductionistic pursuit of detail. Science transcended the simplistic Newtonian ordering of the universe when Einstein introduced his theories of relativity. Modern physics now accepts the limits of a deterministic framework. Since quantum physics plays a crucial role in our comprehension of light, it may also have a role in our understanding of the biological effects of light. Light therapy, which is a process based on the interaction between light quanta and the highly complex nervous system that ultimately evokes a change in human consciousness, may not be totally reliant on a simple hierarchy of cause-and-effect mechanisms. The biological sciences may need to reach beyond the present framework to solve the mysteries of the human psyche and the healing power of light.

References

Adler JS, Kripke DF, Loving RT, et al: Peripheral vision suppression of melatonin. J Pineal Res 12:49–52, 1992

Akerstedt T, Froberg JE, Friberg Y, et al: Melatonin excretion, body temperature and subjective arousal during 64 hours of sleep deprivation. Psychoneuroendocrinology 4:219–225, 1979

American Conference of Governmental Industrial Hygienists: Threshold Limit Values and Biological Exposure Indices for 1991–1992. Cincinnati, OH, American Conference of Govermental Industrial Hygenists, Inc., 1991

American Psychiatric Association: Diagnostic and Statistical Manual of Mental Disorders, 4th Edition. Washington, DC, American Psychiatric Association, 1994

Aschoff J (ed): Handbook of Behavioral Neurobiology, Biological Rhythms. New York, Plenum, 1981

Avery DH, Bolte MA, Dager SR, et al: Dawn simulation treatment of winter depression: a controlled study. Am J Psychiatry 150:113–117, 1993

Bielski RJ, Mayor J, Rice J: Phototherapy with broad spectrum white fluorescent light: a comparative study. Psychiatry Res 43:167–175, 1992

Binkley S: The Pineal: Endocrine and Nonendocrine Function. Englewood Cliffs, NJ, Prentice-Hall, 1988

Binkley S: The Clockwork Sparrow. Englewood Cliffs, NJ, Prentice-Hall, 1990

Birren F: Color Psychology and Color Therapy. Secaucus, NJ, Citadel Press, 1961

Boettner EA, Wolter JR: Transmission of the ocular media. Invest Ophthalmol Vis Sci 1:776–783, 1962

Bojkowski CJ, Aldhous ME, English J, et al: Suppression of nocturnal plasma melatonin and 6-sulphatoxymelatonin by bright and dim light in man. Horm Metab Res 19:437–440, 1987

Brainard GC, Richardson BA, King TS, et al: The suppression of pineal melatonin content and N-acetyltransferase activity by different light irradiances in the Syrian hamster: a dose-response relationship. Endocrinology 113:293–296, 1983

Brainard GC, Richardson BA, King TS, et al: The influence of different light spectra on the suppression of pineal melatonin content in the Syrian hamster. Brain Res 294:333–339, 1984

Brainard GC, Podolin PL, Leivy SW, et al: Near ultraviolet radiation (UV-A) suppresses pineal melatonin content. Endocrinology 119:2201–2205, 1986a

Brainard GC, Vaughan MK, Reiter RJ: Effect of light irradiance and wavelength on the Syrian hamster reproductive system. Endocrinology 119:648–654, 1986b

Brainard GC, Lewy AJ, Menaker M, et al: Dose-response relationship between light irradiance and the suppression of melatonin in human volunteers. Brain Res 454:212–218, 1988

Brainard GC, Rosenthal NE, Sherry D, et al: Effects of different wavelengths in seasonal affective disorder. J Affect Disord 20:209–216, 1990

Brainard GC, Beacham S, Hanifin JP, et al: Ultraviolet regulation of neuroendocrine and circadian physiology in rodents and the visual evoked response in children, in Biological Responses to Ultraviolet-A Radiation. Edited by Urbach F. Overland Park, KS, Valdenmar, 1992, pp 261–271

Brainard GC, Gaddy JR, Barker FM, et al: Mechanisms in the eye that mediate the biological and therapeutic effects of light in humans, in Light and Biological Rhythms in Man. Edited by Wetterberg L. Stockholm, Pergamon Press, 1993, pp 29–53

Brainard GC, Barker FM, Hoffman RJ, et al: Ultraviolet regulation of neuroendocrine and circadian physiology in rodents. Vision Res 34: 1521–1533, 1994a

Brainard GC, Gaddy JR, Ruberg FL, et al: Ocular mechanisms that regulate the human pineal gland, in Advances in Pineal Research, Vol 8. Edited by Møller M, Pévet P. London, John Libby, 1994b, pp 415–432

Brainard GC, Rollag MD, Hanifin JP: Photic regulation of melatonin in humans: ocular and neural signal transductin. J Biol Rhythms 12:537–546, 1997

Brainard G, Hanifin J, Leibowitz S, et al: Constant versus intermittent ocular exposure during light treatment: is there temporal summation of photic stimuli? in SLTBR: Abstracts of the Annual Meeting for the Society for Light Treatment and Biological Rhythms, Vol 6. Wilsonville, OR, SLTBR, 1994c, p 14

Bronstein DM, Jacobs GH, Haak KA, et al: Action spectrum of the retinal mechanism mediating nocturnal light-induced suppression of rat pineal gland N-acetyltransferase. Brain Res 406:352–356, 1987

Campbell SS, Murphy PJ: Extraocular circadian phototransduction in humans. Science 279:396, 1998

Cardinali DP, Larin F, Wurtman RJ: Control of the rat pineal gland by light spectra. Proc Natl Acad Sci USA 69:2003–2005, 1972

Commission Internationale de l'Eclairage: International Lighting Vocabulary, CIE Publication No. 174. Vienna, Commission Internationale de l'Eclairage, 1987

Coohill TP: Action spectra again? Photochem Photobiol 54:859–870, 1991

Czeisler CA, Allan JS, Strogatz SH, et al: Bright light resets the human circadian pacemaker independent of the timing of the sleep-wake cycle. Science 233:667–671, 1986

Czeisler CA, Johnson MP, Duffy JF, et al: Exposure to bright light and darkness to treat physiologic maladaptation to night work. N Engl J Med 322:1253–1259, 1990

Czeisler CA, Shanahan TL, Klerman EB, et al: Suppression of melatonin secretion in some blind patients by exposure to bright light. N Engl J Med 332:6–11, 1995

Daan S, Lewy AJ: Scheduled exposure to daylight: a potential strategy to reduce "jet lag" following transmeridian flight. Psychopharmacol Bull 20:566–568, 1984

Dawson D, Campbell SS: Bright light treatment: are we keeping our subjects in the dark? Sleep 13:267–271, 1990

Eastman CI: Circadian rhythms and bright light: recommendations for shift work. Work and Stress 4:245–260, 1990a

Eastman CI: What the placebo literature can tell us about light therapy for SAD. Psychopharmacol Bull 26:495–504, 1990b

Eastman CI: High-intensity light for circadian adaptation to a 12-h shift of the sleep schedule. Am J Physiol 263:R428–R436, 1992

Eastman CI, Young MA, Fogg LF: A comparison of two different placebo-controlled SAD light treatment studies, in Light and Biological Rhythms in Man. Edited by Wetterberg L. Stockholm, Pergamon Press, 1993, pp 371–393

Evered D, Clark S (eds): Photoperiodism, Melatonin and the Pineal. London, Pitman, 1985

Foster RG, Provencio I, Hudson D, et al: Circadian photoreception in the retinally degenerate mouse (rd/rd). J Comp Physiol (A) 169:39–50, 1991

Foster RG, Argamaso S, Coleman S, et al: Photoreceptors regulating circadian behavior: a mouse model. J Biol Rhythms 8:S17–S23, 1993

Gaddy JR: Sources of variability in phototherapy. Sleep Res 19:394, 1990

Gaddy JR, Edelson M, Stewart K, et al: Possible retinal spatial summation in melatonin suppresion, in Biologic Effects of Light. Edited by Holick MF, Kligman AM. New York, Walter de Gruyter, 1992, pp 196–204

Gaddy JR, Rollag MD, Brainard GC: Pupil size regulation of threshold of light-induced melatonin suppression. J Clin Endocrinol Metab 77: 1398–1401, 1993

Hamilton M: Development of a rating scale for primary depressive illness. British Journal of Social and Clinical Psychology 6:278–296, 1967

Holtz MM, Milette JJ, Takahashi JS, et al: Spectral senstivity of the circadian clock's response to light in Djungarian hamsters. Abstracts of the 2nd Annual Meeting of the Society for Research on Biological Rhythms. Charlottesville, VA, SRBR 1990

Horspool WM, Song P-S (eds): Organic Photochemistry and Photobiology. New York, CRC Press, 1994

Illuminating Engineering Society of North America (eds): IES Lighting Handbook: Reference and Application. New York, Illuminating Engineering Society of North America, 1993

Illuminating Engineering Society of North America: Photobiological Safety for Lamps and Lamp Systems—General Requirements (RP-27.1, Draft Document). New York, Illuminating Ehgineering Society of North America, 1996a

Illuminating Engineering Society of North America: Photobiological Safety for Lamps—Risk Group Classification and Labeling (RP-27.3, Draft Document). New York, Illuminating Engineering Society of North America, 1996b

Jacobs GH: Ultraviolet vision in vertebrates. Am Zool 32:544–554, 1992

Jacobs GH, Deegan JF: Sensitivity to ultraviolet light in the gerbil *(Meriones unguiculatus):* characteristics and mechanisms. Vision Res 34: 1433–1441, 1994

Jimerson DC, Lynch HJ, Post RM, et al: Urinary melatonin rhythms during sleep deprivation in depressed patients and normals. Life Sci 20: 1501–1508, 1977

Joffe RT, Moul DE, Lam RW, et al: Light visor treatment for seasonal affective disorder: a multicenter study. Psychiatry Res 46:29–39, 1993

Kaiser PK: Phototherapy using chromatic, white, and ultraviolet light. Color Research and Application 9:195–205, 1984

Kern HE, Lewy AJ: Corrections and additions to the history of light therapy and seasonal affective disorder. Arch Gen Psychiatry 47:90–91, 1990

Klein DC, Moore RY, Reppert SM (eds): Suprachiasmatic Nucleus: The Mind's Clock. Oxford, Oxford University Press, 1991

Kripke DF: Light regulation of the menstrual cycle, in Light and Biological Rythms in Man. Edited by Wetterberg L. Stockholm, Pergamon, 1993, pp 305–312

Kripke DF, Mullaney DJ, Savides TJ, et al: Phototherapy for nonseasonal major depressive disorders, in Seasonal Affective Disorders and Phototherapy. Edited by Rosenthal NE, Blehar MC. New York, Guilford, 1989, pp 342–356

Lam RW, Buchanan A, Clark CM, et al: Ultraviolet versus non-ultraviolet light therapy for seasonal affective disorder. J Clin Psychiatry 52: 213–216, 1991

Lam RW, Buchanan A, Mador JA, et al: The effects of ultraviolet-A wavelengths in light therapy for seasonal depression. J Affect Disord 24: 237–244, 1992

Lam RW, Goldner EM, Solyom L, et al: A controlled study of light therapy for bulimia nervosa. Am J Psychiatry 151:744–750, 1994

Lerman S: Radiant Energy and the Eye. New York, Macmillan, 1980

Lerman S: Chemical and physical properties of the normal and aging lens: spectroscopic (UV, fluorescence, phosphorescence, and NMR) analyses. Am J Optom Physiol Opt 64:11–22, 1987

Lewy AJ, Wehr TA, Goodwin FK, et al: Light suppresses melatonin secretion in humans. Science 210:1267–1269, 1980

Lewy AJ, Kern HE, Rosenthal NE, et al: Bright artificial light treatment of a manic-depressive patient with a seasonal mood cycle. Am J Psychiatry 139:1496–1498, 1982

Lewy AJ, Sack RL, Miller LS, et al: Antidepressant and circadian phase-shifting effects of light. Science 235:352–354, 1987

Lieberman J: Light: Medicine of the Future. Santa Fe, NM, Bear, 1991

Lowenstein O, Loewenfeld IE: The pupil, in The Eye. Edited by Davson H. New York, Academic Press, 1962, pp 231–267

Lynch HJ, Jimmerson DC, Ozaki Y, et al: Entrainment of rhythmic melatonin secretion in man to a 12-hour phase shift in the light/dark cycle. Life Sci 23:1557–1563, 1978

McIntyre IM, Norman TR, Burrows GD, et al: Human melatonin suppression by light is intensity dependent. J Pineal Res 6:149–156, 1989

Milette JJ, Hotz MM, Takahashi JS, et al: Characterization of the wavelength of light necessary for initiation of neuroendocrine-gonadal activity in male Djungarian hamsters. – Abstract #110 from the 20th Annual Meeting of the Society for Study of Reproduction, Urbana, IL, July, 110, 1987

Minors DS, Waterhouse JM, Wirz-Justice A: A human phase-response curve to light. Neurosci Lett 133:36–40, 1991

Moore RY, Speh JC, Card JP: The retinohypothalamic tract originates from a distinct subset of retinal ganglion cells. J Comp. Neurol 352:351–366, 1995

Nelson DE, Takahashi JS: Comparison of visual sensitivity for suppression of pineal melatonin and circadian phase-shifting in the golden hamster. Brain Res 554:272–277, 1991

Oren DA, Brainard GC, Joseph-Vanderpool JR, et al: Treatment of seasonal affective disorder with green light versus red light. Am J Psychiatry 148:509–511, 1991

Oren DA: Humoral phototransduction: blood is a messenger. Neuroscientist 2:207–210, 1996

Ott JN: Health and Light: The Effects of Natural and Artificial Light on Man and Other Living Things. Old Greenwich, CT, Devin-Adair, 1973

Pickard GE: The afferent connections of the suprachiasmatic nucleus of the golden hamster with emphasis on the retinohypothalamic projection. J Comp Neurol 211:65–83, 1982

Pittendrigh CS, Daan S: A functional analysis of circadian pacemakers in nocturnal rodents, IV: entrainment: pacemaker as clock. J Comp Physiol 106:291–331, 1976

Plautz JD, Kaneko M, Hall JC, et al: Independent photoreceptive circadian clocks throughout drosophila. Science 278:1632–1635, 1997

Podolin PC, Rollag MD, Brainard GC: The suppression of nocturnal pineal melatonin in the Syrian hamster: dose-response curves at 500 nm and 360 nm. Endocrinology 121:266–270, 1987

Reiter RJ: Pineal gland: interface between the photoperiodic enviornment and the endocrine system. Trends Endocrinol Metab 2:13–19, 1991

Riggs LA: Light as a stimulus for vision, in Vision and Visual Perception. Edited by Graham C. New York, Wiley, 1965, pp 1–38

Rosenthal NE: Diagnosis and treatment of seasonal affective disorder. JAMA 270:2717–2720, 1993

Rosenthal NE, Blehar MC (eds): Seasonal Affective Disorders and Phototherapy. New York, Guilford Press, 1989

Rosenthal NE, Sack DA, Gillin JC, et al: Seasonal affective disorder. A description of the syndrome and preliminary findings with light therapy. Arch Gen Psychiatry 41:72–80, 1984

Rosenthal NE, Sack DA, Skwerer RG, et al: Phototherapy for seasonal affective disorder. J Biol Rhythms 3:101–120, 1988

Rosenthal NE, Joseph-Vanderpool JR, Levendosky AA, et al: Phase-shifting effects of bright morning light as treatment for delayed sleep phase syndrome. Sleep 13:354–361, 1990

Rosenthal NE, Moul DE, Hellekson CJ, et al: A multicenter study of the light visor for seasonal affective disorder: no difference in efficacy found between two different intensities. Neuropsychopharmacology 8:151–160, 1993

Ross M, Olson JM: An expectancy-attribution model of the effects of placebos. Psychol Rev 88:408–437, 1981

Ruberg FL, Skene DJ, Hanifin JP, et al: Melatonin regulation in humans with color vision deficiencies. J Clin Endocrinol Metab 81:2980–2985, 1996

Sandord B, Beacham S, Hanifin JP, et al: The effects of ultrviolet-A radiation on visual evoked potential in the young human eye. Acta Ophthalmol Scand 74:553–557, 1996

Sliney D, Wolbarsht M: Safety with Lasers and Other Optical Sources. New York, Plenum, 1980

Smith KC (ed): The Science of Photobiology. New York, Plenum, 1989

Society for Light Treatment and Biological Rhythms: Consensus statements. Light Treatment and Biological Rhythms 3:45–50, 1991

Society for Light Treatment and Biological Rhythms: Questions and Answers About Light Therapy. Wilsonville, OR, Society for Light Treatment and Biological Rhythms, 1994

Stewart KT, Gaddy JR, Benson DM, et al: Treatment of winter depression with a portable, head-mounted phototherapy device. Prog Neuropsychopharmacol Biol Psychiatry 14:569–578, 1990

Stewart KT, Gaddy JR, Byrne B, et al: Effects of green or white light for treatment of seasonal depression. Psychiatry Res 38:261–270, 1991

Takahashi JS, DeCoursey PJ, Bauman L, et al: Spectral sensitivity of a novel photoreceptive system mediating entrainment of mammalian circadian rhythms. Nature 308:186–188, 1984

Tan KEWP: Vision in the ultraviolet (thesis). Utrecht, The Netherlands, University of Utrecht, 1971

Terman M, Terman JS: Light therapy for winter depression, in Biologic Effects of Light. Edited by Holick MF, Kligman AM. Walter de Gruyter, 1992, pp 133–154

Terman M, Terman JS, Quitkin FM, et al: Light therapy for seasonal affective disorder. A review of efficacy. Neuropsychopharmacology 2:1–22, 1989a

Terman M, Schlager D, Fairhurst S, et al: Dawn and dusk simulation as a therapeutic intervention. Biol Psychiatry 25:966–970, 1989b

Terman M, Rem, CE, Rafferty B, et al: Bright light therapy for winter depression: Potential ocular effects and theoretical implications. Photochem Photobiol 51:781–792, 1990

Tessonneaud A, Cooper HM, Caldani M, et al: The suprachiasmatic nucleus in the sheep: retinal projections and cytoarchitectural organization. Cell Tissue Res 278:65–84, 1994

Thiele G, Meissl H: Action spectra of the lateral eyes recorded from mammalian pineal glands. Brain Res 424:10–16, 1987

U.S. Congress, Office of Technology Assessment: Biological Rhythms: Implications for the Worker (OTA-BA-463). Washington, DC, U.S. Government Printing Office, 1991

Vaughan GM, Pelham RW, Pang SF, et al: Nocturnal elevation of plasma melatonin and urinary 5-hydroxyindoleacetic acid in young men: attempts at modification by brief changes in environmental lighting and sleep by autonomic drugs. J Clin Endocrinol Metab 42:752–764, 1976

Vaughan GM, Bell R, de la Pena A: Nocturnal plasma melatonin in humans: episodic pattern and influence of light. Neurosci Lett 14:81–84, 1979

Vision Research (Special Issue): The Biology of Ultraviolet Reception. Vision Res 34:1359–1540, 1994

Wald G: The photoreceptor process in vision. Am J Ophthalmol 40:18–41, 1955

Waxler M, Hitchens VM: Optical Radiation and Visual Health. Boca Raton, FL, CRC Press, 1986

Webb SM, Champney TH, Lewinski AK, et al: Photoreceptor damage and eye pigmentation: influence on the sensitivity of rat pineal N-acetyltransferase activity and melatonin levels to light at night. Neuroendocrinology 40:205–209, 1985

Wehr TA, Skwerer RG, Jacobsen FM, et al: Eye versus skin phototherapy of seasonal affective disorder. Am J Psychiatry 144:753–757, 1987

Wetterberg L: Melatonin in humans: physiological and clinical studies. J Neural Transm Suppl 289–310, 1978

Wetterberg L (ed): Light and Biological Rhythms in Man. Stockholm, Pergamon, 1993

Zajonc A: Catching the Light: The Entwined History of Light and Mind. New York, Bantam Books, 1993

TWO

Light Therapy
for Seasonal Affective Disorder

Virginia A. Wesson, M.D.
Anthony J. Levitt, M.D.

Seasonal affective disorder (SAD) is a subtype of recurrent mood disorder with a characteristic pattern of onset and remission (American Psychiatric Association 1987, 1994; Rosenthal et al. 1984, 1985). The first diagnostic criteria for SAD were published by Rosenthal et al. (1984), and SAD first appeared as a diagnostic entity in DSM-III-R (American Psychiatric Association 1987). The definition was updated for inclusion in DSM-IV (American Psychiatric Association 1994). Table 2–1 summarizes the changes in the diagnostic criteria over time. Episodes of SAD, which may develop within a unipolar or bipolar mood disorder, begin at a particular period of the year, typically fall/winter, and remit with the change of season, unrelated to seasonal stressors. Nonseasonal episodes may occur, but seasonal episodes must predominate. The current DSM-IV definition requires consecutive episodes in the last 2 years without any intervening nonseasonal episodes. The DSM-III-R definition differs from the other diagnostic definitions in that it allows either major depressive or manic episodes, while both the Rosenthal and DSM-IV definitions allow only major depressive episodes.

TABLE 2-1

Comparison of diagnostic criteria for SAD

	Rosenthal criteria[1]	DSM-III-R criteria[2]	DSM-IV criteria[3]
Diagnostic prerequisites	Lifetime history of major affective disorder, depressed, meeting RDC[4] criteria	Lifetime history of bipolar disorder or recurrent major depression	Lifetime history of bipolar I, bipolar II, or major depressive disorder, recurrent
Specific criteria			
Type of mood disorder	Major depressive episode	Major depressive episode *or* episode of bipolar disorder	Major depressive episode
Onset	Recurrent winter depressions	Regular temporal relationship between onset of an episode of bipolar disorder *or* recurrent major depression and a particular 60-day period of the year	Regular temporal relationship between onset of major depressive episode in bipolar I, bipolar II, or major depressive disorder (recurrent), and time of year
Remission	Full remissions by the following spring or summer	Full remissions (or change from depression to mania or hypomania) within a particular 60-day period of the year	Full remissions (or change from depression to mania or hypomania) at a characteristic time of year
Frequency	Major depressive episode in two consecutive winters	Three episodes of mood disturbance in three separate years that demonstrate seasonal relationship, two in consecutive years	Two major depressive episodes in last 2 years meeting criteria above, and no nonseasonal major depressive episodes in the same period
Predominant season		Seasonal episodes outnumber nonseasonal by 3:1 or more	Seasonal episodes substantially outnumber nonseasonal episodes

[1] Rosenthal et al. 1984. [2] American Psychiatric Association 1987. [3] American Psychiatric Association 1994. [4] Research Diagnostic Criteria, Spitzer et al 1978.

The prevalence of SAD is estimated to be between 2.4% (Levitt 1994) and 9.7% (Rosen et al. 1990), depending on latitude and methodology. Prevalence appears to increase with increasing distance from the equator (Rosen et al. 1990). Women are more commonly affected, in a ratio of women to men of about 3:1 to 4:1 (Booker and Hellekson 1992; Hellekson 1989), which is higher than the 2:1 ratio observed in nonseasonal depression (Weissman et al. 1984). In addition, SAD patients tend to be younger than other depressed patients (Booker and Hellekson 1992; Kasper et al. 1989; Rosen et al. 1990). The typical SAD patient has had about 10 episodes of depression, with each episode lasting approximately 4 months (Lam 1994). "Atypical" symptoms of depression, such as hypersomnia with difficulty waking and daytime fatigue, hyperphagia, carbohydrate craving, and weight gain are characteristic of SAD (Booker and Hellekson 1992; M. Terman et al. 1989a).

SAD patients often respond to bright artificial light, frequently within a few days (Lewy et al. 1982; Rosenthal et al. 1984). Consequently, light therapy for this disorder has been the focus of considerable research effort. It is the purpose of this chapter to review this work, including a description of light therapy, its efficacy and side effects, and controversial issues concerning light therapy for SAD.

Light therapy is the current treatment of choice for patients with SAD (American Psychiatric Association 1993; Rosenthal 1993; Society for Light Treatment and Biological Rhythms 1990). In general, treatment entails daily exposure to light, but guidelines for specific treatment parameters, such as the intensity and wavelength of light used and the time of day when it is administered, vary considerably. Much effort has been made to determine which parameters influence response, and investigations aimed at defining optimal treatment conditions continue. In excess of 700 subjects have participated in published clinical trials of light therapy, and response rates to active treatment conditions in the range of 53%–67% have been achieved (Tam et al., 1995; Terman et al. 1989).

Among the technologies developed to deliver the light, two have been used most extensively: the light box and the head-mounted light unit (HMU). In the following sections, the therapeutic effects of each of these devices, as well as less thoroughly studied technologies such as dawn simulators, will be summarized. Second, side effects of light therapy and issues of safety will be examined. Third, current controversies regarding light therapy research and the effectiveness of light therapy as a specific treatment for SAD will be addressed. Particular attention will be given in this last section to sample size, duration of treatment course, and the difficulty of finding a suitable placebo for light therapy.

Therapeutic Effects of the Light Box

Introduction and History

In 1982, the first published report appeared describing the successful use of a light box in the treatment of winter depression in a bipolar patient (Lewy et al. 1982). The light unit was constructed of several fluorescent lamps mounted in a box behind a translucent plexiglass screen. The treatment, which consisted of 6 hours of bright light exposure daily (2,000 lux from 6:00 A.M. to 9:00 A.M., and 4:00 P.M. to 7:00 P.M.), extended the day to its usual spring length of 13 hours. The theoretical basis for the treatment protocol was the observation that animals had seasonal rhythms governed by day length, or photoperiod (Blehar and Rosenthal 1989; Lewy et al. 1982). Thus, it was hypothesized that humans may have similar rhythms that could be manipulated with artificial light. Within 4 days, the patient began to recover, both objectively and subjectively. In addition, nighttime melatonin secretion declined by 88%, suggesting that the treatment was biologically as well as clinically active. This initial case report was followed by numerous other studies involving the light box, which will be reviewed below.

The first pilot study of light therapy, which outlined in some detail the clinical and biological characteristics of SAD and provided the first systematic definition of the disorder, was published by Rosenthal et al. in 1984. Eleven patients out of a group of 29 who underwent extensive evaluation were selected to participate in a comparison of the efficacy of bright, white, full-spectrum fluorescent light (2,500 lux at 90 cm) versus dim, yellow fluorescent light (100 lux at 90 cm), both delivered by a light box. Patients were randomly assigned to receive either bright or dim light for 6 hours daily (3 hours before dawn and 3 hours after dusk) for 2 weeks. At the end of the second week, patients were evaluated clinically. If the patient was judged to be improved, the lights were withdrawn for 1 week or more, following which the second treatment condition was begun, again for 6 hours daily for 2 weeks. If no improvement had occurred, the second treatment was started immediately. "Improvement" required both a clinical change and a fall in Hamilton Rating Scale for Depression score (HAM-D; Hamilton 1961) 0 of 4 points or more to a total of less than 15. The authors predicted that bright white light would be biologically active, but dim yellow light would be inactive and serve as a control condition. The patients, however, were not aware of these hypotheses.

Among the nine patients who completed both courses of light exposre, there was a significant fall in the group mean HAM-D score following bright light treatment but not following dim light treatment. In addition, all patients showed some improvement while receiving bright light, usually within the first 3–7 days. Of six patients questioned prior to treatment regarding efficacy, four felt that the bright white light would be superior to the dim light, but five expected some benefit from both conditions. The authors concluded that bright light therapy, given before dawn and after dusk, had significant antidepressant properties and showed promise in the treatment of SAD. They suggested that extension of the photoperiod was critical to response.

This pilot study was followed by a second trial by the same group (Rosenthal et al. 1985). A larger sample of subjects ($N = 13$) completed a similar counterbalanced crossover comparison of a bright and a dim light; six of the participants were in a structured inpatient setting. An effort was made to choose a more homogeneous group of patients with typical depressive symptoms. Two control conditions were used. A very dim control (5 lux) was given to the inpatients to maximize the possibility of detecting differences in response to the control and active treatments. A brighter control (300 lux), which more closely resembled the active condition (2,500 lux), was given to outpatients to provide a more plausible placebo. Sleep was monitored to address the possibility that the effect of light therapy was secondary to sleep deprivation rather than a specific effect of the light itself. In an attempt to remove expectation of greater benefit from the brighter light, subjects were told that the study was designed to examine the antidepressant effects of sleep deprivation and/or light therapy. One-tailed Wilcoxon signed rank tests demonstrated a significant difference between pre- and post–bright light 21-item HAM-D scores for inpatients ($P < .025$) and outpatients ($P < .01$). Significantly greater changes in HAM-D scores were seen with bright light as compared to dim light for both inpatients ($P < .025$) and outpatients ($P < .025$). Dim light had no significant effect on HAM-D scores. Relapse occurred after withdrawal of bright light treatment, whereas there was no significant deterioration in depressive symptoms after withdrawal of the dim light. Hours of sleep were similar before, during, and after treatment for both conditions. Within each condition, subjects slept less during the treatment phase than before or after, as a result of earlier wakening. When questioned at the conclusion of the trial, inpatients acknowledged that the very dim control treatment was not credible and engendered less hope of benefit than the bright light condition. Outpatients had similar expectation of both conditions but in some cases could not distinguish the two intensities of light.

Eleven patients, including seven who participated in the main portion of the trial, were subsequently treated with bright evening light alone. Seven showed some improvement, although of a more modest degree than with the morning plus evening light regime.

Several conclusions were reached on the basis of these findings. First, bright light appeared to be superior to dim in the treatment of SAD, with morning exposure tending to be more beneficial than evening. Sleep deprivation did not account for the effectiveness of the treatment. The inpatients, who were exposed to the very dim placebo, did not consider it to be a plausible treatment and were less hopeful of benefit from it. Nonetheless, based on the pattern of response and relapse, the authors concluded that a nonspecific placebo response to bright light was an unlikely explanation for the experimental findings.

Terman and Co-Workers' Pooled Analysis

Following these earliest light box studies, many other controlled trials of the light box appeared in the literature. In 1989, M. Terman and colleagues reviewed light box studies published up to the winter of 1986–1987, involving 332 patients in 14 research centers located in 11 cities in the Northern Hemisphere (M. Terman et al. 1989a). Although individual studies involved small numbers of subjects, (median 10, range 6–25), entry criteria and treatment paradigms were similar. Therefore, the data were pooled. Despite the small number of subjects in any individual study, the combined sample allowed meaningful comparisons to be made between different light therapy regimes: bright light was given in the morning, midday, evening, and both morning and evening; and two control treatments consisted of dim light and brief, bright light exposure. The definition of response was a reduction in the 21-item HAM-D score of 50% or more to a total score of less than 8.

On the basis of their elegant pooled analysis, M. Terman et al. concluded that bright light (2,500 lux) given for a least 2 hours daily in the morning for 1 week was an effective treatment for about 53% of SAD sufferers (Table 2–2). Mean response of morning plus evening exposure (51%) was no better than morning light alone. Both treatments involving morning exposure had a superior response rate to evening light alone (38%), midday light alone (32%), and brief, bright light exposure (31%). Response rates to all five bright light conditions were superior to that of dim light (11%). The results of this pooled analysis form the basis of the American Psychiatric Association guidelines regarding light therapy for SAD (American Psychiatric Association 1993).

Patients entered into the studies in Terman and co-workers' pooled analysis generally scored 14 or higher on the 21-item HAM-D. There was a great deal of variation in pretreatment scores; in fact, some subjects entered with scores of less than 8, defined by M. Terman et al. (1989a) to be within the normal or subclinical range. To determine whether their conclusions regarding the efficacy of light therapy applied to patients at all levels of severity, they reanalyzed their data for morning light, evening light, morning plus evening light, and the dim light control, with patients split into 2 groups: mild cases (HAM-D score 10–16) and moderate to severe cases (HAM-D score > 16). Patients with baseline scores less than 10 were omitted because the mildness of their symptoms might make it harder to assess the effectiveness of the treatment. These patients had

TABLE 2-2

Results from a grouped analysis of light therapy studies

	Morning (53%)	Evening (38%)	Morning and evening (51%)	Midday (32%)	Brief (31%)	Dim (11%)
Morning (53%[1])						
Evening (32%)	*					
Morning and evening (51%)	NS	*				
Midday (32%)	*	NS	NS			
Brief (31%)	**	NS	*	NS		
Dim (11%)	***	***	***	*	**	

Note. Number of subjects in each cell: morning = 172; evening = 143; morning and evening = 136; midday = 34; brief = 65; dim = 77.
[1] Percent response.
Post hoc test of significance for proportions (SSTAT program). *$P = .05$; **$P = .01$; ***$P = .001$; NS = not significant.
Source. Adapted from Terman et al., 1989.

been included in the original meta-analysis, but their removal did not alter the results to a statistically significant degree.

When mildly affected subjects were considered separately, the response rate to morning light (67%) was significantly greater than that to evening light (39%; $P < .01$). However, among patients with moderate to severe symptoms, the response rate to morning light (43%) was dramatically lower than in mildly depressed subjects, and not significantly greater than the response to evening light (41%). (Response rates were obtained from M. Terman et al. 1989a, page 17, Figure 2–3, and did not appear in the text.) Therefore, time of day of treatment appeared to be important in mildly affected SAD patients, and light therapy appeared to be relatively less effective for those with moderate to severe symptoms. M. Terman et al. (1989a) also noted that baseline severity did not appear to influence response rates to evening or dim light, suggesting that treatments delivered at these times were nonspecific or inactive treatments.

Parameters of Light Box Treatment

M. Terman et al. (1989a) focused on time of day of exposure, but they noted that other treatment parameters, including intensity, wavelength of light used, the duration of daily exposure, and the length of the treatment course, may influence response. Studies have since been undertaken to determine which of these parameters are influential to outcome, and to define optimal treatment conditions. Experimental findings regarding each of these parameters are described.

Intensity

A number of more recent studies not cited by M. Terman et al. have confirmed that bright light is superior to dim light (Lam et al. 1991; Magnusson et al. 1991; J. S. Terman et al. 1990; Winton et al. 1989) (Table 2–3). Winton et al. (1989) compared three treatment conditions, each of which was given to 10 patients for 5 days in a triple crossover design that examined both intensity and duration of exposure. With regard to intensity, 2,500 lux was compared to 300 lux, each given from 7:00 A.M. to 10:00 A.M., and 8:00 P.M. to 11:00 P.M. The mean percent reduction in the 21-item HAM-D score was significantly greater with 2,500 lux (53% reduction) than with 300 lux (25% reduction). In another crossover study, a high-intensity fluorescent lighting system capable of emitting 10,000 lux was used to compare light doses of 10,000 lux to doses of 3,000 lux. Both exposures were given for 30 minutes in the morning (J. S. Terman et al. 1990). The same light source was employed for both treatments, with distance between patient and source altered to achieve the two intensities. Patients were assigned randomly to one level of exposure, treated for 10 to 14 days, and then given a washout phase. Subjects were rated using the 29-item modified HAM-D (Williams et al. 1991) that includes the 21-item HAM-D ("typical" items) as well as an 8-item subscale that assesses the atypical depressive symptoms

TABLE 2-3

Controlled studies of bright versus dim light using light boxes in the treatment of SAD

	Design	N	Trial length (days)	Exposure duration	Timing	Intensity (lux)	HAM-D Pre[1,2]	HAM-D Post	Notes
Grota et al. 1989	Parallel	8	7	2 h	Evening	2,000 / 300	– / –	– / –	Bright and dim equally effective
Winton et al. 1989	Crossover	10	5	6 h	Morning and evening	2,500 / 300	18.5 / 18.5	53% fall / 25% fall	Bright superior to dim
J.S. Terman et al. 1990[3]	Crossover	12	10–14	30 min	Morning	10,000 / 3,000	16.2 ± 0.7 / 16.2 ± 0.7	$8.3^* \pm 2.4$ / $19.3^* \pm 3.3$	Remission: bright (83%) superior to dim (25%)
Lam et al. 1991	Crossover	11	7	2 h	Morning	2,500 / 500	$21.3^* \pm 3.5$ / 21.6 ± 5.5	$8.9^* \pm 7.8$ / 15.6 ± 8.8	Bright superior to dim
Magnusson et al. 1991	Crossover	10	8	40 min	–	10,000 / 400	22.6^{****} / 23.9^{**}	$6.4^{***,*****}$ / $18.9^{**,***}$	Bright superior to dim

Note. HAM-D, 21-item Hamilton Rating Scale for Depression.
[1]Numbers represent mean ± SD.
[2]Numbers sharing the same superscript within any study are significantly different.
[3]Posttreatment scores represent SIGH-SAD scores.
$*P < .05$; $**P < .02$; $***P < .01$; $****P < .005$.

characteristic of SAD. Using strict criteria for response, 7 of 12 subjects (58%) responded to 10,000 lux only, whereas none responded to 3,000 lux only, a difference that was significant. Overall, mean ± SD posttreatment Structured Interview Guide for the Hamilton Depression Rating Scale, Seasonal Affective Disorders (SIGH-SAD) (Williams et al. 1991) scores were significantly lower following 10,000 lux (8.3 ± 2.4) than 3,000 lux treatment (19.3 ± 3.3; P < .01). In a second crossover study, 10,000 lux of white light was compared to 400 lux of dim red light given to 10 SAD patients for 40 minutes daily for 8 days (Magnusson et al. 1991). Again, treatment with very bright light resulted in significant improvement in both typical and atypical depressive symptomatology, whereas treatment with dim light did not. In a trial that examined both intensity and wavelength, Lam et al. (1991) compared bright, full-spectrum fluorescent light (2,500 lux), with and without the ultraviolet (UV) range blocked, to dim light (500 lux). Eleven patients were treated for 1 week in the morning in a triple crossover design. No significant improvement in depression, as measured by the 21-item HAM-D, Beck Depression Inventory (BDI) (Beck et al. 1961) and atypical subscale score, was produced by the dim light. In contrast, the UV-containing bright light treatment produced significant improvement in all measures, and the UV-blocked bright light treatment produced significant improvement in atypical symptoms.

Not all studies have demonstrated that bright light is more effective than dim. Grota et al. (1989) compared two intensities of light (2,000 lux and 300 lux) in a study of 16 patients treated for 2 hours daily for 1 week. They observed a reduction in the HAM-D among all patients, regardless of which intensity of light the patients received. At 2 weeks post treatment, females who had been given bright light maintained their improvement, whereas females who received dim light, and all male subjects, showed signs of relapse. The authors concluded that response may not depend on intensity. However, they suggested that intensity may be an important determinant of length of remission. They noted the similarities between their results and those of Wirz-Justice et al. (1987) who found that both bright white and dim yellow light alleviated symptoms of SAD, but improvement lasted longer among bright light responders. It should be noted that the study by Grota et al. may not be directly comparable to other trials that examine intensity because treatment was given in the evening only.

Duration of daily exposure

Table 2–4 summarizes the results of studies that examined the effect of duration of exposure on response. In early studies of light therapy for SAD, treatment was administered for 5–6 hours daily, with the total amount commonly split between morning and evening. This protocol was chosen to extend the day to approximate a spring photoperiod beause this was thought necessary for response (Lewy et al. 1982; Rosenthal et al. 1985). In contrast, bright white light of 2,500 lux given for 30 minutes was considered a "brief exposure control." This notion was supported by M. Terman and co-workers' pooled cross-center analysis (1989a) in which a lower response rate of 31% was observed among a group of 65 patients treated with a brief, bright light control. In one of the first studies to directly examine the issue of duration of daily exposure, Winton et al. (1989) found that 3 hours of 2,500-lux exposure in the morning plus 3 hours in the evening was superior to 1-hour sessions twice daily.

Other reports have suggested that a plateau may be reached at 2,500 lux given for 2 hours, beyond which further treatment is of no additional benefit (Wirz-Justice et al. 1987). For example, 4 hours of daily exposure to 2,500 lux was no more effective than 2 hours at the same intensity in 6 patients treated in the evening (Doghramji et al. 1990). More recently, even shorter exposures have been used in conjunction with brighter light sources. Magnusson et al. (1991) demonstrated that a 40-minute treatment with a 10,000-lux source had significant antidepressant effects. Similarly, 30 minutes of exposure to 10,000 lux has proven to be as effective as 2 hours of exposure to 3,000 lux (J. S. Terman et al. 1990). These results have led to the conclusion that there may be an interaction between intensity and duration of exposure, with maximal response at 5,000 lux-hours (Magnusson et al. 1991, J. S. Terman et al. 1990).

Wavelength

In most light box studies, "broad-spectrum" or white light has proven to be more effective than light of restricted wavelength (see

TABLE 2–4

Controlled studies of duration of light exposure using light boxes in the treatment of SAD

	N	Trial length (days)	Timing	Intensity (lux)	Exposure duration (hours)	Dose[1] (lux × h)	HAM-D Pre[2,3]	Post	Notes
Winton et al. 1989[4]	10	5	Morning and evening	2,500 2,500	6 2	15,000 5,000	18.5 18.5	53% fall 25% fall	6 h superior to 2 h
Doghramji et al. 1990	6	7	Evening	2,500 2,500	4 2	10,000 5,000	21* ± 5.2 20.3* ± 4.8	9.8* ± 5.9 9.3* ± 5.2	Both equally effective

Note. HAM-D, 21-item Hamilton Rating Scale for Depression.
[1] Dose is the product of intensity and duration of exposure in units of lux × hours.
[2] Numbers represent mean ± SD.
[3] Numbers sharing the same superscript within any study are significantly different.
[4] Both studies employed a crossover design.
*$P < .05$.

Table 2–5). Brainard et al. (1990) compared white, red, and blue light of equal photon density (2.3×10^{15} photons/sec/cm^2) in the treatment of 18 SAD patients. Subjects were randomly assigned in a balanced, incomplete block crossover design to receive 2 of the 3 wavelengths for 2 hours in the morning and 2 hours in the evening for 1 week. With response defined as a greater than 50% reduction in 21-item HAM-D scores, there were significantly more responders to white light (58%) than there were to either red (17%) or blue (17%; P < .01). However, the three conditions produced mean changes in HAM-D scores that were not statistically different. Pretreatment expectation scores for the three conditions were similar. On the basis of the response rate data, the investigators concluded that narrowing the spectrum of light provided to patients is unlikely to improve efficacy.

Oren et al. (1991) treated 14 patients with green or red light (half peak bandwidths of 505–555 nm and 615–685 nm, respectively) of equal photon density (2.3×10^{15} photons/sec/cm^2) for 2 hours in the morning for 1 week, in a balanced crossover comparison. Overall, there was a main effect of wavelength, with only green light producing a significant decline in HAM-D scores. However, there was also an interaction between order of treatment and wavelength that renders conclusions regarding the superiority of green over red light tentative. Among patients who received red light first, the two conditions were equally effective. In contrast, the green light condition was superior among patients who received it first. Expectations of benefit did not correlate with changes in HAM-D scores.

In another investigation of green light, 12 subjects were exposed to either green or white light of equal photon density (1.23×10^{15} photons/sec/cm^2) for 2 hours daily for 1 week in a randomized crossover design (Stewart et al. 1991). Both white and green light produced significant reductions in all depression scores. White light was significantly more effective than green in reducing "typical" 21-item HAM-D scores (P < .05) but there were no differences between the two conditions in their effect on atypical subscale scores or on 29-item modified HAM-D scores. *Sequence* (white before green or green before white) appeared to influence response but *color* did not, a complex finding that prevents firm conclusions. The authors acknowledged that the sample size may have been too small to detect

TABLE 2-5

Studies of the effect of time of day of light box treatment of SAD

	Design	N	Time of day	HAM-D Pre[1,2]	HAM-D Post	Notes
Avery et al. 1990	Crossover	7	Morning	18.4 ± 4.7	5.0 ± 4.8	Morning superior to evening
		7	Evening	19.3 ± 5.0	15.1 ± 5.2	
Sack et al. 1990	Crossover	8	Morning	12.4 ± 1.7	3.8* ± 1.0	Morning superior to evening
		8	Evening	12.4 ± 1.7	7.8* ± 1.4	
J.S. Terman et al. 1990[3]	Crossover	16	Morning	16.2 ± 0.7	10.9* ± 2.3	Remission: morning (69%) superior to evening (19%)
		17	Evening	16.2 ± 0.7	17.8* ± 2.3	
Avery et al. 1991	Crossover	19	Morning	21.7 ± 4.6	5.5* ± 7.6	Morning superior to evening
		19	Evening	21.5 ± 5.2	12.2* ± 8.6	
Wirz-Justice et al. 1993	Parallel	18	Morning	18.1** ± 3.9	7.7** ± 3.3	Morning and evening equally effective
		21	Evening	18.3** ± 2.4	8.8** ± 5.4	
Lafer et al. 1994	Parallel	9	Morning	26.1 ± 4.7	13.1 ± 7.1	Morning, evening, and alternating equally effective
		8	Evening	27.5 ± 2.9	12.2 ± 7.3	
		14	Alternating	28.1 ± 4.4	14.7 ± 9.2	

Note. All trials used 2,000 lux for 2 hours daily for 7 days except J. S. Terman et al. (10,000 lux for 10–14 days) and Wirz-Justice et al. (1 hour daily). HAM-D, 21-item Hamilton Rating Scale for Depression.
[1] Numbers represent mean ± SD.
[2] Numbers sharing the same superscript within any study are significantly different.
[3] J. S. Terman et al. posttreatment results represent SIGH-SAD scores.
*P < .05. **P < .01.

differences in atypical and 29-item HAM-D scores. However, the white light was also more aesthetically pleasing to patients, which may have led to a greater placebo response to white light.

Not all studies have concluded that wavelength influences response. For example, Wirz-Justice et al. (1986) found that yellow light was as effective as white light. In a series of studies, Lam et al. (1991, 1992) first reported that white light with UV was superior to light of similar intensity with UV filtered out. In a follow-up study involving a larger group of subjects, there was no difference in outcome between bright light with or without UV-A (Lam et al. 1992). On balance, wavelength may influence response, with white light appearing to be superior to any specific wavelength. However, important order effects in many of these trials have confounded the issue of the influence of wavelength on response.

Time of day

Table 2–6 summarizes results from studies evaluating the influence of time of day of exposure. M. Terman and co-workers' pooled analysis (1989a) revealed that morning light was superior to midday or evening light, and that morning plus evening light was no more effective than morning light alone. Several crossover studies published more recently have confirmed that morning was superior to evening light (Avery et al. 1990, 1991; Sack et al. 1990; J. S. Terman et al. 1990). However, two studies employing a parallel design failed to show any difference between morning and evening exposure (Lafer et al. 1994; Wirz-Justice et al. 1993). The apparent contradiction between results from crossover and parallel studies may be due to carryover effects in the crossover studies. Morning light, when given first, may alter baseline severity (Blehar and Lewy 1990; M. Terman et al. 1989a) and reduce the efficacy of evening light given subsequently (M. Terman and Terman 1992; M. Terman, this volume). However, the weight of evidence suggests that morning light is superior, and most clinicians continue to recommend morning treatment.

Duration of treatment course

Most light box studies have been 1–2 weeks long, based partly on the observation that most of the therapeutic effect is obtained in the

TABLE 2-6

Controlled studies of the effect of wavelength of light in the treatment of SAD

	Design	N	Color	Intensity (lux)	HAM-D Pre[1,2]	Post	Order effects	Notes
Brainard et al. 1990[3]	Crossover	12 12 12	White Red Blue	2,236 603 638	— — —	9.6[3] ±6.8 4.3 ±6.9 5.6 ±6.8	Not reported	More responded to white than to red or blue; all equally effective in reducing HAM-D scores
Lam et al. 1991	Crossover	11 11	White UV-blocked	2,500 2,500	21.3* ±3.5 17.8 ±3.2	8.9* ±7.8 12.8 ±9.5	Not reported	White plus UV superior to UV-blocked
Lam et al. 1992	Parallel	16 17	White + UV-A UV-A-blocked	2,500 2,500	20.7* ±4.0 17.4* ±4.5	10.0* ±6.0 8.2* ±4.7	Not applicable (parallel design)	Both treatments equally effective
Oren et al. 1991	Crossover	20 20	Green Red	2,500 2,500	19* ±6 17 ±4	9* ±6 12 ±7	Treatments equally effective if red received first	Green superior to red overall
Stewart et al. 1991	Crossover	12 12	Green White	2,367 1,103	21* ±5.8 23.6* ±4.9	16.3* ±8.0 12.8* ±5.4	Greater fall in scores if green received first	Equally effective, white superior in reducing "typical" item scores

Note. All trials used 2 hours of morning exposure daily for 2 weeks. HAM-D, 21-item Hamilton Rating Scale for Depression.
[1] Numbers represent mean ± SD.
[2] Numbers sharing the same superscript within any study are significantly different.
[3] Brainard et al. report change in HAM-D scores.
*P < .05.

first week. Studies of longer duration would provide useful information regarding the time course of improvement and optimal treatment duration.

Some anecdotal reports of maintained improvement after withdrawal of treatment have been made. In a prospective investigation, Meesters et al. (1993) followed SAD patients beginning in September until their weekly BDI score was 13 or greater, which indicated the first appearance of winter depression. Subjects were then randomly assigned to treatment or a no-treatment control group. The treatment consisted of 2,500-lux light therapy, 9:00 A.M. to 12:00 noon, for 5 days. Among 16 patients treated in this way, none became severely depressed during the remainder of the winter, whereas 5 of 11 control patients did. Although limited in scope and sample size, this study suggests that it may be possible to prevent the full development of a severe episode of SAD if prophylactic light therapy is provided. Unfortunately, a rigorous study conducted by J. S. Terman et al. (1994) was unable to replicate this result; all 17 patients relapsed within the 8-week follow-up period after light therapy discontinuation. Therefore, most investigators recommend continuing light therapy throughout the winter.

Conclusions

In summary, bright white light given in the morning for 2 hours at 2,500 lux remains the best-studied treatment for SAD. Although formal dosing studies have yet to be done, studies examining the intensity-duration relationship suggest that 5,000 lux-hours may produce maximal clinical response. In clinical practice, a protocol of 10,000 lux for 30 minutes is the most commonly used. Studies with parallel designs and lasting longer than 1–2 weeks, with sufficient numbers of subjects, are warranted to provide definitive guidelines for treatment.

Therapeutic Effects of the Head-Mounted Light Unit

The head-mounted light unit (HMU) was developed in the late 1980s (Moul et al. 1990; Stewart et al. 1990) and carries several theoretical advantages over the light box for both clinical management and research. First, it is portable and allows patients to be mobile during treatment. Second, the HMU allows a fixed distance between the light source and the eye to be maintained; theoretically this may provide more consistency in dosage. With the light box it is difficult to maintain a constant distance between eye and source because of patients' movements. Because intensity of light, as measured by lux, falls off exponentially with increasing distance from the source (Dawson and Campbell 1990), the dose of light received in the eye while using the light box may be unpredictable. Several versions of the HMU have been used in published studies. A number of differences in the pattern of response to the HMU and the light box have been noted and are described in the following section.

Parameters of HMU Treatment

Intensity

Several studies comparing bright and dim HMUs have been published (Joffe et al. 1993; Levitt et al. 1996; Rosenthal et al. 1993; Teicher et al. 1995). Rosenthal et al. (1993) first tested an HMU capable of emitting light of two intensities, one theoretically greater than that required for therapeutic efficacy with the light box (6,000 lux), and one substantially less (400 lux). The two intensities were compared in a multicenter trial at three sites with a total of 55 patients. After a 1-week, no-treatment, baseline phase, subjects received one of the two intensities for 1 week in a single-blind design, followed by a 1-week withdrawal phase. Both bright and dim HMUs produced a significant fall in HAM-D scores and there was no significant difference in efficacy between the two conditions, although the rate of relapse was higher following withdrawal of the dim HMU.

Joffe et al. (1993) conducted a study to meet two principal objectives: first, to determine the optimal intensity of light for use with the HMU; and second, to address methodological difficulties with many light box studies, particularly small sample size and crossover design. This study, involving 105 subjects at five sites, is the largest single light therapy trial completed to date. Three intensities of light, 3,500 lux ($n = 34$), 600 lux ($n = 38$), and 60 lux ($n = 33$), were compared in a randomized, parallel design. Subjects were aware that there were three intensities and that there may be differences in their effectiveness. However, neither subjects nor raters were aware of the intensity received by any individual subject.

After a 1-week baseline phase, subjects underwent a 2-week active phase that consisted of treatment for 30 minutes each morning, followed by a 1-week withdrawal phase. All three intensities led to significant declines in total 29-item modified HAM-D scores, but there were no significant differences in efficacy between the three intensities. With response defined as a 50% fall in the 29-item modified HAM-D score to a score of 8 or less, the frequencies of response were not significantly different between 60 lux (67% response), 600 lux (58%), and 3,500 lux (65%). The 60-lux HMU was designed to be an inactive dim light control because it emitted light at an intensity likely to be below that of ambient light. Nevertheless, the response was not different from those of the two brighter HMUs. Patients' expectations, measured after brief exposure to their HMU but before treatment began, did not differ between treatments.

Levitt et al. (1996) examined the efficacy of two intensities of red light (mean 4,106 lux and 96 lux) from an HMU containing light-emitting diode (LED) light sources. Forty-three patients were randomly assigned to receive 2 weeks of treatment with either bright (n = 24) or dim (n = 19) HMUs for 30 minutes in the morning, followed by a 1-week withdrawal period. By ANOVA, mean HAM-D, atypical subscale, and 29-item modified HAM-D scores at baseline, week 2, and withdrawal were not significantly different in subjects receiving bright or dim light. With response defined as a greater than 50% decline in a 17-item HAM-D score to a final score less than 8, and a Clinical Global Impression of Improvement (CGI-I) (Guy 1976) score of 2 (moderately improved) or better, the response rates were not significantly different between bright light (67% response) and dim light (74%). In addition, no variable, including pretreatment expectations, initial symptom severity, or illuminance, was predictive of response.

Most recently, Teicher et al. (1995) investigated an incandescent light visor similar to that used in the Joffe et al. (1993) and Rosenthal et al. (1993) studies. After a 2-week baseline period, 57 SAD patients were randomly assigned to 2 weeks of morning treatment with a 30-lux red light visor ($n = 28$) or a 600-lux white light visor ($n = 29$) in a two-center, parallel design study. Again, there were no significant differences between conditions in the depression scores or percentage improvement from baseline. The remission rates (defined as greater than 50% reduction in the 21-item HAM-D and a final score less than 8) were also not significantly different between the 30-lux red light (39%) and the 600-lux white light (41%).

In summary, four methodologically rigorous studies have not shown any differences in therapeutic response to HMUs with light intensities ranging from 30 lux to 6,000 lux. In contrast to the light box studies where "bright" light exposure has been clearly shown to be superior to "dim" light, an intensity-response relationship has not been demonstrated by the HMU studies.

Duration of daily exposure

Rosenthal et al. (1993) initially treated subjects for 60 minutes daily. However, when the first 21 patents showed good response to the dim light HMU, the exposure time was shortened to 30 minutes to maximize the possibility of detecting a difference between the two intensities. In spite of this change, no differences were observed between the 30- and 60-minute exposures. In fact, the four treatment combinations (bright and dim intensities given for 30 or 60 minutes) were equally effective. Thus, subsequent HMU trials have also used the 30-minute exposure time. Other treatment durations have not been studied.

Wavelength

Both white light (Joffe et al. 1993; Rosenthal et al. 1993) and red light (Levitt et al. 1994, 1996; Teicher et al. 1995) have been used in HMU studies. Comparison of results across studies is problematic because there may be differences in patient populations, entry and response criteria, and light units. Within studies, in addition to wavelength, there were also differences in light intensity between conditions. Nonetheless, response rates to white and red light from the HMU are similar. Overall, current evidence suggests that white and red light given by HMU produce similar response rates, and both continue to be used clinically. It should be noted that the spectral characteristics of the LED treatment, which may or may not influence its therapeutic effects, have not yet been described.

Time of day

All HMU studies to date have used morning treatment times.

Duration of treatment course

HMU trials of both 1 (Rosenthal et al. 1993) and 2 (Joffe et al. 1993; Levitt et al. 1994, 1996) weeks have been conducted. In the 2-week studies, improvement continued across both weeks of treatment, followed by deterioration after withdrawal (Joffe et al. 1993; Levitt et al. 1994, 1996). As illustrated in Figure 2–1, the rate of reduction of HAM-D scores is not slowed in week 2. These results suggest that additional benefit is obtained with 2 weeks of treatment, although 1 week is sufficient to show significant improvement during therapeutic trials. Further improvement in response rates with longer treatment periods has not been studied.

Comparison of the Light Box and the HMU

Several possible explanations for the differences in intensity-response patterns between the light box and HMU have been suggested. One possibility is that the HMU is an active treatment that is effective across a wider range of intensities and wavelengths. Light as dim as 29 lux is capable of suppressing melatonin production in normal subjects (Brainard et al. 1988; Brainard, this volume), suggesting that even a dim light HMU of 30 lux may be biologically and therapeutically active. Therefore, illuminance may be important in the HMU, but only at intensities below 60 lux (a "ceiling" effect); above 6,000 lux (a "floor" effect); at a specific illuminance between 60 and 6,000 lux (a "therapeutic window"); only with treatment course longer than 2 weeks (a "lag" effect); or if longer than 30 minutes daily ("underdosing") (Levitt et al. 1996).

Alternatively, although illuminance (whose unit of measure is the lux) is commonly used to describe intensity in light therapy trials, it may not be the appropriate measure for the therapeutic effect of light. Light may be characterized by a number of other measures in-

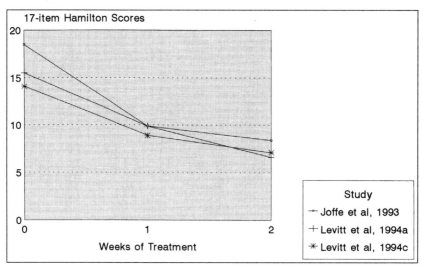

FIGURE 2–1. Severity of depression scores across 2 weeks of light treatment.

cluding luminance, spectral distribution, contrast, and radiant energy, one or more of which may provide a better measure of the biological activity of light than illuminance (Brainard, this volume; Joffe et al. 1993; Levitt et al. 1996).

Another possibility is that the HMU elicits a greater placebo response compared to the light box (Teicher et al. 1995). However, the absence of a dose effect neither supports nor discounts a placebo effect, because it is known that a dose effect may be observed even with placebo treatments (Eastman 1990).

Another possible explanation for the apparent differences in the results of light box and HMU studies may be the methodological limitations of many light box studies. M. Terman et al. (1989a) calculated that, in studies comparing bright light to a dim light control, 24 patients are required in each treatment cell to allow statistically meaningful conclusions to be drawn; however, no individual light box study has included this number in a parallel design. Although light box studies published following M. Terman and co-workers' (1989a) pooled analysis have almost all demonstrated the same dose effect, all have used a small sample size (Grota et al. 1989; Lam et al. 1991; Magnusson et al. 1991; J. S. Terman et al. 1990; Winton et al.

1989); the dose effect may no longer be observed if a sufficiently large sample of subjects is studied. Arguing against this possibility, however, are the numerous independent replications of the light box findings.

A further possibility is that differences in response to the light box and HMU are the result of different retinal exposures (Stewart et al. 1990). Patients' movements during treatment, the pupil diameter, the position of the light source, its distance from the eye, or the width of the light beam may lead to differences in the amounts of light reaching the retina or the illumination of different retinal areas (Stewart et al. 1990). However, there is no evidence to support or refute these hypotheses, and they remain unproved. It should be noted that HMUs equipped with broad-spectrum incandescent or fluorescent light sources, which have a diffuse beam, do not result in a different pattern of response from that found with HMUS equipped with red LEDs, which have a narrower, more focused light beam (Joffe et al. 1993; Levitt et al. 1996; Rosenthal et al. 1993).

One way of addressing differences between the light box and the HMU is to compare them directly to each other, and each to a credible placebo. In a preliminary study involving a small number of patients, Stewart et al. (1990) compared bright, white fluorescent light (4,000 lux) delivered by a light box or HMU in a randomized crossover protocol. Six patients received 1 week of treatment, consisting of 2 hours of morning exposure, with each type of unit. The two active phases were separated by a withdrawal period, and relapse to a HAM-D score of 10 or greater was required before the second treatment was commenced. Both the light box and HMU led to significant decreases in both HAM-D and 29-item modified HAM-D scores, but there were no significant differences between the two devices. Expectation of benefit did not differ between the two types of unit. The correlation between expectation scores and changes in 29-item modified HAM-D scores just reached statistical significance ($r = 0.566$, $P = .049$). In other words, pretreatment expectations may have influenced response but likely affected the two treatments equally.

In a larger study, Levitt et al. (1996) randomly assigned 21 subjects to 2 weeks of treatment given for 30 minutes in the morning, with either a light box emitting white light ($n = 9$, mean illuminance 7,600 lux) or an HMU emitting red light ($n = 12$, mean illuminance 646 lux). There was no significant difference in response rates between patients treated with the light box (38%) compared to the HMU (50%). Although a Type II error is possible because of the small sample size, these results suggest that response rates to the two treatment modalities are similar. However, neither of these studies included a putative placebo condition.

Conclusions

A number of conclusions can be drawn from these results. First, the HMU has yet to be shown effective against a placebo condition. However, the HMU appears to produce response rates in SAD similar to the light box, both when the results of separate HMU and light box studies are compared and when the two technologies are compared directly in a single study. Second, the dose-response relationship seen in light box studies has not been replicated with the HMU. Finally, the therapeutic effect of the HMU does not appear to depend on the wavelength of light used. Results obtained with both the light box and HMU are internally consistent with respect to the apparent importance of intensity and wavelength, but not consistent with each other. The results with the HMU may be more statistically powerful because individual studies have involved larger samples of patients than light box trials, but the results of light box studies have been independently replicated by many different groups.

Other Technologies

A novel treatment modality, the dawn simulator, has been tested in SAD. This therapy was based on the fact that, at dawn and dusk, the intensity of light changes gradually compared to the on-off characteristic of artificial light sources (Avery and Norden, this volume; M. Terman et al. 1989b). Thus, technology was developed that gradually increased the intensity of light over 2 hours while the patient slept, to levels below those commonly used in light therapy. It showed some promise in early open trials that employed a peak intensity of 1,000 lux (M. Terman et al. 1989b) or 2,000 lux (M. Terman and Schlager 1990). However, in a follow-up controlled comparison with the light box, a 2-hour dawn signal peaking at 1,700 lux failed to match the standard therapy (Avery et al. 1992a), and a 2.5-hour dawn signal peaking at 275 lux was no more effective than a 10-minute placebo signal of equal intensity (Avery et al. 1992b). More recent studies have shown that a 2-hour dawn signal peaking at 250 lux was more effective than a 30-minute 0.2-lux placebo treatment (Avery et al. 1993), and a 1.5-hour 250-lux signal was more effective than a 1.5-hour 2-lux signal (Avery et al. 1994). Thus further studies of the dawn simulator are warranted. The results of dawn simulator trials are summarized in Table 2–7.

Side Effects of Light Therapy

Most side effects of light therapy are mild, transient, and cause few patients to discontinue treatment (Labbate et al. 1994; Levitt et al. 1993). A side-effects questionnaire has been developed to quantify the frequency of emergent side effects (Levitt et al. 1993; Rosenthal et al. 1993). Headache, eyestrain, feeling "wired," nausea, and dizziness may occur in up to 20% of patients but usually diminish during the course of treatment and appear to be, at least in the case of the HMU, unrelated to the intensity of light used (Levitt et al. 1993). The frequency of the most common emergent side effects is outlined in Table 2–8. Light therapy may also alleviate these same symptoms in patients experiencing them prior to treatment (Levitt et al. 1996). Figure 2–2 shows the proportion of subjects with improvement or worsening in physical symptoms during HMU treatment and demonstrates that, for most patients, the benefits of treatment with respect to side effects outweigh the disadvantages.

In another study using a prospective side-effects questionnaire, 30 patients received 2 hours of bright light (2,500 lux) daily from a light box for 2 weeks (Labbate et al. 1994). Patients were randomized to morning ($n = 11$), evening ($n = 8$), or alternating morning and evening ($n = 11$) light exposure. The most common side effects

TABLE 2-7

Controlled studies of the dawn simulator in the treatment of SAD

	N	Trial length (days)	Exposure duration	Intensity (lux)	HAM-D Pre[1,2]	HAM-D Post
Avery et al. 1992a	7	7	2 h	1,700	18.0 ± 3.8	11.3** ± 4.3
	7	7	2 h	1,700 box	18.9* ± 4.1	6.6*,*** ± 4.3
Avery et al. 1992b	9	7	2.5 h	275	17.7** ± 6.2	5.9** ± 4.7
	9	7	10 min	275	17.2* ± 3.8	7.0* ± 8.0
Avery et al. 1993	13	7	2 h	250	17.1** ± 4.6	5.5*,*** ± 4.5
	9	7	30 min	0.2	18.6 ± 7.0	11.1* ± 4.9
Avery et al. 1994	10	7	1.5 h	250	20.7*** ± 4.9	8.0*** ± 5.1
	9	7	1.5 h	2	20.4 ± 4.6	15.6 ± 8.0

Note. HAM-D, 21-item Hamilton Rating Scale for Depression.
[1]Numbers represent mean ± SD.
[2]Numbers sharing the same superscript within any single study are significantly different.
*$P < .01$. **$P < .05$. ***$P < .001$.

TABLE **2–8**

Emergent side effects following treatment with light box and head-mounted unit

	Light box			Head-mounted unit		
	Active N (%)	Placebo N (%)	Total N (%)	Active N (%)	Placebo N (%)	Total N (%)
Eyestrain	2 (22)	1 (8)	3 (14)	3 (25)	4 (40)	7 (32)
Headache	1 (11)	1 (8)	2 (10)	3 (25)	1 (10)	4 (18)
Feeling "wired"	1 (11)	2 (17)	3 (14)	1 (8)	2 (20)	3 (14)
Nausea	1 (11)	0 (0)	1 (5)	2 (17)	1 (10)	3 (14)
Dizziness	0 (0)	1 (8)	1 (5)	2 (17)	0 (0)	2 (9)
Insomnia	0 (0)	0 (0)	0 (0)	1 (8)	2 (20)	3 (14)
Total with no side effects	6 (66)	7 (58)	13[1] (62)	4 (33)	3 (30)	7[1] (32)

Note. Only side effects reported by greater than 5% of subjects treated with either technology are included.

[1] Significantly more subjects who received the HMU (active or placebo) experienced one or more side effects than those subjects who received the light box (active or placebo; Fisher's exact test, $P = 0.047$).

Source. Adapted from Levitt et al. 1994b.

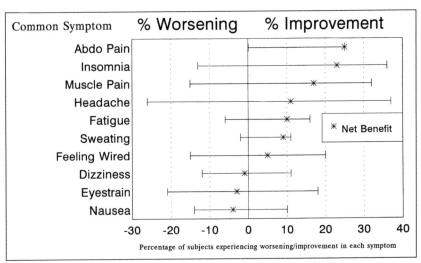

FIGURE 2–2. Worsening or improvement in common symptoms during HMU treatment of SAD.

Source. Adapted from Levitt et al, 1994c

Note. "Net benefit" reflects the difference between percent improvement and percent worsening.

were visual, including eyestrain, blurred vision, and photophobia (experienced by 26% of all subjects), and sleep related (experienced by 62% of patients receiving evening light).

More serious and of greater concern are potential ocular complications secondary to prolonged bright light exposure, particularly if light of higher intensity is used. Although no serious eye damage has been reported to date, this question has received only limited attention (Gallin et al. 1995; Gorman et al. 1993; M. Terman et al. 1990b). It is generally agreed that light therapy is relatively contraindicated in patients with known eye pathology such as retinal or optic nerve disorders, glaucoma, cataracts, and aphakic states. For the majority of patients, routine ophthalmological examination may be advisable (M. Terman et al. 1990b; Reme and Terman 1992; Vanselow et al. 1991), although some investigators consider it necessary only for selected patients (Lam 1994; Rosenthal 1993; Waxler et al. 1992).

Concern has been expressed regarding UV emissions from light therapy apparatus because of the demonstrated association between UV exposure and cataract formation (Taylor et al. 1988) and retinal damage (W. R. Ham et al. 1982; W. T. Ham et al. 1976; Lam et al. 1991). The "full-spectrum" fluorescent light sources used in light boxes emit small amounts of UV light, with the amount reaching the eye modified by filters placed on the light source. Cool-white fluorescent bulbs emit less UV-A radiation (wavelengths 315–400 nm) (Blehar and Lewy 1990; Lam et al. 1991). However, UV-B radiation (285–325 nm) may be responsible for cataract formation (Bochow et al. 1989), and the two types of bulbs emit similar amounts of UV-B (Lam et al. 1991; Oren et al. 1990). Two small studies suggested that UV wavelengths had beneficial effects during light therapy (Docherty et al. 1988; Lam et al. 1991). However, greater experience with light of restricted wavelength suggests that UV-free light sources can be used for greater safety without compromising efficacy (Lam et al. 1992; Levitt et al. 1994, 1996; Oren et al. 1991; J. S. Terman et al. 1990).

Another serious consideration is the potential for light therapy to cause patients to develop hypomania or mania. Although a number of case reports have been published (Chan et al. 1994; Kantor et al.

1991; Kasper et al. 1990; Kripke 1991; Labbate et al. 1994; Levitt et al. 1993;), the incidence of hypomania or mania is probably low.

In summary, light therapy does not appear to lead to significant short-term side effects. However, its long-term safety, particularly with respect to eye toxicity, has yet to be established. Therefore, patients using light therapy should be monitored over time. Further research is required in this area given the increasing numbers of patients using this treatment.

Controversial Issues in Light Therapy Research

Placebo Response

It has been difficult to establish conclusively the efficacy of light therapy, in part because of the difficulty in finding an appropriate placebo. Compounding this difficulty is the belief among patients with SAD that the disorder is due to lack of light, and the knowledge that light therapy is an effective treatment. Thus, treatments other than bright light are less likely to be credible to patients. Because expectation of benefit may influence response to light therapy (Wehr et al. 1987), an implausible treatment may not be suitable for use as a placebo.

The most appropriate placebo for light therapy is one that is similar in every way to light therapy but does not involve the emission of light. Such a "no-light" or "sham light" condition is difficult to engineer because treatment with light cannot be "blind" (Brown 1990; Eastman 1990; Stewart 1990). A variety of potential placebos have been employed, including dim light (Lam et al. 1991; Rosenthal et al. 1984, 1985; Stinson and Thompson 1990; M. Terman et al. 1989a), light of restricted wavelength (Brainard et al. 1990; Oren et al. 1991; Wirz-Justice et al. 1986), evening light, and brief exposure (M. Terman et al. 1989a; Wirz-Justice et al. 1987), but some of these "placebos" may be active and, therefore, might best be called control treatments.

Several groups have devised placebos that do not involve the emission of light and yet are credible to patients. Eastman et al.

(1992) employed a deactivated negative ion generator as a placebo treatment for comparison with 7,000-lux light box treatment in a crossover trial. The negative ion generators had been deactivated by altering an internal circuit, and subjects were aware that the generator they received might be active or inactive. (Data reported concerned the deactivated generators only.) As the fan and pilot light still functioned, subjects could not determine which type of generator they received. The study lasted 5 weeks: a baseline week was followed by 2 weeks each of light and placebo treatments given for 1 hour upon wakening. Thirty-two subjects completed the protocol and experienced a significant reduction in depression scores on both the active and placebo treatments, regardless of the scale used: 17-item HAM-D, a composite HAM-D scale including the 17 original and 7 atypical items, and the BDI. In addition, there were no differences between the two treatments in their antidepressant effects, although response rates were low. With response defined as a 50% fall in composite HAM-D score to a score less than 16, 31% were light responders and 19% were placebo responders. Subjects expected to benefit from both treatments but felt that the light box would be superior to the negative ion generator, which they knew might be a placebo.

Given that no difference was detected between the active and placebo treatments, the authors considered whether the sample size was too small. They concluded that the effect size was so small as to be clinically irrelevant even if shown to be statistically significant with a larger sample. They also addressed the issue of the low response rate, noting that an inadequate dose of light (in duration, intensity, or timing), the inclusion of a placebo, or the selection of a less light-sensitive patient sample could account for the observed results. Although this placebo did not involve the emission of light, the ion generator and light box clearly appeared different, and patients therefore were not blind to all treatment conditions. Further, patients expected to derive slightly more benefit from the active condition.

More recently, a study employing a no-light placebo has been completed (Levitt et al. 1996). Light boxes and HMUs emitting visible light were compared with others that emitted no light. Deception was used to make plausible a treatment unit that emitted no light and to remove expectation of benefit from the presence of visible light. The no-light condition allowed the comparison of light with a genuine placebo differing from the active treatment only in the absence of the active ingredient (Horvath 1988).

Forty-three subjects were randomly assigned in a double-blind manner to receive 2 weeks of active treatment with a light box ($n = 9$) or HMU ($n = 12$) that emitted visible light, or 2 weeks of placebo treatment with a light box ($n = 12$) or HMU ($n = 10$) that emitted no visible light. Response was defined as a 50% reduction in both the 17-item "typical" score and 8-item "atypical" score on the SIGH-SAD. Using ANOVA for repeated measures, with change in total SIGH-SAD score as the dependent measure, there was no significant main effect of treatment condition (active vs. placebo; $F = 0.20$, $P = $ NS) or unit (light box vs. HMU; $F = 0.50$, $P = $ NS), and no interaction ($F = 0.21$, $P = $ NS). Using χ^2 analysis, there was no significant difference in response rates between patients who received light (48%) versus patients who received no light (41%; $\chi^2 = 0.2$, $P = $ NS).

There are several possible explanations for the failure to detect a difference in outcome between the two groups. First, the inability to find a difference between the active and placebo treatments may be due to the small number of patients studied. The sample size was small, which raises the possibility of Type II error. A second explanation for the observed findings is that the study and treatments were not credible, and so subjects had a universally low response rate, equal across both groups. However, subjects had very positive expectations even after exposure to the treatments, and expectations of benefit did not predict eventual outcome. In addition, when subjects were asked whether they believed they had received active or placebo treatment, their reply depended more on whether they had responded to treatment, than on the treatment condition. These findings suggest that the deception was effective in making both treatment conditions plausible. Third, it may be that the inclusion of a placebo reduced overall response rates (Eastman et al. 1992), an effect observed in both antidepressant drug (Wechsler et al. 1965) and light therapy (Eastman et al. 1992; M. Terman and Terman 1991) trials. Fourth, the entry criteria may have been too lenient, leading to the inclusion of mildly depressed patients, and, therefore, response patterns may be different from those in previous studies. However, subjects in this study were about as depressed as subjects in a variety of previous light therapy studies (M. Terman et al. 1989a), which makes this an unlikely explanation for the observed results. Furthermore, more mildly depressed patients appear to respond more readily to light treatment (M. Terman et al. 1989a). Thus, a relatively larger difference in response rates to the bright and dim conditions might have been expected if the subjects were less severely depressed than those in other studies. Fifth, the "dose" of light, that is, some function of intensity and duration of treatment, may have been inadequate. This seems unlikely, because similar methodology has been used in nonplacebo controlled trials of light therapy in which response rates were well above 50% (Joffe et al. 1993; Levitt et al. 1991, 1994). In addition, the results were in keeping with previous findings in controlled trials (M. Terman et al. 1989a). Therefore, the failure to detect a difference in response rates between the treatments was not likely due to relative "underdosing." Last, the failure to demonstrate a difference in response rates between the active and placebo conditions may indicate that light therapy is not superior to no light, as observed in earlier studies involving no-light placebo treatments (Eastman et al. 1992; M. Terman and Terman 1994). Because the majority of experimental results to date suggest that light therapy does have specific therapeutic effects in SAD beyond any nonspecific effects, it is premature to suggest that light therapy is a nonspecific or placebo treatment. Further investigation is required to establish the efficacy of light therapy more conclusively. These studies will most likely have to be of the multicenter type in order to provide adequate numbers of patients for sufficient power analysis and will also depend on the development of an appropriate control condition or a credible no-light placebo. For further comments on the placebo and sample size issues, see Chapter 12.

Other Research Issues

Inadequate sample size has plagued research in the area of light therapy for SAD. M. Terman et al. (1989a) calculated that more than 24 patients per treatment cell (active and placebo) were required in any individual trial to draw statistically meaningful conclusions regarding the efficacy of light treatment. No published investigation of the light box has included 24 subjects per cell. To reduce sample size requirements, many light box studies employed crossover designs. However, the strength of findings from studies using this design may be diminished because treatment order appears to influence response to light therapy (Oren et al. 1991; Stewart et al. 1991; M. Terman et al. 1990a), and carryover effects may alter baseline severity and expectations of benefit (Blehar and Lewy 1990; M. Terman et al. 1989a). Thus, caution must be exercised in the interpretation of the results of individual light therapy trials that have small sample size or crossover design. With regard to the HMU, a number of studies have appeared in the literature, each of which involved in excess of 25 patients per treatment cell (Joffe et al. 1993; Levitt et al. 1996; Rosenthal et al. 1993; Teicher et al. 1995). For example, the largest (Joffe et al. 1993) included 105 subjects in three treatment cells. Consequently, the results of these individual trials may be more statistically powerful than the results of previous light box studies that involved smaller sample sizes.

Another methodological issue that has impacted the field is the duration of light therapy trials. Most studies have been of short duration (1–2 weeks). To conclusively establish the effectiveness of any treatment, including light therapy, longer trials are likely required, particularly because placebo response tends to occur early but is not sustained (Brown 1990). Therefore, light box and HMU studies that use larger samples, parallel designs, and extend beyond 2 weeks are clearly needed.

Finally, only a few centers report standardized measurement of the properties of light, such as luminance, illuminance, irradiance, and photon density. Standardization across all centers is essential to assess the significance of experimental findings and allow meaningful comparisons to be made between work done at different centers.

Clinical Management of Seasonal Affective Disorder

Light therapy is the current treatment of choice for SAD (American Psychiatric Association 1993; Rosenthal 1993; Society for Light

Treatment and Biological Rhythms 1990) and may be used safely in patients in whom the diagnosis has been confirmed and active eye pathology excluded. Clinical guidelines for the use of light therapy will be outlined and followed by a description of alternative therapies for treatment nonresponders.

Light Therapy

Standard treatment involves a 7- to 14-day trial of daily exposure to 10,000 lux of white light for 30 minutes upon wakening (Figure 2–3). The effects of light therapy are usually brisk, with some response often evident after 1 day and usually within the first week.

For treatment responders, it is recommended that light therapy be continued throughout the entire winter until the time at which patients usually experience a spontaneous remission in their symptoms. During this continuation phase, it may be possible for some

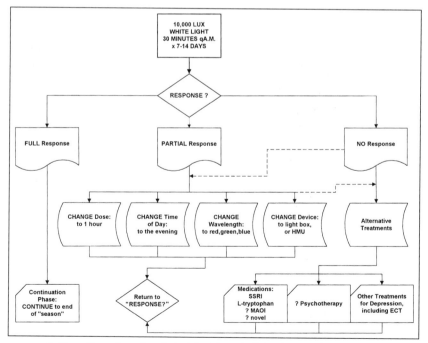

FIGURE 2–3. Flow chart for clinical decisions in light therapy for seasonal depression.

patients to lower the dose of light received by reducing daily exposure time or taking treatment on alternate days. The onset of response and relapse is so rapid during light therapy, that this type of "titration" is relatively common and appropriate. Such modification in treatment parameters, if undertaken in a systematic way with appropriate monitoring, will allow patients to avoid relapse while receiving lower levels of light exposure.

If there is only a partial response after 7–14 days, there are several treatment options to consider.

1. *Increase the dose.* Dose increase can be achieved by increasing the duration of exposure time to 1 hour daily or adding a second light treatment in the evening, or by increasing the intensity of the light being received. There is no empirical evidence to support either strategy, but clinicians often report success following dose increases.

2. *Change the timing.* As demonstrated by M. Terman and co-workers' (1989a) meta-analysis and confirmed by more recent crossover studies (Avery et al. 1990, 1991; Sack et al. 1990; J. S. Terman et al. 1990), morning light appears to be superior to evening light for most patients. However, a small number of patients may be preferential evening light responders (J. S. Terman et al. 1990). Therefore, switching from morning to evening exposure may be considered.

3. *Change the spectrum (color).* Another strategy for partial responders may be to narrow the spectrum of light delivered from white light to light of a specific wavelength or color. However, light box studies (Brainard et al. 1990; Stewart et al. 1991) appear to demonstrate the superiority of white light, and HMU studies (Joffe et al. 1993; Levitt et al. 1994 1996; Rosenthal et al. 1993; Teicher et al. 1995) suggest that response rates to red and white light are similar. Further, little is known about the effect of changing to a specific wavelength in the treatment of nonresponders. Nonetheless, such a trial may be warranted in some cases, when time and the clinical situation allow.

4. *Change the technology.* Another possibility to consider for partial responders is switching from one means of delivering light to another. The two most commonly used technologies, the light box

and the HMU, appear to produce similar response rates whether one compares the results of separate light box and HMU studies or when the two are compared directly in a single study. We have treated 11 patients who failed to respond to 2 weeks of red light from an HMU, with bright white light from a light box, using the same 2-week design, and found that 7 of the 11 (63%) had full response, and 1 (9%) had partial response (Levitt AJ et al., unpublished data, 1994).

5. *Try alternative therapies.* A final option for partial responders or patients who experience recurrence of symptoms after an initial response to light is the addition of an antidepressant medication. The use of pharmacotherapy is described later.

If there is no response after a 14-day trial of light therapy, it may still be possible to consider the these five options. However, many clinicians recommend that if there is complete lack of response, light therapy be discontinued and alternate treatment commenced. This recommendation is based on the clinical observations that a majority of patients who eventually respond to light therapy show some response in the first week and that, among patients who fail to show even a partial response at 14 days, few will respond if treatment is extended. Further, such an extension must be balanced against the risk of continued depression. Alternative treatments are discussed in the following section.

Alternative Treatments

Although antidepressant medications are the treatment of choice for depression, many patients with SAD do not wish to take them. They may have the expectation that they will receive and benefit from light therapy or may have had previous unsatisfactory medication trials. Few studies have investigated the use of pharmacological treatments for SAD, but those that have suggest that antidepressants may be helpful. Two preliminary trials of fenfluramine, a serotonin agonist, have demonstrated its effectiveness in SAD when compared to a pill placebo (O'Rourke et al. 1987, 1989). In a small ($N = 13$), 1-week crossover study, McGrath et al. (1990) showed that L-tryptophan, an amino acid involved in the formation of several neurotransmitters including serotonin, was equivalent to bright evening light and superior to a pill placebo. In a 3-week trial, moclobemide was shown to be no more effective than a pill placebo among 31 SAD patients (Lingjaerde et al. 1993). In two recent, multicenter trials, fluoxetine ($N = 68$) (Lam et al. 1995) and sertraline ($N = 190$) (Moscovitch et al. 1995) were superior to a pill placebo. Based on the results of these large, randomized, double-blind, placebo-controlled studies, serotonin reuptake inhibitors are currently the recommended antidepressant medications for SAD. These drugs may be prescribed using guidelines similar to those used for patients with nonseasonal depression.

Much is known about the efficacy of psychotherapy for depression. In contrast, little is known about its use for patients with SAD. Clinical experience suggests that psychotherapy may be of benefit to some patients, although evidence of seasonal variation in mood usually persists. Firm recommendations regarding the use of psychotherapy in the management of SAD await further study.

Conclusions

Light therapy has been consistently shown to alleviate the symptoms of SAD in well over 50% of subjects, although its mechanism of action or therapeutic ingredient is, as yet, unknown. With regard to light box treatment, bright white light given in the morning appears to be the most effective modality. Treatment with the light box allows the use of control conditions (evening light, dim light, or brief exposure), whereas all treatment conditions with the HMU thus far produce similar results. A number of clinical issues regarding light therapy for SAD remain to be resolved and are the focus of continued research effort.

References

American Psychiatric Association: Diagnostic and Statistical Manual of Mental Disorders, 3rd Edition. Revised. Washington, DC, American Psychiatric Association, 1987.

American Psychiatric Association: Practice guideline for major depressive disorder in adults. Am J Psychiatry 150(suppl):1–26, 1993

American Psychiatric Association: Diagnostic and Statistical Manual of Mental Disorders, 4th Edition. Washington, DC, American Psychiatric Association, 1994

Avery DH, Khan A, Dager SR, et al: Bright light treatment of winter depression: morning versus evening light. Acta Psychiatr Scand 82:335–338, 1990

Avery DH, Khan A, Dager SR, et al: Morning or evening bright light treatment of winter depression? The significance of hypersomnia. Biol Psychiatry 29:117–126, 1991

Avery DH, Bolte MA, Millet M: Bright dawn simulation compared with bright morning light in the treatment of winter depression. Acta Psychiatr Scand 85:430–434, 1992a

Avery DH, Bolte MA, Cohen S, et al: Gradual versus rapid dawn simulation treatment of winter depression. J Clin Psychiatry 53:359–363, 1992b

Avery DH, Bolte MA, Dager SR, et al: Dawn simulation treatment of winter depression: a controlled study. Am J Psychiatry 150:113–117, 1993

Avery DH, Bolte MA, Wolfson JK, et al: Dawn simulation compared with a dim red signal in the treatment of winter depression. Biol Psychiatry 36:181–188, 1994

Beck AT, Ward CH, Mendelson M, et al: An inventory for measuring depression. Arch Gen Psychiatry 4:561–571, 1961

Blehar MC, Lewy AJ: Seasonal mood disorders: consensus and controversy. Psychopharmacol Bull 26:465–494 1990

Blehar MC, Rosenthal NE: Seasonal affective disorders and phototherapy. Report of a National Institute of Mental Health sponsored workshop. Arch Gen Psychiatry 46:469–474, 1989

Bochow TW, West SK, Azar A, et al: Ultraviolet light exposure and risk of posterior subcapsular cataracts. Arch Ophthalmol 107:396–372, 1989

Booker JM, Hellekson CJ: Prevalence of seasonal affective disorder in Alaska. Am J Psychiatry 149:1176–1182, 1992

Brainard GC, Lewy AJ, Menaker M, et al: Dose-response relationship between light irradiance and the suppression of melatonin in human volunteers. Brain Res 454:212, 1988

Brainard GC, Sherry D, Skwerer RG, et al: Effects of different wavelengths in seasonal affective disorder. J Affect Disord 20:209–216, 1990

Brown WA: Is light treatment a placebo? Psychopharmacol Bull 26: 527–530, 1990

Chan PKY, Lam RW, Perry KF: Mania precipitated by light therapy for patients with SAD (letter). J Clin Psychiatry 55:454, 1994

Dawson D, Campbell SS: Bright light treatment: are we keeping our subjects in the dark? Sleep 13:267–271, 1990

Docherty JP, Hafez HM, Frank AF, et al: Wavelength study of phototherapy for seasonal affective disorder, in CME Syllabus and Proceedings Summary. Edited by American Psychiatric Association. Washington, DC, American Psychiatric Association, 1988

Doghramji K, Gaddy JR, Stewart KT, et al: 2 versus 4 hour evening phototherapy of seasonal affective disorder. J Nerv Ment Dis 178:257–260, 1990

Eastman CI: What the placebo literature can tell us about light therapy for SAD. Psychopharmacol Bull 26:495–504, 1990

Eastman CI, Lahmeyer HW, Watell LG, et al: A placebo-controlled trial of light treatment for winter depression. J Affect Disord 26:211–222, 1992

Gallin PF, Terman M, Reme CE, et al: Ophthalmologic examination of patients with seasonal affective disorder, before and after bright light therapy. Am J Ophthalmology 119:202–210, 1995

Gorman CP, Wyse PH, Demjen S, et al: Ophthalmological profile of 71 SAD patients: a significant correlation between myopia and SAD (abstract), in Abstracts of the 5th Annual Meeting. Edited by Society for Light Treatment and Biological Rhythms. Wilsonville, OR, Society for Light Treatment and Biological Rhythms, 1993

Grota LJ, Yerevanian BI, Gupta K, et al: Phototherapy for seasonal major depressive disorder: effectiveness of bright light of high or low intensity. Psychiatry Res 29:29–35, 1989

Guy W: ECDEU Assessment Manual for Psychopharmacology, Revised (DHEW Publ No ADM-76-338) Rockville, MD, National Institute of Mental Health, 1976

Ham WT, Mueller HA, Sliney DH: Retinal sensitivity to damage from short wavelength light. Nature 260:153–155, 1976

Ham WR, Mueller HA, Ruffolo JJ Jr, et al: Action spectrum for retinal injury from near-ultraviolet radiation in the aphakic monkey. Am J Ophthalmol 83:299–306, 1982

Hamilton M: A rating scale for depression. J Neurol Neurosurg Psychiatry 23:56–62, 1960

Hellekson CJ: Phenomenology of seasonal affective disorder: an Alaskan perspective, in Seasonal Affective Disorders and Phototherapy. Edited by Rosenthal NE, Blehar. New York, Guilford Press, 1989

Horvath P. Placebos and common factors in two decades of psychotherapy research. Psychol Bull 104:214–225, 1988

Joffe RT, Moul DE, Lam RW, et al: Light visor treatment for seasonal affective disorder: amulticenter study. Psychiatry Res 46:29–39, 1993

Kantor DA, Browne M, Ravindran A, et al: Manic-like response to phototherapy (letter). Can J Psychiatry 36:697–698, 1991

Kasper S, Wehr T, Bartko JJ, et al: Epidemiological findings of seasonal changes in mood and behavior: a telephone survey of Montgomery County, Maryland. Arch Gen Psychiatry 46:823–833, 1989

Kasper S, Rogers SL, Madden PA, et al: The effects of phototherapy in the general population. J Affect Disord 18:211–219, 1990

Kripke DF: Timing of phototherapy and occurrence of mania (letter). Biol Psychiatry 29:1156, 1991

Labbate LA, Lafer B, Thibault A, et al: Side effects induced by bright light treatment for seasonal affective disorder. J Clin Psychiatry 55:189–191, 1994

Lafer BLA, Sachs GS, Labbate LA, et al: Phototherapy for seasonal affective disorder: a blind comparison of three different schedules. Am J Psychiatry 151:1081–1083, 1994

Lam RW: Seasonal affective disorder: Emerging from the dark. Can J Diagnosis 11:53–64, 1994

Lam RW, Buchanan A, Clark CM, Remick RA: Ultraviolet versus non-ultraviolet light therapy for seasonal affective disorder. J Clin Psychiatry 52:213–216, 1991

Lam RW, Buchanan A, Mador JA, et al: The effects of ultraviolet-A wavelengths in light therapy for seasonal depression. J Affect Disord 24: 237–243, 1992

Lam RW, Gorman CP, Michalon M, et al.: A multi-centre, placebo-controlled study of fluoxetine in seasonal affective disorder. Am J Psychiatry 152:1765–1770, 1995

Levitt AJ: Prevalence of seasonal and non-seasonal depression (abstract), in New Research Abstracts of the 150th Annual Meeting. Edited by

American Psychiatric Association. Philadelphia, PA, American Psychiatric Association, 1994

Levitt AJ, Joffe RT, Kennedy SH. Bright light augmentation in antidepressant non-responders. J Clin Psychiatry 52:336–337, 1991

Levitt AJ, Joffe RT, Moul DE, et al: Side effects of light therapy in seasonal affective disorder. Am J Psychiatry 150:650–652, 1993

Levitt AJ, Joffe RT, King EF: Dim versus bright (LED) light in the treatment of seasonal affective disorder. Acta Psychiatr Scand 89:341–345, 1994

Levitt AJ, Wesson VA, King EF, et al: A controlled comparison of light box and head mounted units in teh treatment of seasonal depression. J Clin Psychiatry, 57:105–110, 1996

Lewy AJ, Kern HA, Rosenthal NE, et al: Bright artificial light treatment of a manic-depressive patient with a seasonal mood cycle. Am J Psychiatry 139:1496–1498, 1982

Lingjaerde O, Reichborn-Kjennerud T, Haggag A, et al.: Treatment of winter depression in Norway, II: a comparison of the selective monoamine oxidase A inhibitor moclobemide and placebo. Acta Psychiatr Scand 88:372–380, 1993

Magnusson A, Kristbjarnarson H: Treatment of seasonal affective disorder with high-intensity light. A phototherapy study with an Icelandic group of patients. J Affect Disord 21:141–147, 1991

McGrath RE, Buckwald B, Resnick EV: The effect of L-tryptophan on seasonal affective disorder. J Clin Psychiatry 51:162–1633, 1990

Meesters Y, Lambers PA, Jansen JHC, et al: Can winter depression be prevented by light treatment? J Affect Disord 23:75–79, 1993

Moscovitch A, Blashko C, Wiseman R, et al.: A double-blind, placebo-controlled study of sertraline in patients with seasonal affective disorder (abstract), in New Abstracts of the 148th Annual Meeting. Edited by American Psychiatric Association. Washington, DC, American Psychiatric Association, 1995

Moul DE, Hellekson CJ, Oren DA, et al: Treating SAD with a light visor: a multicenter study (abstract), in Abstracts of the 2nd Annual Meeting. Edited by Society for Light Treatment and Biological Rhythms. Wilsonville, OR, Society for Light Treatment and Biological Rhythms, 1990

Oren DA, Rosenthal FS, Rosenthal NE, et al: Exposure to ultraviolet B radiation during phototherapy. Am J Psychiatry 147:675–676, 1990

Oren DA, Brainard GC, Johnston SH, et al: Treatment of seasonal affective disorder with green light and red light. Am J Psychiatry 148:509–511, 1991

O'Rourke D, Wurtman JJ, Brzezinski A, et al.: Serotonin implicated in etiology of seasonal affective disorder. Psychopharmacol Bull 23: 358–359, 1987

O'Rourke D, Wurtman JJ, Wurtman RJ, et al.: Treatment of seasonal depression with d-fenfluramine. J Clin Psychiatry 50:343–347, 1989

Reme CE, Terman M: Does light therapy present an ocular hazard (letter)? Am J Psychiatry 149:1762–1763, 1992

Rosen LN, Targum SD, Terman M, et al: Prevalence of seasonal affective disorder at four latitudes. Psychiatry Res 31:131–144, 1990

Rosenthal NE: Diagnosis and treatment of seasonal affective disorder. JAMA 270:2717–2720, 1993

Rosenthal NE, Sack DA, Gillin C, et al: Seasonal affective disorder. A description of the syndrome and preliminary findings with light therapy. Arch Gen Psychiatry 41:72–80, 1984

Rosenthal NE, Sack DA, Carpenter CJ, et al: Antidepressant effects of light in seasonal affective disorder. Am J Psychiatry 142:606–608, 1985

Rosenthal NE, Moul DE, Hellekson CJ, et al: A multicenter study of the light visor for seasonal affective disorder: no difference in efficacy found between two different intensities. Neuropsychopharmacology 8:151–160, 1993

Sack DL; Lewy AJ, White DM, et al: Morning vs. evening light treatment for winter depression. Evidence that the therapeutic effects of light are mediated by circadian phase shifts. Arch Gen Psychiatry 47:343–351, 1990

Society for Light Treatment and Biological Rhythms: Consensus statement on the efficacy of light treatment for SAD. Light Treatment and Biological Rhythms Bulletin 3:5–9, 1990

Stewart J: Placebos in evaluating light therapy for seasonal affective disorder. Psychopharmacol Bull 26:525–526, 1990

Stewart KT, Gaddy JR, Benson DM, et al: Treatment of winter depression with a portable, head-mounted phototherapy device. Prog Neuropsychopharmacol Biol Psychiatry 14:569–578, 1990

Stewart KT, Gaddy JR, Byrne B, et al: Effects of green or white light for treatment of seasonal depression. Psychiatry Res 38:261–270, 1991

Stinson D, Thompson C: Clinical experience with phototherapy. J Affect Disord 18:129–135, 1990

Tam EM, Lam RW, Levitt AJ: Treatment of seasonal affective disorder: a review. Can J Psychiatry 40:457–466, 1995

Taylor HR, West SK, Rosenthal NE, et al: Effect of ultraviolet radiation on cataract formation. N Engl J Med 319:1429–1433, 1988

Teicher MH, Glod CA, Oren DA, et al: The phototherapy light visor: more to it than meets the eye. Am J Psychiatry 152:1197–1202, 1995

Terman JS, Terman M, Schlager D, et al: Efficacy of brief, intense light exposure for treatment of winter depression. Psychopharmacol Bull 26:3–11, 1990

Terman JS, Terman M, Amira L: One-week light treatment of winter depression near its onset: the time course of relapse. Depression 2:20–31, 1994

Terman M, Schlager D: Twilight therapeutics, winter depression, melatonin, and sleep, in Sleep and Biological Rhythms. Edited by Montplasir J, Godbout R. New York, Oxford University Press, 1990, pp 113–128

Terman M, Terman JS. Light Therapy for Seasonal Affective Disorder: Report to the Depression Guidelines Panel (U.S. Public Health Service Agency for Health Care Policy and Research). New York, New York Psychiatric Institute, 1991

Terman M, Terman JS: Light therapy for winter depression, in Biological Effects of Light. Edited by Holick MF, Kligman AM. Berlin, de Gruyter, 1992, pp 171–187

Terman M, Terman JS: A controlled trial of light therapy and negative ions (abstract), in Abstracts of the 6th Annual Meeting. Edited by Society for Light Treatment and Biological Rhythms. Wilsonville, OR, Society for Light Treatment and Biological Rhythms, 1994

Terman M, Terman JS, Quitkin FM, et al: Light therapy for seasonal affective disorder. A review of efficacy. Neuropsychopharmacology 2:1–22, 1989a

Terman M, Schlager D, Fairhurst S, Perlman B: Dawn and dusk simulation as a therapeutic intervention. Biol Psychiatry 25:966–970, 1989b

Terman M, Terman JS, Rafferty B: Experimental design and measures of success in the treatment of winter depression by bright light. Psychopharmacol Bull 26:505–510, 1990a

Terman M, Reme CE, Rafferty B, et al: Bright light therapy for winter depression: potential ocular effects and theoretical implications. Photochem Photobiol 51:781–792, 1990b

Vanselow W, Dennerstein L, Armstrong S, et al: Retinopathy and bright light therapy. Am J Psychiatry 148:1266–1267, 1991

Waxler M, James RH, Brainard GC, et al: Retinopathy and light therapy (letter). Am J Psychiatry 149:1610–1611, 1992

Wechsler H, Grosser GH, Greenblatt M. Research evaluating antidepressant medications on hospitalized mental patients: a survey of published reports during a five-year period. J Nerv Ment Dis 141:231–239, 1965

Wehr TA, Skwerer RG, Jacobsen FM, et al: Eye versus skin phototherapy of seasonal affective disorder. Am J Psychiatry 144:753–757, 1987

Weissman MM, Leaf PJ, Holzer CE III, et al: The epidemiology of depression: an update on sex differences in rates. J Affect Disord 7:178–188, 1984

Williams JBW, Link M, Rosenthal NE, et al.: Structured Interview Guide for the Hamilton Depression Rating Scale, Seasonal Affective Disorders Version (SIGH-SAD). New York, New York Psychiatric Institute, 1991

Winton F, Corn T, Huson LW, et al: Effects of light treatment upon mood and melatonin in patients with seasonal affective disorder. Psychol Med 19:585–590, 1989

Wirz-Justice A, Bucheli C, Graw P, et al: Light treatment of seasonal affective disorder in Switzerland. Acta Psychiatr Scand 74:193–204, 1986

Wirz-Justice A, Schmid AC, Graw P, et al: Dose relationships of morning bright white light in seasonal affective disorder. Experientia 43:574–576, 1987

Wirz-Justice A, Graw P, Kräuchi K, et al: Light therapy in seasonal affective disorder is independent of time of day or circadian phase. Arch Gen Psychiatry 50:929–937, 1993

THREE

On the Specific Action and Clinical Domain of Light Treatment

Michael Terman, Ph.D.

Studies of light treatment have been driven both by clinical successes (e.g., the antidepressant effect) and the discovery of associated physiological effects (e.g., melatonin suppression and circadian phase shifting). Although there are tantalizing connections across these levels of analysis, each has had a life of its own. Clinical results stand even when the mechanism of action is unknown, and physiological responses to light are of intrinsic interest even when their therapeutic relevance is uncertain. Although there is heuristic value in designing clinical studies around hypothesized underlying mechanisms, one senses a certain despair in the literature—even loss of interest in the therapeutic result—when the connection seems absent or imperfect. Thus, for example, a failure to obtain contrasting results for morning and evening light in treatment of winter depression may lead to abandonment of the circadian rhythm explanation, and a perilous assertion of the null hypothesis that overlooks or disputes other positive

Research supported by NIMH MH-42931. I thank Jiuan Su Terman for her collaboration in this work. Copies of the complete *Task Force Report on Light Treatment for Sleep Disorders,* cited earlier, are available from the Society for Light Treatment and Biological Rhythms, 10200 West 44th Avenue, Suite 304, Wheat Ridge, CO 80033; Tel 303-424-3697, Fax 303-422-8894, E-mail sltbr@resourcenter.com.

data. An investigator may be motivated by a search for a unique solution. However, adherence to an exclusive hypothesis in the face of other productive leads—for example, increased central nervous system serotonin availability—discounts the possibility of multiple underlying factors. As one result, laboratories begin ignoring each others' work.

The ubiquitous placebo factor complicates the analysis of specific mechanisms of action. Given substantial antidepressant placebo effects, it is inevitable that as more experiments are performed, some will fail to distinguish active from control conditions. As the list of negative results for light therapy has grown, some investigators have begun to ignore or downplay successful demonstrations of differential effects, and citations of the literature have become overly selective. It is discouraging to expend effort on a clinical trial and not be able to distinguish between the trial's groups. Investigators who find no differential effect may conclude that the placebo was itself active; it is unfortunate that lighting technology has been commercially disseminated on the basis of such arguments. This is a dangerous development for the field, one that undermines or obscures the application of treatments with demonstrated specific benefits.

The number of successful controlled trials has been sufficient to establish that the results are not flukes. Heuristically, I believe, the field needs to focus on what was "right" in studies that have shown differential effects, whether this involves the choice of controls, lighting conditions and circadian phase, treatment durations, scheduling of treatment relative to episode onset, location of treatment (hospital or home; individual or group), ancillary instructions to subjects concerning sleep timing and outdoor light exposure, loading of subjects' (and experimenters') expectations, medication exclusions, diagnostic profile, baseline symptom severity, consistency of untreated symptoms, course of symptoms during withdrawal, ascertainment of compliance, or measures of effect. One problem of earlier research—small sample size—has been overcome by a series of ambitious multiyear and multicenter studies, although it must be said that the added confidence of larger numbers has not consistently led to the conclusion that active treatment results in a response superior to a placebo.

The formidable complexity of outpatient trials—with imperfect control of light exposure and sleep patterns, and reliance on subjective reports of mood state and somatic symptoms—certainly creates an obstacle to generating clear-cut results. There have been few rigorous studies of inpatient populations receiving light treatment, and a large-scale clinical trial for a syndrome such as seasonal affective disorder (SAD)—for which patients rarely need hospitalization—might well be unfeasible. Regardless of the potential benefits of inpatient studies, demonstrations of clinical effect have to be made in the real world because that is where a proven treatment would be disseminated. A successful result with outpatients depends on being able to override many confounding factors. Although some outpatient studies have shown only subtle effects of questionable clinical significance, the thrust of data for light therapy of winter depression is powerful. This motivates the search for new arenas of application, and—as this book attests—the list of candidate syndromes is growing rapidly.

Circadian and Placebo Factors

Whether the primary mechanism of action of light in winter depression is circadian is still debatable. For certain other maladies—an example being the sleep disturbances of jet lag—a central therapeutic principle is the reentrainment of the circadian system by light. Circadian factors will remain prominent in new applications even as additional physiological effects of light may be discovered. For a comprehensive review, see the recent consensus report *Light Treatment for Sleep Disorders* (Boulos et al. 1995; Campbell et al. 1995a, 1995b, 1995c; Dijk et al. 1995; Eastman et al. 1995; Terman et al. 1995).

A basic question is whether there will be light-treatable syndromes, diseases, or disturbances that do *not* implicate circadian involvement—for example, through direct alerting/energizing effects, potentiation of serotonin availability, or photoimmune response. SAD is a prime candidate for such analysis, given experiments that have failed to find circadian phase shifts despite therapeutic response, and others that have found phase shifts that are not correlated with therapeutic response. In this context, the serotonin hypothesis (Jacobsen et al. 1989; O'Rourke et al. 1989) has received greatest attention as an alternative (e.g., Joseph-Vanderpool et al. 1993; Tam et al., this volume), although recent data for animals show an interaction between serotonin availability in the suprachiasmatic nuclei (SCN), and susceptibility of the SCN circadian pacemaker to phase shifting by light (Glass et al. 1995). In view of the extensive literature demonstrating phase shifts to light, a negative result might be caused by inadequate scheduling or intensity of light, unspecified conflicting light exposure at alternate times of day, conflicting non-photic zeitgebers (stimuli that phase-shift circadian rhythms), measurement of circadian markers vulnerable to masking by noncircadian factors, or insensitive measurement of the phase marker. An additional confound common in data analysis is group averaging of results for subjects who differ in baseline circadian phase, and whose individual responses to light would be expected to differ.

An ongoing experiment in my laboratory illustrates one approach to teasing out circadian from other influences on therapeutic response. Outpatients with winter depression were assigned to 10- to 14-day sequences of morning light (10,000 lux, 30 minutes on awakening) followed by evening light (30 minutes, 1–2 hours before bedtime), or vice versa. A subgroup (n-38) received plasma melatonin sampling in the laboratory immediately before and at the end of one or both treatment intervals. Blood samples were taken every 30 minutes for 5 hours to determine the onset of melatonin secretion under dim-light conditions; in several cases, the complete nocturnal secretory episode was measured in 15-hour sessions. Melatonin levels were ascertained by a direct radioimmunoassay, and the onset phase was specified as the time when the curve reached 10 pg/ml. At baseline (while depressed), onset phases ranged widely, from 7:45 P.M. to 12:24 A.M. (mean of 9:34 P.M.). Clinical response was measured as percent change relative to the depressed baseline, using the 29-item *Structured Interview Guide to the Hamilton Depression Rating Scale—Seasonal Affective Disorder Version* (SIGH-SAD) (Williams et al. 1994).

Although morning light reliably elicited circadian phase advances (mean of 0.69 hours in treatment 1, and 1.23 hours in treatment 2), and evening light produced phase delays (0.74 hours and 1.24 hours, respectively), the overall proportion of patients showing SIGH-SAD score improvements of at least 50% was similar given phase delays or advances (0.67 vs. 0.77, $\chi^2 = 0.76$, NS). Thus, one might conclude that although light elicited the anticipated phase shifts, these shifts did not contribute to the clinical effect. Furthermore, the clinical effect might have been caused by placebo factors alone, or by the placebo in combination with other active antidepressant properties of the light. A pure placebo explanation seems unlikely given the far lower response rate (0.15) in an independent group that had been randomized into low-density negative ion treatment (Terman and Terman 1995).

However, a circadian factor *is* involved. Clinical response was significantly correlated with the magnitude of melatonin phase advances ($r = 0.41, P < .05$). Nonresponders (those with less than 50% improvement) showed a mean phase advance of 0.56 hours, while responders showed an advance of 1.12 hours ($P < .01$). Furthermore, there was no significant correlation between clinical improvement and phase delays ($r = -0.11$). This selective circadian effect is illustrated in Figure 3–1, which shows 1) a group mean overnight melatonin secretion profile at baseline while subjects were depressed, and 2) individual improvement scores obtained with light exposure at various times across evening and morning hours. Both the melatonin curve and clinical data are anchored, at 0 hours, to each individual's pretreatment melatonin onset phase. Evening light exposures were distributed before and after melatonin onset, whereas morning light exposures were confined to the declining segment of secretion (6–12 hours after melatonin onset) and did not occur after melatonin offset. For evening light, there was no significant correlation between time of treatment and percent improvement ($r = 0.09$); the response to morning light declined the later the light was received ($r = -0.52, P = .01$).

These results suggest a model reminiscent of the hypothesis of Lewy et al. (1988; Hughes and Lewy, this volume), in which morning light elicits circadian phase advances according to the phase response curve (PRC), and these phase advances subserve the antidepressant effect. Such a hypothesis may apply to a subset of our data ($n = 17$) that excludes cases in which there were small dim light melatonin onset (DLMO) phase delays to morning light ($n = 3$), symptoms were exacerbated after treatment ($n = 1$), or the timing of light was so early (approximately 6 hours post-DLMO, $n = 2$) that it may have coincided with the PRC crossover region, causing smaller phase

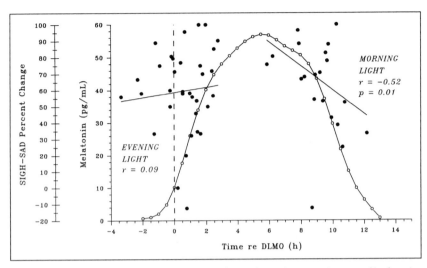

FIGURE 3-1. *Continuous curve:* Overnight melatonin secretion profile for six patients with winter depression. Individual curves were smoothed and averaged, and each was anchored to t_0, the dim light melatonin onset (DLMO), when secretory levels in plasma first reached 10 pg/ml. *Filled data points:* Baseline-to-posttreatment change in depression rating scale (29-item SIGH-SAD) scores for 30-minute exposure intervals of morning light (which produced phase advances of the melatonin cycle) or evening light (which produced delays), with treatment durations of 10–14 days. Data are positioned on the abscissa according to the time difference between the scheduled light exposure and each individual's pretreatment DLMO. (The correlation between treatment time and morning light response, $r = -0.52$, excludes the outlying nonresponder; inclusion of this subject lowers r to $-0.34, P = 0.07$.)

advances and poorer clinical response relative to treatment given later. As tested by MANOVA for the restricted subset of 17 cases (specified earlier), the data indicate that the circadian time of morning light jointly affects the magnitude of the melatonin phase advances and improvement on the SIGH-SAD scale (Wilks' lambda $= 0.603$, $F = 4.61$, $P = .029$). By contrast, in the case of evening light ($n = 34$), there is no significant relationship between the size of phase delays and clinical response (Wilke's lambda $= 0.974$, $F = 0.42$, $P = .66$).

Light exposure at a constant clock time (e.g., 6:00 A.M., as has been common in group studies of winter depression) will vary with respect to circadian time for individuals across an expected range of about 5 hours, to judge by the distribution of melatonin onset times at baseline. If the circadian time of light exposure determines the magnitude of clinical effect, results will be suboptimal if exposure is anchored to a standard external clock time, and thereby introduce a noise factor that could obfuscate group differences in otherwise controlled studies. However, without a simple way for clinicians to determine circadian phase, it would be impossible to specify the recommended hour of morning light administration, apart from guesswork and individual empirical adjustment. Both experimenters and clinicians would benefit from a commercial service that provides rapid turnaround of salivary melatonin profiles to guide the timing of light treatment.

According to the data in Figure 3–1, maximal clinical improvement is obtained by using a 30-minute, 10,000-lux light exposure approximately 8 hours post-DLMO. Even without direct measurement, one can roughly estimate an individual's baseline DLMO phase from daily sleep logs that record the times of habitual sleep onset and awakening. In a group of 36 patients who were depressed in winter, we found a high correlation between the sleep midpoint and DLMO ($r = 0.53$, $P = .0004$), which exceeded the correlations of DLMO with the sleep onset and awakening. The regression equation yields the DLMO phase estimate as

$$Y_{DLMO} = 0.91\, X_{midpoint} + 18.73,$$

where X is expressed as time of day in decimal hours (e.g., 3.76 A.M.). Although estimates will deviate substantially from the true DLMO in individual cases, the average error will be smaller than that obtained by using arbitrary clock time assignments for morning light exposure. If the formula is applied for 2-hour, 2,500-lux light treatment, care should be taken to specify the light onset phase, rather than the midpoint, in order to avoid excessively early exposure that coincides with the PRC crossover region and a risk of phase delays.

According to the simple circadian hypothesis, evening light should be ineffective, except for a minority of patients who are relatively phase advanced at baseline. The observed similar overall efficacy of morning and evening light remains a puzzle. If morning light is a specific antidepressant—as evidenced by the correlation of phase advances with clinical improvement—evening light must act either by another specific mechanism or by a powerful placebo effect (cf., Eastman et al. 1993). Clinically, the use of evening light might be advantageous in that its timing does not appear to be a significant dosing parameter. However, do we really want to prescribe a powerful placebo?

There is another line of evidence for evening light as a placebo, which derives from crossover studies in which patients receive a sequence of lighting conditions that permits within-subject comparisons of clinical response. Data from my laboratory—and pooling of data from other laboratories—indicate a reduced antidepressant effect when a trial of evening light follows a trial of morning light (for a review, see Terman 1993). We have not found such reduction when morning light follows a trial of evening light. Nor have we found between-group differences between morning and evening light in the initial treatment period, which corroborates a host of parallel-group studies that have not provided for a crossover. The reduced period 2 response to evening light may indicate a placebo effect in period 1. Under initial treatment, it can be reasoned that the placebo factor overwhelms any contrast in antidepressant response between morning and evening light. However, once a patient has experienced the specific action of morning light, the efficacy of evening light diminishes.

The morning × evening crossover provides an incomplete picture, however, because the diminished effect of evening light in period 2 must be expressed, indirectly, as a time-of-day × period interaction. An expansion of the experiment into a "balanced" crossover design (in progress in my laboratory) serves to clarify the effect. Additional groups receive morning or evening light in both periods 1 and 2. In this way we can directly compare response to evening light, given prior exposure at either time of day (i.e., morning-evening versus evening-evening). The placebo hypothesis predicts that patients will sustain their positive response under the evening-evening sequence because they lack prior experience with the specifically active

TABLE 3-1

Response rate to morning and evening light following positive response in period 1 of a balanced crossover

Treatment sequence	Continued positive response*	Reduced response
Morning-morning	82%	18%
Evening-morning	90%	10%
Evening-evening	80%	20%
Morning-evening	37%	63%

*At least 67% improvement in SIGH-SAD score relative to baseline.

treatment. Table 3-1 summarizes preliminary results for the balanced crossover. We restricted the analysis to patients who responded in period 1 with at least 67% improvement in SIGH-SAD score ($n = 57$), which is a high threshold indicative of clinical remission. (Inclusion of period 1 nonresponders obfuscates the results by adding a major noise factor.) While only 37% of patients responded to evening light following exposure to morning light, 80%–90% of patients responded to all other period 2 conditions ($\chi^2 = 12.78, P = .005$).

Previously I described an alternative to the evening-placebo hypothesis: The elicitation of circadian phase delays as a result of evening light exposure following exposure to morning light—as described above—might be depressogenic (Terman 1993). If that were true, light at either time of day would be effective as long as large phase delays are avoided. However, this explanation seems unlikely now that we have been unable to find a correlation between phase delays and clinical response. Pending completion of the study, we conclude provisionally that morning light is a specific antidepressant by virtue of 1) the correlation of phase advances with clinical response and 2) the reduced effect of evening light following exposure to morning light. Unfortunately, experiments that do not specify the circadian time of light administration (e.g., by reference to the time of melatonin onset at baseline), or tease out reduced response to placebo following exposure to active treatment, may be vulnerable to negative results.

Casting a Net for Candidate Syndromes

Circadian phase disorders provide the most obvious jumping point for new applications of light treatment, and the man-made disturbances of jet lag and shift work (Boulos, this volume) provide the simplest models. The potential etiologic role of circadian phase disturbances in primary medical syndromes is still an open question. In some situations, circadian disturbances might result from changes in the pattern or intensity of daily light exposure during an illness. An altered sleep pattern will change the timing of light exposure, as will confinement to the bedroom or hospitalization. The delayed sleep phase syndrome (Hughes and Lewy, this volume), for example, may be triggered inadvertently by the absence of early morning light, and not necessarily reflect abnormal clock function (cf., Terman et al. 1995).

Mood disorders and a growing list of other psychiatric syndromes provide a second jumping point for which a circadian phase disorder may not be obvious. As in SAD, it is interesting that several of the promising syndromes are cyclic. Seasonality may be a key, as in winter-exacerbated bulimia nervosa (Lam and Goldner, this volume) and chronic fatigue syndrome (Lam 1991), or summer depressive episodes in bipolar illness (Bauer 1993). Syndromes that show non-seasonal cyclicity also show promise, for example, premenstrual dysphoric disorder (Parry, this volume) and rapid-cycling bipolar disorder (Kusumi et al. 1995). Cyclicity may not be an exclusive key, however, as illustrated by some successes using light therapy for treatment of chronic depressive disorders (Kripke, this volume). For nonwinter seasonal syndromes especially, one must ask whether symptoms are secondary to behaviorally or architecturally induced light deprivation. Does light therapy simply serve to bring these patients "outdoors"? Abnormalities of sleep phase and sleep continuity may provide another key. Indeed, there have been positive responses to light therapy in sleep-disordered patients with Alzheimer's disease (Mishima et al. 1994; Satlin et al. 1992), Parkinson's disease (Mosbach et al. 1993), and pediatric brain damage with mental retardation (Guilleminault et al. 1993).

Light therapy saw its genesis in psychiatry, but perhaps this was a historic accident, and nonpsychiatric medical applications will be discovered. A provocative literature, which predates light therapy and SAD, has implicated circadian disturbances in a wide range of medical illness (see, for example, Touitou and Haus 1992), but the bridge to light treatment has yet to be drawn. Here, too, seasonal variation may provide a key, particularly with regard to the status of the immune system, which may be light responsive (Kasper et al. 1991; Roberts et al. 1991).

One empirical approach for identifying seasonal patterns of potential interest—"casting the net"—would be to survey a broad range of physical symptoms in various clinical populations. An applicable tool is the *Systematic Assessment for Treatment Emergent Effects* (SAFTEE) (National Institute of Mental Health, 1986). It was originally designed to identify drug side effects but can be administered to patients on or off treatment and to contrasting patient groups. The list is categorized according to organ system and body part (e.g., head, eyes/vision, ears/hearing, mouth, chest, heart, stomach) and includes 88 core symptoms and 8 additional symptoms specifically related to the menstrual cycle. Each symptom is rated on a 5-point scale (1, absent; 3, moderate; 5, severe).

Seasonal Effects as Determined by the SAFTEE

Using SAD as an example, it is interesting to see how the SAFTEE can be used empirically to extract a syndromal definition and to identify which symptoms are affected by light treatment. Eighty-six patients who met the National Institute of Mental Health (NIMH) criteria for SAD (Rosenthal et al. 1984) completed a checklist based on the SAFTEE when depressed in winter, and again in spring. Table 3–2 lists 1) the frequency of symptom occurrence at the winter assessment, 2) the frequency with which each symptom was rated more prominent in winter than spring, and vice versa, and 3) the effect size of changes (based on McNemar's χ^2), which gauges the magnitude of seasonal difference and forms the basis for rank ordering of the symptoms in the table. It is important to note that this

TABLE **3–2**

Winter symptom frequency and changes from winter to spring ($n = 86$)

Symptom	Winter frequency[1] (%)	Seasonal contrast			Effect size (w)
		Winter > spring	Spring > winter	Unchanged	
Feeling depressed/"down"/"blue"	**100.0**	93.8	0.0	2.5	0.99
Thought/concentration/memory problems	**81.0**	76.2	0.0	21.4	0.98
Fatigue	**94.1**	90.6	1.2	5.9	0.96
Drowsiness	**91.7**	82.1	1.2	13.1	0.96
Irritability	**88.2**	81.9	1.2	14.5	0.96
Decreased sexual interest	**67.1**	61.7	1.2	30.9	0.94
Hypersomnia	**60.0**	58.8	1.2	37.6	0.94
Fever/chills	13.1	13.1	0.0	84.5	0.91
Change in stool color	12.8	11.6	0.0	87.2	0.90
Difficulty moving	30.6	29.4	1.2	67.1	0.88
Appetite increase	**70.9**	65.1	3.5	30.2	0.88
Anxiety	**78.8**	72.9	4.7	20.0	0.86
Weight gain	**57.0**	53.5	3.5	41.9	0.86
Gas	**57.0**	50.0	3.5	45.3	0.85
Middle insomnia	48.2	47.1	3.5	47.1	0.84
Dizziness/faintness	21.2	20.0	1.2	77.6	0.83
Diarrhea	18.6	17.4	1.2	80.2	0.81
Initial insomnia	42.4	37.6	3.5	56.5	0.80
Muscle/bone/joint pain	**56.5**	47.6	4.8	45.2	0.80
Heartburn	24.4	22.4	2.4	74.1	0.76
Rapid heartbeat	15.1	12.8	1.2	84.9	0.75
Dry mouth	34.9	27.9	3.5	67.4	0.74
Jumpiness/jitteriness	35.3	32.9	4.7	60.0	0.72
Abdominal discomfort	38.4	30.2	4.7	64.0	0.70
Frequent urination	27.1	22.6	3.6	71.4	0.68
Increased thirst	36.0	32.9	5.9	60.0	0.67
Headaches	**51.2**	40.7	8.1	50.0	0.64
Unsteady on feet	17.6	14.1	2.4	81.2	0.64
Difficulties with orgasm	22.5	15.5	2.8	69.0	0.62

(continued)

TABLE 3–2

Winter symptom frequency and changes from winter to spring ($n = 86$)
Continued

Symptom	Winter frequency (%)	Seasonal contrast			Effect size (w)
		Winter > spring	Spring > winter	Unchanged	
Nausea	15.1	12.8	2.3	83.7	**0.62**
Change in taste	16.5	16.5	3.5	78.8	**0.59**
Nasal congestion	47.7	33.7	9.3	55.8	**0.54**
Restlessness	31.3	28.9	8.4	60.2	**0.52**
Hand/foot numbness	20.2	13.1	3.6	79.8	**0.50**
Shortness of breath	20.0	15.3	4.7	78.8	**0.47**
Constipation	23.3	19.8	7.0	72.1	**0.43**
Skin rash/itch/irritation	23.5	16.5	5.9	75.3	**0.42**
Poor vision	14.1	12.9	4.7	81.2	**0.40**
Bleeding gums	14.0	12.9	4.7	81.2	**0.40**
Increased sexual interest[2]	12.2	9.9	**24.7**	59.3	**0.39**
Eye irritation	27.9	22.1	9.3	67.4	0.37
Weight loss[2]	10.5	9.3	**22.1**	67.4	0.37
Late insomnia	29.4	25.9	11.8	60.0	0.34
Coughing	19.8	15.1	7.0	76.7	0.32
Chest pain	10.6	10.6	4.7	83.5	0.31
Sore throat	25.6	20.9	11.6	66.3	0.25
Light bothersome to eyes	16.5	10.6	5.9	81.2	0.21
Dental problems	8.4	6.0	9.6	83.1	0.15
Blurred vision	15.1	9.3	5.8	83.7	0.15
Overactive/excited/elated[2]	16.7	9.5	**14.3**	73.8	0.15
Wheezing	8.2	5.9	5.9	87.1	0.10
Appetite decrease[2]	19.8	16.3	**14.0**	68.6	0.04
Breast tenderness	16.5	9.4	8.2	81.2	0.00
Excessive energy[2]	9.4	7.1	6.0	84.5	0.00
Difficulty with erection ($n = 20$ males)	35.0	**35.3**	0.0	64.7	–[3]
Noise/ringing in ears	12.0	8.4	1.2	86.7	–
Leg/arm swelling	10.7	9.5	0.0	86.9	–
Difficulty swallowing	10.5	9.3	0.0	89.5	–

(continued)

TABLE **3–2**

Winter symptom frequency and changes from winter to spring (n = 86)
Continued

Symptom	Winter frequency (%)	Seasonal contrast			Effect size (w)
		Winter > spring	Spring > winter	Unchanged	
Hemorrhoids	9.4	8.2	0.0	90.6	–
Irregular heartbeat	9.3	8.1	2.3	88.4	–
Mouth sores	9.3	7.0	3.5	88.4	–
Rigidity/stillness	8.4	8.4	0.0	89.2	–
Eye swelling	8.1	8.1	2.3	88.4	–
Hearing loss	8.1	3.5	1.2	94.2	–
Shaking	7.2	7.2	0.0	90.4	–
Sweating	7.1	6.0	4.8	88.1	–
Laryngitis	7.0	7.0	0.0	91.9	–
Double vision	5.9	4.7	0.0	94.1	–
Swollen/sore tongue	5.8	5.8	2.3	90.7	–
Genital discomfort	4.9	3.7	2.5	87.7	–
Genital swelling/discharge	4.9	3.7	0.0	90.1	–
Change in urine color	4.7	4.8	1.2	91.7	–
Bruising	4.7	4.7	2.4	90.6	–
Breast pain/discharge	4.7	4.7	3.5	90.7	–
Excess salivation	4.7	3.5	1.2	94.2	–
Unwanted body movements	3.6	3.6	0.0	94.0	–
Sunlight irritation	3.5	2.4	3.5	91.8	–
Painful bowel movements	3.5	3.5	0.0	95.3	–
Vomiting	3.5	3.5	0.0	95.3	–
Earache	3.5	2.3	2.3	94.2	–
Difficulty urinating	2.4	2.4	1.2	94.0	–
Decreased urinary pressure	2.4	2.4	0.0	95.2	–
Ear discharge	2.3	2.3	2.3	94.2	–
Nasal bleeding	2.3	2.3	1.2	95.3	–
Painful urination	1.2	1.2	0.0	96.4	–
Urinary burning	1.2	1.2	1.2	95.2	–
Loss of consciousness	0.0	0.0	0.0	98.8	–
Seizures	0.0	0.0	0.0	98.8	–

[1] All symptoms reported, mild to severe (boldfaced items, frequency >50%).
[2] Symptoms characteristic of hypomania.
[3] Change frequencies too low to calculate χ^2 and w.

analysis uses each subject as its own control (increased, decreased, or unchanged in the alternate season) and thus differs from a mere comparison of population symptom frequencies at the two assessment points.

In winter, 13 symptoms were registered by more than half the group (Table 3–2, first data column, boldfaced items). Taken together, they describe the SAD patient in a way that overlaps the classic syndromal description (i.e., depressed mood, fatigue and drowsiness, and atypical symptoms of hypersomnia, appetite increase, and weight gain). The prominence of irritability (88%), cognitive problems (81%), and anxiety (79%) is striking, however. Additionally, there is a small, specific set of somatic symptoms (gas and headaches) that falls within Hamilton's (1986) anxiety spectrum; and muscle/bone/joint pain may correspond to his characterization of "diffuse muscular achings." Decreased sexual interest ranks high (67%) as a typical symptom of depression.

The symptoms most prominent in winter are not exclusively the ones that show the greatest seasonal contrast, as gauged by the effect size of changes between winter and spring (for comparison, w = 0.1, small; 0.3, medium; 0.5, large) (cf., Cohen 1988). Other symptoms with medium-to-large effect size were found for subsets of the group, and the winter frequencies of these symptoms ranged from 10.6% to 48.2%. Some of these symptoms, for example, nasal congestion (47.7%), fever and chills (13.1%), and change in stool color (12.8%), are of particular interest because they fall outside the depressive cluster. Others, for example, digestive and abdominal problems, dry mouth, and increased thirst, are conventionally classified as somatic symptoms of anxiety, but are not necessarily anxiety-related.

One defining symptom of nonseasonal atypical depression, leaden paralysis (Klein 1974), is akin to the SAFTEE item "difficulty moving," which has a winter frequency of 30.6%. Although other data indicate that patients with nonseasonal atypical depression more frequently show leaden paralysis than do patients with winter depression (47% vs. 35%, χ^2 = 4.58, P = .032) (Terman et al., in press, in patients with SAD this symptom nonetheless shows large seasonal variation (w = 0.88).

When the objective is an empirical symptom screen untied to the conventional syndromal definition, low-frequency items are also of interest for identifying the presence or absence of seasonal variation. A given low-frequency symptom may strongly characterize a functionally distinct subgroup (e.g., unipolar or bipolar, male or female, menstrual or postmenopausal, and specific comorbid Axis I or Axis III disorders). In the present sample, symptoms with an effect size of seasonal change as small as $w = 0.39$ would show statistically significant differences at $P < .05$, according to McNemar's χ^2, (uncorrected for multiple tests). (Table 3–2, right-hand column, shows in boldface the range of symptoms with $w \geq 0.39$.) For example, "bleeding gums" is present in winter at a frequency of only 14% and yet shows moderate-to-large seasonal variation ($w = 0.40$). By contrast, sore throat shows twice the frequency (25.6%), but only small-to-moderate seasonal variation ($w = 0.25$). Eye irritation is reported by 27.9% of untreated patients in winter, with small-to-moderate improvement in spring ($w = 0.37$). Other low-frequency symptoms, which are characteristic of hypomania (third data column, boldface), show relatively higher frequencies in spring than in winter, although none shows a high effect size.

Difficulty with erection was present in winter in 35% of males. One patient spontaneously reported total inability to achieve erection throughout every winter, and no such problem in spring or summer. For him this was of greater concern than the depression; it preceded the onset of depressed mood in fall and persisted till spring, regardless of variations in mood state. Of the 20 males in this sample, 6 showed worsening of this symptom in winter, whereas none showed worsening in spring. Although the sample size is insufficient to express this change in terms of effect size the seasonal contrast is significant by a binomial test ($P = .016$, one-tailed).

The SAFTEE survey of patients with SAD has the advantage of a broader scope than the standard psychiatric diagnostic interview. The most prominent seasonal symptoms are closely associated with the established syndromal definition, although the dominance of irritability and anxiety over atypical symptoms is striking. The results provide a validation of the diagnostic profile, strengthened by the systematic discrimination of nonseasonal symptoms. There are few surprises within this well-studied population. However, such results provide a springboard for comprehensive descriptive comparisons with other clinical groups whose seasonality is not well documented, and who might be light responsive. In this respect the SAFTEE casts a broader net than the Seasonal Pattern Assessment Questionnaire (SPAQ) (Rosenthal et al. 1987), which focuses on a limited set of SAD-associated symptoms (mood, energy, sleep length, appetite and weight, and social activity). For example, a SPAQ study of patients with chronic fatigue syndrome (CFS) showed significant global seasonal variation in which winters were worse in 22% of cases (Zubieta et al. 1994). CFS shares several features with SAD but is also characterized by somatic symptoms such as low-grade fever, myalgias, stiffness, arthralgia, and rash (Komaroff and Buchwald 1991). As shown in Table 3–2, similar symptoms—which show seasonal variation—are reported by patients with SAD.

An obvious question arises: With regard to symptoms that do or do not "fit" the syndromal definition of SAD, to what extent is the spring-summer state achieved under light treatment? As one example, it appears that light may provide substantial benefit to CFS patients (Lam 1991; Terman M et al., in press), a group that has been historically treatment refractory and for which the syndromal definition accommodates considerable variability across cases (Fukuda et al. 1994).

Treatment effects

The SAFTEE can also be used, according to its original design, to monitor symptom change following treatment—improvement as well as side effects. The wide scope of the instrument provides an opportunity to identify responses to light treatment that might be overlooked in syndromally confined psychiatric assessments (e.g., the SIGH-SAD). Using SAD as a model, Table 3–3 lists the symptoms in order of decreasing effect size between pre- and posttreatment evaluations for 83 patients who received 10,000 lux, 30-minute light therapy in morning or evening. The group of subjects overlaps those that completed the winter and spring assessments (Table 3–2), and the highest-frequency symptoms at baseline are necessarily in close agreement. Middle insomnia joins the list of symptoms reported by

TABLE **3–3**

Winter symptom frequency and baseline-to-posttreatment change ($n = 83$)

Symptom	Baseline frequency[1] (%)	Treatment response			Effect size (w)
		Decreased	Increased	Unchanged	
Poor vision	14.6	13.4	0.0	86.6	0.91
Feeling depressed/ "down"/"blue"	100.0	76.9	6.4	12.8	0.83
Thought/concentration/ memory problems	80.0	61.3	5.0	31.3	0.83
Drowsiness	93.9	72.5	6.3	20.0	0.83
Fatigue	92.7	66.7	7.4	24.7	0.78
Increased thirst	33.7	30.1	3.6	66.3	0.75
Change in taste	13.6	13.6	1.2	85.2	0.75
Bleeding gums	13.3	10.8	1.2	88.0	0.70
Dry mouth	33.7	24.1	3.6	72.3	0.70
Irritability	82.9	63.0	11.1	24.7	0.68
Restlessness	37.8	28.4	4.9	65.4	0.67
Decreased sexual interest	60.0	49.3	9.3	36.0	0.66
Difficulty moving	26.8	21.0	3.7	74.1	0.65
Dizziness/faintness	17.1	14.6	2.4	81.7	0.64
Hypersomnia	56.8	45.7	11.1	40.7	0.59
Anxiety	79.3	56.8	14.8	27.2	0.57
Rapid heartbeat	21.7	15.7	3.6	80.7	0.56
Light bothersome to eyes	19.3	15.7	3.6	80.7	0.56
Initial insomnia	45.1	28.4	7.4	63.0	0.55
Hand/foot numbness	20.0	15.0	3.8	80.0	0.53
Middle insomnia	51.2	30.9	8.6	59.3	0.53
Eye irritation	26.5	21.7	6.0	72.3	0.52
Gas	49.4	28.9	8.4	62.7	0.52
Appetite increase	65.1	56.6	18.1	25.3	0.50
Headaches	53.0	34.9	10.8	54.2	0.50
Constipation	24.1	16.9	4.8	78.3	0.50
Skin rash/itch/irritation	20.7	16.0	4.9	77.8	0.47
Jumpiness/jitteriness	35.4	30.0	10.0	58.8	0.47
Frequent urination	29.6	22.2	7.4	69.1	0.46

(continued)

TABLE **3–3**

Winter symptom frequency and baseline-to-posttreatment change ($n = 83$) Continued

Symptom	Baseline frequency %	Treatment response			Effect size (w)
		Decreased	Increased	Unchanged	
Weight gain	**51.8**	41.0	14.5	44.6	**0.46**
Muscle/bone/joint pain	45.0	27.5	10.0	61.3	**0.43**
Difficulties with orgasm	20.0	17.5	6.3	63.5	0.40
Weight loss[2]	9.6	8.4	**19.3**	72.3	0.35
Heartburn	19.3	13.6	6.2	80.2	0.31
Unsteady on feet	14.6	11.1	4.9	82.7	0.31
Abdominal discomfort	37.3	24.1	12.0	63.9	0.30
Nasal congestion	49.4	31.7	17.1	51.2	0.28
Increased sexual interest[2]	12.0	10.8	**18.9**	64.9	0.23
Mouth sores	8.4	4.8	8.4	86.7	0.18
Late insomnia	32.9	21.0	13.6	64.2	0.18
Nausea	12.2	11.0	**17.1**	72.0	0.17
Chest pain	13.3	9.6	6.0	84.3	0.15
Overactive/excited/elated[2]	15.9	9.9	**13.6**	75.3	0.11
Laryngitis	9.6	7.2	4.8	88.0	0.10
Dental problems	7.4	7.4	4.9	86.4	0.10
Diarrhea	20.5	17.1	13.4	69.5	0.08
Shortness of breath	18.1	9.6	7.2	83.1	0.07
Breast tenderness	14.5	7.2	9.6	83.1	0.07
Coughing	20.7	19.5	15.9	64.6	0.07
Sore throat	20.5	13.3	13.3	73.5	0.05
Appetite decrease[2]	24.1	21.7	**19.3**	59.0	0.03
Fever/chills	11.0	8.6	9.9	80.2	0.00
Difficulty with erection ($n = 22$ males)	31.8	20.0	10.0	65.0	—[3]
Blurred vision	14.5	8.4	0.0	91.6	—
Noise/ringing in ears	11.3	6.4	5.1	85.9	—
Change in stool color	10.8	7.2	2.4	90.4	—
Rigidity/stillness	9.8	4.9	3.7	90.1	—
Eye swelling	9.6	9.6	1.2	89.2	—

(continued)

TABLE **3–3**

Winter symptom frequency and baseline-to-posttreatment change (n = 83)
Continued

Symptom	Baseline frequency %	Treatment response			Effect size (w)
		Decreased	Increased	Unchanged	
Wheezing	9.6	7.2	3.6	89.2	—
Hemorrhoids	9.6	6.0	1.2	92.8	—
Excessive energy**	8.8	5.1	**6.3**	86.1	—
Leg/arm swelling	8.6	6.2	1.2	91.4	—
Irregular heartbeat	8.5	6.1	2.4	91.5	—
Decreased urinary pressure	6.2	3.7	2.5	92.6	—
Difficulty swallowing	6.1	3.7	3.7	92.7	—
Excess salivation	6.0	4.8	1.2	94.0	—
Hearing loss	6.0	2.4	4.8	92.8	—
Shaking	4.9	2.5	4.9	90.1	—
Sweating	4.9	3.7	4.9	90.1	—
Swollen/sore tongue	4.8	4.8	0.0	95.2	—
Double vision	4.8	3.6	0.0	96.4	—
Genital swelling/discharge	4.0	4.0	1.3	89.3	—
Genital discomfort	4.0	2.7	2.7	89.3	—
Change in urine color	3.7	3.7	2.5	91.4	—
Difficulty urinating	3.7	1.2	4.9	92.6	—
Sunlight irritation	3.7	3.7	1.2	93.8	—
Bruising	3.7	2.5	2.5	93.8	—
Painful bowel movements	3.7	2.4	0.0	97.6	—
Earache	3.6	3.6	3.6	92.8	—
Painful urination	2.5	1.2	2.5	95.1	—
Unwanted body movements	2.5	0.0	2.5	96.3	—
Nasal bleeding	2.4	2.4	1.2	96.3	—
Vomiting	2.4	2.4	6.1	91.5	—
Ear discharge	2.4	1.2	1.2	97.6	—
Breast pain/discharge	1.2	1.2	1.2	97.6	—
Urinary burning	0.0	0.0	2.5	96.3	—
Loss of conciousness	0.0	0.0	0.0	98.8	—
Seizures	0.0	0.0	0.0	98.8	—

[1] All symptoms reported, mild to severe (boldfaced items, frequency >50%.
[2] Symptoms characteristic of hypomania.
[3] Change frequencies too low to calculate χ^2 and w.

more than half the group. For this sample, symptoms with pre- to posttreatment effect sizes as small as w = 0.43 can show statistically significant values of McNemar's χ^2 for change.

The rank ordering by effect size of treatment (Table 3–3) shows several major contrasts with that for season (Table 3–2). Several symptoms outside the SAD cluster showed major improvement. Notably, "poor vision," with a baseline frequency of only 14.6%, showed the largest effect size of all symptoms (w = 0.91), with 13.4% showing improvement and none showing exacerbation. Similarly, bleeding gums (13.3%, w = 0.70), change in taste (13.6%, w = 0.75), "light bothersome to eyes" (19.3%, w = 0.56), eye irritation (26.5%, w = 0.52), and skin rash/itch/irritation (20.7%, w = 0.47) showed large improvement. Statistically, it is difficult to demonstrate posttreatment change for symptoms that have a low baseline frequency; indeed, a minimum of 10 change scores is needed to calculate McNemar's χ^2 and the size of effect. Nonetheless, a low-frequency symptom in the group as a whole can cause distress in a subgroup, and a positive response to light therapy might be of great importance. Analyses of non-SAD populations are needed to determine whether such symptoms are syndromally associated with SAD or are independently responsive to light. Indeed, other clinical populations may show light-treatable symptoms whose frequencies exceed those of SAD patients.

The ocular symptoms are of particular interest. Considering the therapeutic modality, the reported improvement in "poor vision," "light bothersome to eyes," and eye irritation is both surprising and reassuring (cf., Gallin et al. 1995). Bright light treatment of certain visual sensory or ocular problems, beyond SAD, may be worth investigation using more precise, objective measures than self-reports on the SAFTEE. Bright light effects on retinal physiology have been reported in animals, and connections to etiology and treatment of SAD have been hypothesized (Remé et al. 1990). (Different lighting configurations, spectral distribution, and intensity could introduce ocular side effects not found in the present study. For example, with respect to eyestrain—a symptom that is not specifically probed by the SAFTEE—Levitt et al. (1993) found approximately equal frequencies of improvement and worsening following use of a krypton-halogen light visor.)

In contrast to the seasonal analysis, there were, however, many bothersome symptoms that showed posttreatment exacerbation (frequencies of 10% or more). These exacerbations could be true side effects or could reflect the flowering of symptoms during the natural episode course in patients who did not respond to light treatment. (Separate analyses of responders and nonresponders will be presented elsewhere.) In almost all such cases, however, the frequency of improvement exceeded that of exacerbation, often with moderate to large effect size (e.g., anxiety, appetite increase, headaches, and weight gain). Nausea, which occurred at a frequency of 12.2% at baseline, stands out as a symptom that showed greater exacerbation than improvement (17.1% vs. 11.0%), and this was identified selectively as an emergent symptom among responders to light, perhaps reflecting autonomic activation.

Conclusion

Our field has developed a potent treatment intervention, and we have at least a preliminary understanding of its mechanisms of action. The domain of light treatment will surely expand in the years ahead, and collaboration with colleagues outside the specialties of circadian rhythms and psychiatry will be key.

References

Bauer MS: Summertime bright-light treatment of bipolar major depressive episodes. Biol Psychiatry 33:663–665, 1993

Boulos Z, Campbell SS, Lewy AJ, et al: Light treatment for sleep disorders: consensus report, VII: jet lag. J Biol Rhythms 10:167–176, 1995

Campbell SS, Dijk D-J, Boulos Z, et al: Light treatment for sleep disorders: consensus report, III: alerting and activating effects. J Biol Rhythms 10:129–132, 1995a

Campbell SS, Eastman CI, Terman M, et al: Light treatment for sleep disorders: consensus report, I: chronology of seminal studies in humans. J Biol Rhythms 10:105–109, 1995b

Campbell SS, Terman M, Lewy AJ, et al: Light treatment for sleep disorders: consensus report, V: age-related disturbances. J Biol Rhythms 10: 151–154, 1995c

Cohen J: Statistical Power Analysis for the Behavioral Sciences, 2nd Ed. Hillsdale, NJ, Lawrence Erlbaum Associates, 1988

Dijk D-J, Boulos Z, Eastman CI, et al: Light treatment for sleep disorders: consensus report, II: basic properties of circadian physiology and sleep regulation. J Biol Rhythms 10:113–125, 1995

Eastman CI, Young MA, Fogg LF: A comparison of two different placebo-controlled SAD light treatment studies, in Biological Rhythms and Light in Man. Edited by Wetterberg L. Oxford, Pergamon, 1993, pp 371–384

Eastman CI, Boulos Z, Terman M, et al: Light treatment for sleep disorders: consensus report, VI: shift work. J Biol Rhythms 10:157–164, 1995

Fukuda K, Straus SE, Hickie I, et al: The chronic fatigue syndrome: a comprehensive approach to its definition and study. Ann Int Med 121: 953–959, 1994

Gallin PF, Terman M, Remé CE, et al: Ophthalmologic examination of patients with seasonal affective disorder before and after light therapy. Am J Ophthal 119:202–210, 1995

Glass JD, Selim M, Srkalovic G, Rea MEA: Tryptophan loading modulates light-induced responses in the mammalian circadian system. J Biol Rhythms 10:80–90, 1995

Guilleminault C, McCann CC, Quera-Salva M, et al: Light therapy as treatment of desynchronosis in brain impaired children. Eur J Pediat 152: 754–759, 1993

Hamilton M: The Hamilton Rating Scale for Depression, in Assessment of Depression. Edited by Sartorius N, Ban TA. New York, Springer-Verlag, 1986, pp 143–152

Jacobsen FM, Murphy DL, Rosenthal NE: The role of serotonin in seasonal affective disorder and the antidepressant response to phototherapy, in Seasonal Affective Disorders and Phototherapy. Edited by Rosenthal NE, Blehar MC. New York, Guilford, 1989, pp 333–341

Joseph-Vanderpool JR, Jacobsen FM, Murphy DL, et al: Seasonal variation in behavioral responses to m-CPP in patients with seasonal affective disorder and controls. Biol Psychiatry 33:496–504, 1993

Kasper S, Rosenthal NE, Barberi S, et al: Immunological correlates of seasonal fluctuations in mood and behavior and their relationship to phototherapy. Psychiatry Res 36:253–264, 1991

Klein DF: Endogenomorphic depression: a conceptual and terminological revision. Arch Gen Psychiatry 31:447–451, 1974

Komaroff AL, Buchwald D: Symptoms and signs of chronic fatigue syndrome. Rev Infect Dis 13:S8–11, 1991

Kusumi I, Ohmori T, Kohsaka M, et al: Chronobiological approach for treatment-resistant rapid cycling affective disorders. Biol Psychiatry 37: 553–559, 1995

Lam RW: Seasonal affective disorder presenting as chronic fatigue syndrome. Can J Psychiatry 36:680–692, 1991

Levitt AJ, Joffe RT, Moul DE, et al: Side effects of light therapy in seasonal affective disorder. Am J Psychiatry 150:650–652, 1993

Lewy AJ, Sack RL, Singer CM, et al: Winter depression and the phase-shift hypothesis for bright light's therapeutic effects: history, theory, and experimental evidence. J Biol Rhythms 3:121–134, 1988

Mishima K, Okawa M, Hishikawa Y, et al: Morning bright light therapy for sleep and behavior disorders in elderly patients with dementia. Acta Psychiatr Scand 89:1–7, 1994

Mosbach P, Auerbach A, St. Hilaire M: Phototherapy as a treatment for sleep disorder in Parkinson's disease: a case study (abstract). Neurology 43:A302, 1993

National Institute of Mental Heath: Systematic Assessment for Treatment Emergent Effects (SAFTEE). Rockville, MD, National Institute of Mental Health, 1986

O'Rourke D, Wurtman JJ, Wurtman RJ, et al: Treatment of seasonal depression with d-fenfluramine. J Clin Psychiatry 50:343–347, 1989

Remé CE, Terman M, Wirz-Justice A: Are deficient retinal photoreceptor mechanisms involved in the pathogenesis of winter depression? (letter) Arch Gen Psychiatry 47:878–879, 1990

Roberts JE, Lawless D, Terman JS, et al: Cellular immune response to visible light treatment of SAD (abstract). Photoderm Photoimmunol Photomed 8:48, 1991

Rosenthal NE, Sack DA, Gillin JC, et al: Seasonal affective disorder: a description of the syndrome and preliminary findings with light therapy. Arch Gen Psychiatry 41:72–80, 1984

Rosenthal NE, Bradt GH, Wehr TA: Seasonal Pattern Assessment Questionnaire (SPAQ). Bethesda, MD, National Institute of Mental Health, 1987

Satlin A, Volicer L, Ross V, et al: Bright light treatment of behavioral and sleep disturbances in patients with Alzheimer's disease. Am J Psychiatry 149:1028–1032, 1992

Terman M: Problems and prospects for use of bright light as a therapeutic intervention, in Biological Rhythms and Light in Man. Edited by Wetterberg L. Oxford, Pergamon, 1993, pp 421–436

Terman M, Terman JS: Treatment of seasonal affective disorder with a high-output negative ionizer. Journal of Alternative and Complementary Medicine 1:87–91, 1995

Terman M, Lewy AJ, Dijk D-J, et al: Light treatment for sleep disorders: consensus report, IV: sleep phase and duration disturbances. J Biol Rhythms 10:135–147, 1995

Terman M, Levine SM, Terman JS, et al: Chronic fatigue syndrome and seasonal affective disorder: comorbidity, diagnostic overlap, and implications for treatment. Am J Med (in press)

Touitou Y, Haus E (eds): Biologic Rhythms in Clinical and Laboratory Medicine. Berlin, Springer-Verlag, 1992

Williams JBW, Link MJ, Rosenthal NE, et al: Structured Interview Guide for the Hamilton Depression Rating Scale—Seasonal Affective Disorder Version, Revised. New York, New York State Psychiatric Institute, 1994

Zubieta JK, Engleberg NC, Yargic LI, et al: Seasonal symptom variation in patients with chronic fatigue syndrome: comparison with major mood disorders. J Psychiatr Res 28:13–22, 1994

FOUR

Psychobiological Effects of Light Therapy in Seasonal Affective Disorder

Edwin M. Tam, M.D.
Raymond W. Lam, M.D.
Lakshmi N. Yatham, M.D.
Athanasios P. Zis, M.D.

The efficacy of light therapy in seasonal affective disorder (SAD) has been well demonstrated (Tam et al., 1995; Terman et al. 1989; Wehr and Rosenthal 1989; Wesson and Levitt, this volume), but its mechanism of action is still poorly understood. The original rationale for the therapeutic use of light lay in the fact that bright light (>2,000 lux), but not dim light (<500 lux), could suppress nocturnal secretion of melatonin, a pineal hormone that helps regulate circadian rhythms (Lewy et al. 1980). Seasonal changes in animal behaviors are mediated by changes in the daily photoperiod that act through alterations of circadian rhythms. If seasonal mood changes were analogous to these animal models of photoperiodicity, then bright light should treat winter depression through a corrective effect on abnormal circadian rhythms in SAD.

The authors' research is supported, in part, by the Canadian Psychiatric Research Foundation (Dr. Tam) and the Medical Research Council of Canada (Dr. Lam and Dr. Zis).

Since the first bright light studies, however, research appears to show that human pineal melatonin can be suppressed by a wide range of light intensities, and that the suppression is dependent on other parameters in addition to light intensity (Brainard, this volume). Although bright light clearly shifts circadian rhythms (as discussed by Hughes and Lewy, Boulos, and Campbell, this volume), there is still conflicting evidence for the etiologic role of circadian rhythm disturbances in SAD, and for the mechanism of action of light therapy in SAD. Indeed, many studies have shown that light has a number of biological effects that should be considered in its therapeutic mode of action. In this chapter, we review other psychobiological effects of light therapy in SAD, beginning with neurophysiological aspects and then proceeding to neurochemical aspects. We focus on our recent studies of the retinal and serotonergic effects of light.

Neurophysiological Studies

Retinal Electrophysiologic Measures

Light acts as a *zeitgeber* (synchronizer) of circadian rhythms, and its effects are mediated through the retinohypothalamic tract leading from the retina to the suprachiasmatic nucleus of the hypothalamus, which is the circadian pacemaker in mammals (Moore 1983). It is possible that circadian rhythm abnormalities may be caused by improper processing of light at the level of the retina, resulting in alterations of the light signal to the suprachiasmatic nucleus. Changes in retinal light sensitivity have been hypothesized for the etiology of SAD, with both subsensitivity and supersensitivity hypotheses proposed (Beersma 1990; Reme et al. 1990).

We have been investigating retinal light sensitivity by means of electrooculography (EOG) and electroretinography (ERG), which are well-studied clinical electrophysiologic measures of retinal function. The EOG records eye movement potentials between electrodes placed near the lateral canthi of each eye; the potential increases when the retina is exposed to light (Arden and Kelsey 1962; Arden er al. 1962). The EOG ratio is represented by the peak electric potential in the light-adapted eye divided by the lowest potential found during dark adaptation; it is therefore an indirect measure of light-induced retinal change. In our initial study, we found that 19 depressed, medication-free patients with SAD had significantly lower EOG ratios than comparison subjects (Lam et al. 1991). This finding was replicated by Ozaki et al. (1993) in an EOG study of 16 patients with SAD. These EOG data indicate that SAD patients are less sensitive to a standardized light stimulus, and are consistent with our hypothesis that SAD patients are subsensitive to light at the level of the retina. However, abnormalities in the EOG cannot point to pathology in a specific retinal cell layer. The EOG arises from the retinal pigmented epithelium, which is intimately associated with retinal photoreceptors and is important for daily photoreceptor renewal. Although a normal EOG requires an intact photoreceptor layer, it predominantly assesses the retinal pigmented epithelium.

ERG is more specific than EOG in its physiologic origin, because ERG responses are mediated through neuroglial cells that reflect retinal photoreceptor activity (Berson 1975). Individual retinal layers and groups of rod or cone photoreceptors can be assessed by varying the type of light stimulus presented to the eye and measuring the potential response via corneal electrodes. The ERG yields a waveform with a and b waves that can be analyzed for amplitude and implicit time (time from stimulus to peak of waveform). Typically, the b wave is used as the index of photoreceptor activity. The pattern ERG (PERG) uses an alternating striped pattern as the stimulus to elicit the ERG response. The PERG response is thought to arise from the inner ganglion cell layer of the retina (Maffei and Fiorentini 1981). The flash ERG consists of presenting standardized single flashes of light to the dark-adapted eye, and the response arises from the bipolar Müeller cells in the mid-retinal cell layer (Miller and Dowling 1970; Witkovsky 1980).

Using PERG, Oren et al. (1993) found no differences in 12 patients with SAD and matched controls; however, the sample size was small and the output of the PERG has marked intersubject variability. In contrast, the flash ERG has less variability of response. We studied the flash ERG response in 24 depressed, drug-free SAD patients (18 women and 6 men) and 22 age- and sex-matched normal control subjects (Lam et al. 1992). The ERG showed significant differences between males and females in the b-wave amplitude. The female patients with SAD (all of whom were premenopausal) had significantly lower ERG b-wave amplitudes, whereas male patients with SAD had higher amplitudes than their matched controls. This suggests that there is physiologic heterogeneity between female and male SAD patients. The reduced retinal sensitivity to light (as suggested by a low b-wave amplitude) may be limited to premenopausal females.

Effects of Light Therapy on EOG and ERG

We have also recently completed a study on the effects of light therapy on both EOG and ERG in SAD (Lam et al., unpublished data, June 1995). We studied 23 patients (16 women and 7 men) diagnosed with recurrent major depressive episodes with a seasonal pattern by DSM-III-R criteria (American Psychiatric Association 1987). Six of the 23 patients (26%) met criteria for bipolar disorder type II (with hypomania). The rest of the patients had unipolar depression. The mean age of patients was 38.3 years (SD = 10.7, range 20–63 years). Patients were drug-free for at least 2 weeks (5 weeks if they had previously been treated with fluoxetine) and had scores greater than 14 on the 21-item Hamilton Depression Rating Scale (HAM-D) (Hamilton 1967). Patients were excluded if they had a history of retinal disease, cataracts, or severe myopia, or if they had any abnormalities on clinical ophthalmologic examination including fundoscopy and slit-lamp examination. Patients were assessed weekly with the 29-item modified HAM-D, which includes 8 items rating atypical depressive symptoms (Williams et al. 1991). After a baseline observation week, they were treated for 2 weeks with a cool-white fluorescent light box rated at 2,500 lux. Patients used the light box at home for 2 hours/day between 6:00 A.M. and 8:00 A.M.

EOG and ERG testing were conducted by technicians blind to the diagnosis and treatment condition during the baseline week, and then repeated following the light therapy. During testing, pupils were dilated and eyes were dark adapted for at least 25 minutes. For the ERG, corneal gold foil electrodes were carefully placed over the lower eyelids, and a ground electrode was placed on the forehead.

ERG signals were recorded in response to single flashes of white light, which elicit mixed rod and cone photoreceptor responses. Data were analyzed by multivariate analysis of variance on two repeated measures: time (before and after light therapy) and eye (right and left), and one between-groups measure: sex (male and female).

Results are shown in Table 4–1. There were significant main effects of time for the EOG ratios ($F = 11.4$, df = 1,21, $P < .005$) and ERG b-wave amplitudes ($F = 11.4$, df = 1,21, $P < .005$), but not for the ERG b-wave implicit times ($P > .40$). In this study there were no main effects of sex, or significant interaction effects involving time, sex, or eye. The EOG ratios increased after light therapy to a mean of 2.3, which was the mean ratio for the normal comparison subjects in our previous study using the same protocol (Lam et al. 1991). The ERG b-wave amplitude also showed a small but significant increase after light therapy.

These results suggest that the EOG and ERG abnormalities found in our previous studies of SAD appear to normalize after treatment

TABLE 4–1

Depression scores and retinal measures ($\pm$ SD) before and after light therapy (N = 23 SAD patients)

Measure	Pretreatment	Posttreatment
Depression scores		
21-item Ham-D[1]	19.4 ± 4.4	8.9 ± 5.6
29-item Ham-D[1]	34.5 ± 6.8	16.4 ± 9.4
EOG ratio[2]		
Left eye	2.07± 0.24	2.25 ± 0.35
Right eye	2.08 ± 0.27	2.31 ± 0.40
ERG b-wave amplitude		
Left eye[2]	340 ± 57 mv	375 ± 61 mv
Right eye[2]	323 ± 66 mv	350 ± 50 mv
ERG b-wave implicit time		
Left eye	43.8 ± 1.6 ms	44.9 ± 3.0 ms
Right eye	44.1 ± 1.9 ms	44.8 ± 2.3 ms

[1] Paired t- tests, significant difference between pre- and posttreatment, $P < .001$.
[2] MANOVA, significant difference between pre- and posttreatment, $P < .005$.

with light, indicating a state-dependent abnormality. Since dopamine is the major neurotransmitter involved in the ERG b-wave amplitude and the EOG retinal light response (as reviewed in Iuvone 1986), it is plausible to suggest that bright light increases abnormally low retinal dopaminergic activity in SAD. Alternatively, it is possible that these findings indicate changes in retinal melatonin or serotonin, which can also be involved in the retinal light response by complex feedback mechanisms (Oren 1991). Of interest to a hypodopaminergic hypothesis are our ERG results showing low b-wave amplitudes in premenopausal women but not in men. The positive studies showing results consistent with low central dopaminergic function in SAD involved only premenopausal women (Arbisi et al. 1989, 1994; Depue et al. 1988, 1989, 1990), whereas the negative studies have involved mixed gender groups (Barbato et al. 1993; Rudorfer et al. 1993). One negative study (using eye blink rates as a putative measure of central dopaminergic activity) found on post hoc testing that the SAD subgroup of premenopausal women did show significant reduction of eye blink rates following light therapy (Barbato et al. 1993), a finding similar to the positive results from the study of eye blink rates (Depue et al. 1988). Similarly, a treatment study of SAD that used levodopa/carbidopa to test a hypodopaminergic hypothesis found no significant overall effects, but a post hoc analysis showed that the subgroup of premenopausal women had a significant positive response against placebo (Oren et al. 1994).

We must point out, however, that the study of Ozaki et al. (1993) found no change in EOG ratios after light therapy (10,000 lux, 60–90 minutes/day, 1 week). Their results, in contrast to our EOG and ERG data, would suggest that reduced retinal light sensitivity is a trait marker, rather than a state-dependent finding, for SAD.

EEG and Brain-Imaging Studies

Researchers have also looked more centrally for neurophysiological effects of light therapy. Regional electroencephalographic (EEG) asymmetries have been found in nonseasonally depressed patients. Specifically, an excess of left-frontal alpha-band activity and right-parietal alpha-band activity has been noted (Davidson et al. 1985;

Schaffer et al. 1983). A study of eight SAD patients similarly revealed significantly greater left-frontal alpha-band activity, and marginally greater right-parietal alpha-band amplitudes. There was no change after 2 weeks of light therapy at 2,500 lux for 2 hours twice daily; however, there was an increase in right-frontal coherence, which suggests an increased synchronization with ipsilateral frontal and parietal regions after light therapy (Allen et al. 1993). Sleep EEG (baseline and after total sleep deprivation) was measured in 11 female SAD patients and 8 controls before and after light therapy (6,000 lux from 10 A.M. to 2 P.M. for 5 days) (Brunner et al. 1996). The EEG changes found were explainable by normal sleep regulation alone, suggesting that the antidepressant effect of light therapy is not mediated by sleep changes. Event-related brain potential testing in seven patients with SAD revealed significant increases in P300 amplitude to visual but not auditory stimuli after twice daily 2,500-lux light (total of 5.5 hours) for 1 week. No changes were seen in five control subjects with either measure (Rosenthal et al. 1987). Quantitative EEG was used to study functional asymmetries in brain activity in 10 patients with SAD and 8 control subjects (Teicher et al. 1996). SAD patients had a reverse pattern of hemispheric asymmetry with left greater than right power in delta, theta, and beta bands, especially in the posterior region. Light therapy at 10,000 lux for 0.5–1.0 hour/day reversed the posterior abnormality in the delta band, partially reversed the asymmetry in the beta band, and had no effect on the theta band. The same study also used echo-planar MRI to examine $T2^*$ relaxation time in 5 patients with SAD. Asymmetry in $T2^*$ was most prominent in the frontal region; furthermore, this decreased after light therapy.

Positron emission tomography (PET) has been used to study brain metabolic patterns. The PET scans of 7 patients with SAD were compared to those of 38 normal control subjects by examining 60 different brain regions (Cohen et al. 1992). Six patients went on to receive light treatment (2,500 lux, 2.5 hours/day, 10 days) and were again compared to controls. Global metabolic rates in patients with SAD were lower than in normal controls both before and after light treatment, especially in the superior medial frontal cortex. Of interest here is the observation that although there were no significant differences in the occipital cortex between normal control subjects and patients with

SAD before light therapy, there was a significant difference following exposure to light, suggesting activation by light therapy.

In a related study involving a single light treatment session, Murphy examined cerebral blood flow (CBF) with single-photon emission computerized tomography (SPECT). Four patients with SAD were compared to 4 control subjects before and after exposure to 1,500-lux light for 2 hours. Both groups were similar at baseline in terms of global, regional, and hemispheric CBF, but the authors reported that the percentage change in CBF after light exposure was significantly different between the two groups (Murphy et al. 1993). More recently, an examination of regional CBF with SPECT in 10 depressed patients before and after light therapy (>2,500 lux, 0.5–2 hours/day) found that improvement in depressive symptoms was associated with an increase in regional CBF in the frontal, cingulate, and thalamic regions (Matthew et al. 1996).

These preliminary brain-imaging studies suggest that there is a stimulatory effect of light on the brain activity of patients with SAD. More studies are required to replicate these results and to determine their significance in the pathophysiology of SAD and the mechanism of action of light therapy.

Neurochemical Studies

Neuroendocrine Measures

There are relatively few studies examining the effect of light therapy on peripheral measures of central neuroendocrine function. Adrenocorticotropin hormone (ACTH) and cortisol response to corticotropin-releasing hormone were examined in 10 patients with SAD. Initial blunted responses as compared with controls were reversed by light treatment (2,500 lux, 5 hours/day, 9 days) (Joseph-Vanderpool et al. 1991). In contrast, basal cortisol and prolactin plasma levels showed no changes in seven patients with SAD after light therapy (2,500 lux, 5.5 hours/day, 1 week) (Rosenthal et al. 1987).

Changes in thyroid hormone levels have been reported after antidepressant treatment of nonseasonal depression. However, a study of

14 patients with SAD, treated with 5,000-lux light for 1 hour/day over 2 weeks, showed no changes in serum levels of T_4, T_3, TSH, or FTI, or of T_3 resin uptake, despite antidepressant response in 11 of the patients (Joffe et al. 1991).

Neurotransmitter Measures

Of late, there has been a great research focus on neurochemical changes in depression that are more central. Many of the current theories concerning nonseasonal depressive disorders emphasize the role of neurotransmitters, and the mechanisms of action of many antidepressant medications are thought to be related to their effects on serotonin, norepinephrine, and, to a lesser extent, dopamine. The effects of light therapy on these neurotransmitter systems have likewise been studied.

Norepinephrine and dopamine

Several studies have looked at light therapy effects on norepinephrine (NE) and dopamine and their metabolites. Rudorfer et al., in their 1993 study of 17 unmedicated patients with SAD, showed that light treatment (2,500 lux, 5 hours/day, 2 weeks) had no effect on cerebrospinal fluid (CSF) levels of 3-methoxy-4-hydroxyphenylglycol (MHPG), a metabolite of NE, despite clinical response in 14 patients. On the other hand, plasma NE levels showed nonsignificant increases with light treatment that were not correlated to degree of clinical improvement (Rudorfer et al. 1993). However, Rosenthal et al. (1987), using an orthostatic challenge paradigm, found blunted plasma NE responses to orthostatic challenge in eight patients with SAD compared with five normal controls. The abnormal NE responses normalized after treatment with light therapy (2,500 lux, 5.5 hours/day, 1 week).

Urinary levels of NE and its metabolites normetanephrine (NMN), 3-methoxy-4-hydroxymandelic acid (VMA), and MHPG have also been examined. Twenty-four-hour urine-collection samples showed significantly decreased levels of NE, NMN, and VMA, but not MHPG, in nine female patients with SAD after light therapy (>2,500 lux, 1 hour/day, 2 weeks). Unlike the effect seen with desipramine, the ratio of NMN to whole-body NE turnover (the sum of urinary NMN, VMA, and MHPG) was not significantly altered, suggesting that changes in NE output and metabolism were not due to NE reuptake blockade (Anderson et al. 1992).

As for dopamine, Rudorfer et al. (1993) found no difference in levels of CSF homovanillic acid (HVA), a metabolite of dopamine, after light therapy. Dopamine activity modulates the rate of spontaneous eye blinking in humans. In the previous section we mentioned two studies involving eye blink rates. In the first study, light therapy (2,500 lux, 4 hours/day, 2 weeks) decreased the initially high eye blink rates of 4 premenopausal female patients with SAD back to normal control levels (Depue et al. 1988), suggesting that light increases dopaminergic activity. In contrast, the second study found no baseline differences in blink rates, and no change in blink rates in patients with SAD (n = 10) and control subjects (n = 12) receiving 10,000-lux light treatment for 1 hour/day for 1 week (Barbato et al. 1993). However, a post-hoc analysis showed a decreased eye blink rate for the premenopausal female subgroup. Again, these findings are of interest in view of our findings of low ERG b-wave amplitude in premenopausal female patients with SAD and a significant increase in b-wave amplitude after light therapy, and the hypothesized involvement of dopamine in the ERG light response.

In summary, although light therapy has not shown significant effects on basal plasma and CSF NE levels, there is some evidence from orthostatic challenge tests for a subsensitive NE system that is corrected by light therapy. Urinary but not CSF measures of NE turnover are consistent with the possibility that NE turnover decreases as the system sensitivity is restored. Similarly, although there is little evidence from CSF studies to suggest an effect of light therapy on dopamine systems in patients with SAD, there is indirect evidence from eye blink and retinal electrophysiologic studies for a subsensitive dopaminergic system normalized by light therapy. However, these findings may be limited to premenopausal women.

Serotonin

In view of the current interest in the etiologic role of serotonin (also called 5-hydroxytryptamime, or 5-HT) in nonseasonal depression, it is reasonable to postulate that the antidepressant effect of light therapy may act via serotonergic pathways. There is presumptive evidence for a serotonergic hypothesis in SAD because there are consistent seasonal changes in central 5-HT metabolism (for a review, see Lacoste and Wirz-Justice 1989), and serotonergic medications such as d-fenfluramine and fluoxetine have been found effective in SAD (Lam et al. 1995; O'Rourke et al., 1989). An initial study found that CSF levels of 5-hydroxyindoleacetic acid (5-HIAA), the major metabolite of 5-HT, were unchanged in 17 patients with SAD after 2 weeks of light therapy at 2,500 lux for 5 hours/day, even though 14 patients clearly responded to treatment (Rudorfer et al. 1993). However, there have been a number of positive studies suggesting a role for 5-HT in light therapy of SAD.

Platelets show many similarities to central 5-HT neurons, including similar 5-HT receptors, imipramine binding, and active 5-HT transport (Stahl 1985). The density of ^{3}H-imipramine sites (B_{max}) on platelets can potentially be viewed as a peripheral marker of central serotonergic activity because these binding sites are located on the same serotonin transporter in platelet membranes and in serotonergic neurons. The mean B_{max} of patients with SAD ($n = 7$) was significantly lower than controls and increased significantly after light treatment ($>2,000$ lux, 1 hour/day, 1 week) to levels similar to those found in the untreated control subjects (Szadoczky et al. 1989). In a second study with the same light treatment parameters, 17 patients with SAD had significant increases in B_{max} after treatment, whereas no changes were seen in 8 medicated non-SAD depressed patients and 6 control subjects who underwent an identical light regimen (Szadoczky et al. 1991). In both studies, the affinity constant (K_d) did not change with light therapy.

On the other hand, studies with tritiated paroxetine (^{3}H-paroxetine) as a ligand showed different effects. In one study ($n = 26$ patients with SAD), responders to light therapy (2,500 lux, 2 hours/day, 1 week) had a significant decrease in platelet ^{3}H-paroxetine binding, whereas nonresponders had no significant changes (Mellerup et al. 1993). K_d did not change in either group. In contrast, another study ($n = 18$ patients with SAD) found no change in platelet ^{3}H-paroxetine binding, K_d, 5-HT-stimulated Ca^{2+} response, or 5-HT content in platelets after light therapy (10,000 lux, 45 minutes/day, 2 weeks)

(Ozaki et al. 1994). In summary, platelet studies have not shown consistent findings.

Using *meta*-chlorophenylpiperazine (m-CPP) as a probe, Jacobsen et al. (1994) infused participants with this partially selective $5\text{-}HT_{2A}/5\text{-}HT_{2C}$ agonist. Ten depressed patients with SAD experienced activation-euphoria responses and significant decreases in carbohydrate hunger, whereas 11 control subjects felt "slowed down." Treatment with 1 week of light therapy (2,500 lux, 4 hours/day) led to a normalization of responses to m-CPP infusion in the SAD patients, suggesting an effect of light on serotonergic measures. The hormonal responses to m-CPP in this group also produced some interesting findings. Untreated patients with SAD had significantly higher prolactin and cortisol responses to m-CPP compared to control subjects, and these responses were significantly reduced by light treatment (Garcia-Borreguero et al. 1995). Comparison of untreated patients with control subjects in the winter and summer periods revealed that patients had higher cortisol responses than controls in the winter, but lower responses than controls in the summer. The investigators postulate that an underlying reduced serotonin availability produces a supersensitivity of $5\text{-}HT_{2C}$ receptors that is normalized with remission in the summer and by light treatment. A replication study done by the same group involved 17 patients with SAD and 15 controls undergoing successive 3-week periods of light therapy (10,000 lux, 1.5 hours/day) and light avoidance in randomized order (Schwartz et al. 1997). Again, m-CCP produced significant increases in activation-euphoria ratings only in the untreated SAD group. Light treatment in both groups produced significant reductions in core temperature. There were no differences in prolactin and cortisol responses between the groups or light conditions. In contrast, a double-blind placebo-controlled trial using m-CPP or normal saline on 14 untreated patients with SAD and 15 control subjects done during fall/winter months found blunted prolactin responses in the SAD group (Levitan et al. 1996).

Sumatriptan challenge tests in SAD: effects of light therapy

The neuroendocrine and behavioral effects of m-CPP can be considered a measure of net serotonergic activity. More selective agents are now available that are specific to the numerous 5-HT subtypes now known (Yatham and Steiner 1993). Sumatriptan, a drug used in the treatment of migraine, binds to 5-HT_1-receptor subtypes in the following order of affinity: $5\text{-HT}_{1D} > 5\text{-HT}_{1B} > 5\text{-HT}_{1A}$ receptors (Schoeffter and Hoyer 1989). When given subcutaneously at a dose of 6 mg, sumatriptan produces a significant increase in growth hormone levels, which peak about 30 minutes following the administration of the drug and return to baseline within 2 hours. Pretreatment with cyproheptadine abolishes growth hormone release induced by sumatriptan, suggesting involvement of serotonergic systems in this response (Franceschini et al. 1994).

We recently examined growth hormone responses to sumatriptan challenge in 11 patients with SAD (8 females and 3 males) and 9 healthy volunteers (8 females and 1 male) with no lifetime history of psychiatric illness (Yatham et al. 1997). The mean age of the healthy controls was 39.3 (SD = 11.9) and the mean age of the SAD patients was 36.3 (SD = 9.6). SAD patients had a mean score on the 29-item modified HAM-D of 29.3 (SD = 6.6). All participants were drug free for at least 4 weeks prior to the sumatriptan challenge test session. An intravenous blood sample for baseline growth hormone levels was obtained approximately 60 minutes after the insertion of the canula. At this time sumatriptan (6 mg) was given subcutaneously, and additional blood samples were obtained at 30, 60, 90, and 120 minutes to determine growth hormone responses to sumatriptan challenge.

There was no difference in baseline growth hormone levels between the two groups (mean ±SD: SAD patients 2.40 ± 1.56 μg/l, healthy controls 1.71 ±0.41 μg/l; $t = 1.29$, df = 18, $P = .21$). Sumatriptan administration led to significant increase in growth hormone levels in healthy controls, but the response in patients with SAD was blunted. Analysis of variance with repeated measures showed a significant main effect for time ($F = 6.96$, df = 4,72, $P < .001$) and a group-by-time interaction ($F = 2.47$, df = 4,72, $P < 0.05$) (see Figure 4–1 for details).

Patients with SAD were treated with light therapy, 10,000 lux for 30 minutes daily. The sumatriptan challenge test was repeated for 10 of the 11 participants between 2 and 4 weeks after starting

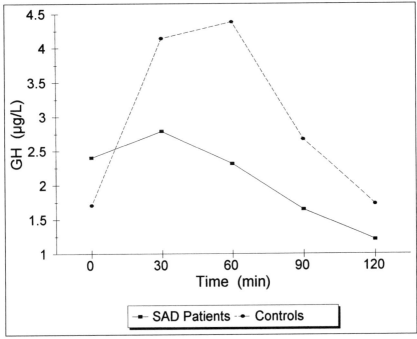

FIGURE 4–1. Growth hormone (GH) response to sumatriptan challenge in patients with SAD ($N = 11$) and control subjects ($N = 9$).

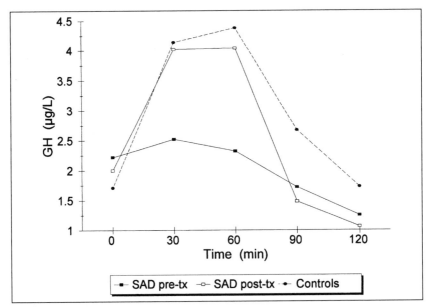

FIGURE 4–2. Growth hormone (GH) response to sumatriptan challenge in patients with SAD ($N = 11$) before and after light therapy as compared with control subjects ($N = 9$).

light therapy. All 10 patients improved significantly after 2 weeks of light therapy. After treatment these patients showed significant enhancement of growth hormone responses to sumatriptan challenge (Figure 4–2). Analysis of variance with repeated measures showed significant interaction between time and condition ($F = 4.22$, df = 4,36, $P < .01$). Similarly, a paired t test comparing the net change (baseline level subtracted from peak level) in growth hormone responses before and after treatment also showed a significant difference ($t = 2.71$, df = 9, $P < .02$), suggesting that recovery following light therapy led to normalization of growth hormone responses to sumatriptan challenge. These data implicate a hypothesis of 5-HT$_{1D}$ receptor subsensitivity in the pathophysiology of SAD that is corrected by light therapy.

Tryptophan depletion studies

Another paradigm for the investigation of serotonergic effects of light is rapid tryptophan depletion. Tryptophan is the dietary amino acid precursor of 5-HT, and blood tryptophan levels are correlated with brain 5-HT function (Curzon 1979; Young et al. 1989). Plasma tryptophan levels can be rapidly reduced by administering an oral tryptophan-free mixture containing high amounts of other amino acids; brain 5-HT can be decreased to 20% of normal levels by this procedure (Moja et al. 1989; Young et al. 1989). Tryptophan depletion in normal subjects produces transient mild, negative mood changes (Delgado et al., 1989; Young et al. 1985). The same procedure done with depressed patients in remission after treatment with serotonergic antidepressants produces transient depressive relapses (Delgado et al. 1990), but patients treated with noradrenergic antidepressants are less likely to experience these relapses (Delgado et al. 1991). This procedure is thus informative for examining the serotonergic effects of antidepressant treatments.

We have studied effects of rapid tryptophan depletion in patients with SAD who were in remission with light therapy (Lam et al. 1996). In this crossover study, our hypothesis was that rapid tryptophan depletion, but not a sham control treatment, would reverse the antidepressant effects of light therapy. Entry criteria included meeting DSM-III-R criteria for major depressive disorder, recurrent, with seasonal pattern (diagnosed using data from the Structured Clinical Interview for DSM-III-R) (Spitzer et al. 1990); being medication free for at least 2 weeks (5 weeks if previously on fluoxetine); and scoring 15 or higher on the 21-item HAM-D. Patients were treated with a light box producing 10,000 lux of cool-white fluorescent light for 30 minutes/day between 7:00 A.M. and 8:00 A.M. Patients were considered in remission if they scored less than 8 on the 21-item HAM-D and less than 12 on the 29-item modified HAM-D for at least 3 weeks.

The remitted SAD patients underwent a randomized, double-blind, counterbalanced protocol with experimental and control test sessions separated by 5 days. The tryptophan depletion session involved a 24-hour low-tryptophan diet (160 mg/day) and a blue placebo capsule given three times a day on the first day, followed by a tryptophan-free 15–amino acid drink on the second day. The control session consisted of the low-tryptophan diet and blue capsules containing 500 mg of tryptophan on the first day, followed by a 16–amino acid drink that included 2.3 g of tryptophan. Patients continued their morning light therapy during the study.

The Hamilton Anxiety Scale (HAM-A) (Hamilton 1959) and a 20-item modified HAM-D (nine items that could not be measured within the same day were excluded from the 29-item modified HAM-D) were administered each morning at 9:00 A.M. on both test days, and at 5 hours after ingestion of the amino acid drink. Blood samples were drawn at those times and assayed for total and free tryptophan concentration. Data were analyzed with repeated measure analysis of variance (ANOVA), with order of sessions as a grouping variable, and time and session (depletion, control) as repeated measures.

Seven women and 3 men completed the study (mean age ±SD 33.0 ± 8.8 years, range 21–49 years). As shown in Figure 4–3, baseline tryptophan levels before depletion and control sessions were similar. The depletion session significantly lowered both the total and free plasma tryptophan levels by a mean of 89% and 72%, respectively, whereas the control session, as expected, increased tryptophan levels (Figure 4–3). Results were significant for both total plasma tryptophan (session-by-time interaction, $F = 230.1$, df = 2,7,

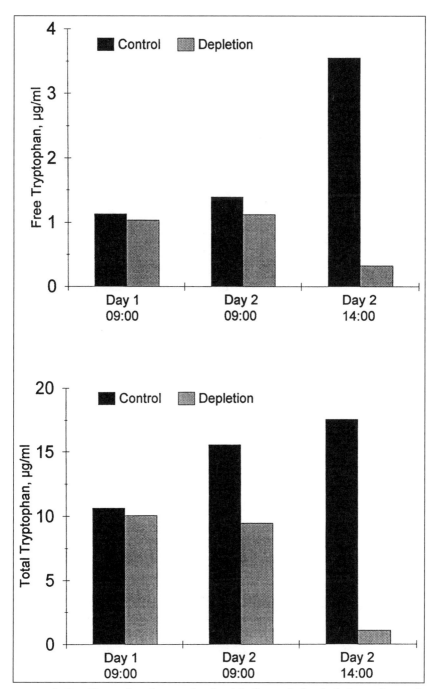

FIGURE 4–3. Free and total tryptophan levels before and after depletion and control sessions in remitted patients with SAD (*N* = 10).

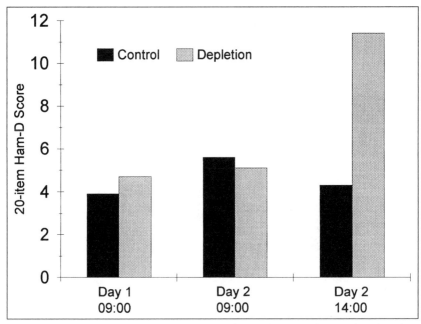

FIGURE 4–4. Depression scores before and after depletion and control sessions in remitted patients with SAD (*N* = 10).

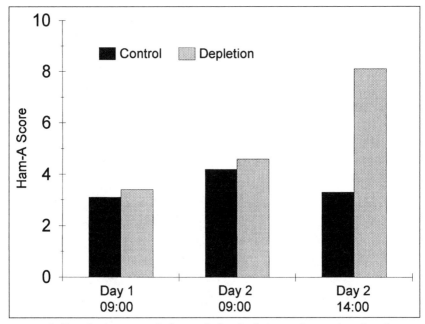

FIGURE 4–5. Anxiety scores before and after depletion and control sessions in remitted patients with SAD (*N* = 10).

$P < .001$) and free plasma tryptophan (session-by-time interaction, $F = 106.1$, df $= 2,7$, $P < .001$).

Figures 4–4 and 4–5 show the HAM-D and HAM-A scores for the participants in the depletion and control sessions. There were significant time-by-session effects for the depression scores ($F = 10.6$, df $= 2,7$, $P < .01$). Post-hoc paired t tests showed modified HAM-D scores to be no different at baseline, but significantly higher in the depletion group at 5 hours postingestion ($t = 6.1$, df $= 9$, $P < .001$). Similar results were found with the HAM-A ratings. During the depletion session, six patients experienced clinically significant depressive symptoms (defined as scores of 12 or greater on the 20-item modified HAM-D), and two other patients had marked increases in depression and anxiety ratings. Symptoms remitted the next day on resumption of normal dietary intake. There was little clinical effect on depression or anxiety scores after the sham control session. Examination of the tryptophan depletion session with Pearson correlations revealed trends for negative correlations between changes in HAM-D scores and changes in both free and total plasma tryptophan levels ($r = 0.55$, $P < .07$, one-tailed test).

Recently, our results were replicated by another laboratory using a similar tryptophan depletion protocol. Neumeister et al. (1997a) also found that depletion led to transient depressive relapses in 12 SAD patients in remission after light therapy (3,000 lux for 2 hours in the evening). These results strongly suggest that the therapeutic effects of light treatment are acutely dependent on tryptophan availability. Alternate mechanisms of light therapy are less compatible with these results. Given the rapidity with which the effects of tryptophan depletion occurred, it is unlikely that these effects resulted from changes in circadian rhythms. Decreases in melatonin levels resulting from changes in its precursor, 5-HT, would also not account for the symptomatic changes, given that very little melatonin is produced during the hours when this study was conducted. Interestingly, tryptophan depletion done during the winter with 11 drug-free depressed patients with SAD did not worsen the depressive symptoms in a placebo-controlled double-blind crossover study (Neumeister et al. 1997b). This is consistent with findings in drug-free non-SAD depressed patients (Delgado et al. 1994), and would suggest that presynaptic serotonergic activity is not the primary cause of winter depression. Together with the m-CPP and sumatriptan results, these studies strongly suggest that light therapy acts via serotonergic mechanisms. However, the exaggerated (or blunted) hormonal responses to m-CPP are contrasted by the blunted responses seen with sumatriptan, suggesting that several 5-HT receptors, or a complex interaction of receptors, may be involved in the therapeutic response to light.

Conclusions

Much of the work investigating the psychobiologic effects of light therapy has been preliminary and needs to be replicated. Thus far, many different areas have been studied, and, in general, the breadth of research far exceeds the depth. Given this state of affairs, we can nonetheless see some consistent patterns emerging. Studies of central neurotransmitter function lend strongest support to serotonergic mechanisms of light therapy. Whereas tryptophan depletion studies show the importance of 5-HT in maintaining the antidepressant effects of bright light, studies with the serotonin agonists m-CPP and sumatriptan point to a complex interaction between various 5-HT subtypes. Hypotheses of noradrenergic and dopaminergic subsensitivity treatable with light, though less validated, remain of interest for further study. Replicated electrophysiologic abnormalities of retinal function have been demonstrated in SAD, but these studies have shown conflicting results of effects of light therapy. It remains unclear whether these retinal findings can lead to (or be caused by) changes in circadian rhythms, or whether they reflect retinal or central neurotransmitter function, such as dopaminergic subsensitivity. Initial EEG and brain-imaging studies point to an acute stimulating effect of bright light. The field thus remains open for much more active research in elucidating the psychobiologic effects of light therapy, which in turn will contribute to a better understanding of the nature of seasonal depressive disorders.

References

Allen JJ, Iacono WG, Depue RA, et al: Regional electroencephalographic asymmetries in bipolar seasonal affective disorder before and after exposure to bright light. Biol Psychiatry 33:642–646, 1993

American Psychiatric Association: Diagnostic and Statistical Manual of Mental Disorders, 3rd Edition, Revised. Washington, DC, American Psychiatric Association, 1987

Anderson JL, Vasile RG, Mooney JJ, et al: Changes in norepinephrine output following light therapy for fall/winter seasonal depression. Biol Psychiatry 32:700–704, 1992

Arbisi PA, Depue RA, Spoont MR, et al: Thermoregulatory response to thermal challenge in seasonal affective disorder: a preliminary report. Psychiatry Res 28:323–34, 1989

Arbisi PA, Depue RA, Krauss S, et al: Heat-loss response to a thermal challenge in seasonal affective disorder. Psychiatry Res 52:199–214, 1994

Arden GB, Kelsey JG: Changes produced by light in the standing potential of the human eye. J Physiol 161:205–226, 1962

Arden GB, Barrada A, Kelsey JH: New clinical test of retinal function based upon the standing potential of the eye. Br J Ophthalmol 46:449–467, 1962

Barbato G, Moul DE, Schwartz P, et al: Spontaneous eye blink rate in winter seasonal affective disorder. Psychiatry Res 47:79–85, 1993

Beersma DGM: Do winter depressives experience summer nights in winter? Arch Gen Psychiatry 47:879–880, 1990

Berson EL: Electrical phenomena in the retina. in Adler's Physiology of the Eye. Edited by Moses RA. St. Louis, MO, Moseby, 1975, pp 453–499

Brunner DP, Krauchi K, Kijk DJ, et al: Sleep electrocephalogram in seasonal affective disorder and in control women: effects of midday light treatment and sleep depreivation. Biol Psychiatry 40:485–496, 1996

Cohen RM, Gross M, Nordahl TE, et al: Preliminary data on the metabolic brain pattern of patients with winter seasonal affective disorder. Arch Gen Psychiatry 49:545–552, 1992

Curzon G: Relationships between plasma, CSF and brain tryptophan. J Neural Transm 15:93–105, 1979

Davidson RJ, Schaffer CE, Saron C: Effects of lateralized presentations of faces on self-reports of emotion and EEG asymmetry in depressed and non-depressed subjects. Psychophysiology 22:353–364, 1985

Delgado PL, Charney DS, Price LH, et al: Neuroendocrine and behavioral effects of dietary tryptophan restriction in healthy subjects. Life Sci 45: 2323–2332, 1989

Delgado PL, Charney DS, Price LH, et al: Serotonin function and the mechanism of antidepressant action. Arch Gen Psychiatry 47:411–418, 1990

Delgado PL, Price LH, Miller HL, et al: Serotonin and the neurobiology of depression: effects of tryptophan depletion in drug-free depressed patients. Arch Gen Psychiatry 51:865–874, 1994

Delgado PL, Price LH, Miller HL, et al: Rapid serotonin depletion as a provocative challenge test for patients with major depression: relevance to antidepressant action and the neurobiology of depression. Psychopharmacol Bull 27:321–330, 1991

Depue RA, Iacono WG, Muir R, et al: Effect of phototherapy on spontaneous eye blink rate in subjects with seasonal affective disorder. Am J Psychiatry 145:1457–1459, 1988

Depue RA, Arbisi P, Spoont MR, et al: Seasonal and mood independence of low basal prolactin secretion in premenopausal women with seasonal affective disorder. Am J Psychiatry 146:989–95, 1989

Depue RA, Arbisi P, Krauss S, et al: Seasonal independence of low prolactin concentration and high spontaneous eye blink rates in unipolar and bipolar II seasonal affective disorder. Arch Gen Psychiatry 47:356–64, 1990

Franceschini R, Cataldi A, Garibaldi P, et al: The effects of sumatriptan on pituitary secretion in man. Neuropharmacology 33:235–239, 1994

Garcia-Borreguero D, Jacobsen FM, Murphy DL, et al: Hormonal responses to the administration of m-chlorophenylpiperazine in patients with seasonal affective disorder and controls. Biol Psychiatry 37: 740–749, 1995

Hamilton M: The assessment of anxiety states by rating. Br J Med Psychol 32:50–55, 1959

Hamilton M: Development of a rating scale for primary depressive illness. Br J Soc Clin Psychol 6:278–296, 1967

Iuvone PM: Neurotransmitters and neuromodulators in the retina: regulation, interactions, and cellular effects, in The Retina: A Model for Cell Biology Studies, Part II. Edited by Adler R, Farber D. Orlando, FL, Academic, 1986, pp 1–72

Jacobsen FM, Mueller EA, Rosenthal NE, et al: Behavioral responses to intravenous meta-chlorophenylpiperazine in patients with seasonal affective disorder and control subjects before and after phototherapy. Psychiatry Res 52:181–197, 1994

Joffe RT, Levitt AJ, Kennedy SH: Thyroid function and phototherapy in seasonal affective disorder (letter; published erratum appears in Am J Psychiatry 148:819, 1991). Am J Psychiatry 148:393, 1991

Joseph-Vanderpool JR, Rosenthal NE, Chrousos GP, et al: Abnormal pituitary-adrenal responses to corticotropin-releasing hormone in patients with seasonal affective disorder: clinical and pathophysiological implications. J Clin Endocrinol Metab 72:1382–1387, 1991

Lacoste V, Wirz-Justice A: Seasonal variation in normal subjects: an update of variables current in depression research, in Seasonal Affective Disorders and Phototherapy. Edited by Rosenthal NE, Blehar MC (eds). New York, Guilford, 1989, pp 167–229

Lam RW, Beattie CW, Buchanan A, et al: Low electrooculographic ratios in patients with seasonal affective disorder. Am J Psychiatry 148: 1526–1529, 1991

Lam RW, Beattie CW, Buchanan A, et al: Electroretinography in seasonal affective disorder. Psychiatry Res 43:55–63, 1992

Lam RW, Gorman CP, Michalon M, et al: A multicenter, placebo-controlled study of fluoxetine in seasonal affective disorder. Am J Psychiatry 152:1765–1770, 1995

Lam RW, Zis AP, Grewal A, et al: Effects of rapid tryptophan depletion in patients with seasonal affective disorder in remission with light therapy. Arch Gen Psychiatry 53:41–44, 1996

Levitan R, Kaplan A, Brown G, et al: Hormonal responses to intravenous m-CPP challenge in seasonal affective disorder (abstract), in SLTBR: Abstracts of the Annual Meeting of the Society for Light Treatment and Biological Rhythms, Vol. 8. Wheat Ridge, CO, Society for Light Treatment and Biological Rhythms, 1996, p 8

Lewy AJ, Wehr TA, Goodwin FK, et al: Light suppresses melatonin secretion in humans. Science 210:1267–1269, 1980

Maffei L, Fiorentini A: Electroretinographic responses to alternating gratings before and after sectioning of the optic nerve. Science 211:953, 1981

Matthew E, Vasile RG, Sachs G, et al: Regional cerebral blood flow changes after light therapy in seasonal affective disorder. Nuclear Medicine Communications 17:475–479, 1996

Mellerup ET, Errebo I, Molin J, et al: Platelet paroxetine binding and light therapy in winter depression. J Affect Disord 29:11–15, 1993

Miller RF, Dowling JE: Intracellular responses of the Müeller (glial) cells of mudpuppy retina: their relation to b-wave of the electroretinogram. J Neurophysiol 33:212, 1970

Moja EA, Cipolla P, Castoda D, et al: Dose-responsive decrease in plasma tryptophan and in brain tryptophan and serotonin after tryptophan-free amino acid mixtures in rats. Life Sci 44:971–976, 1989

Moore RY: Organization and function of a central nervous system circadian oscillator: the suprachiasmatic hypothalamic nuclei. Fed Proc 42: 2783–2789, 1983

Murphy DG, Murphy DM, Abbas M, et al: Seasonal affective disorder: response to light as measured by electroencephalogram, melatonin suppression, and cerebral blood flow. Br J Psychiatry 163:327–331, 1993

Neumeister A, Praschak-Rieder N, Heßelmann B, et al: Effects of tryptophan depletion on drug-free patients with seasonal affective disorder during a stable response to bright light therapy. Arch Gen Psychiatry 54:133–138, 1997a

Neumeister A, Praschak-Reider N, Hesselmann B, et al: Rapid tryptophan depletion in drug-free depressed patients with seasonal affective disorder. Am J Psychiatry 154:1153–1155, 1997b

Oren DA: Retinal melatonin and dopamine in seasonal affective disorder. J Neural Transm 83:85–95, 1991

Oren DA, Moul DE, Scwartz PJ, et al: An investigation of ophthalmic function in winter seasonal affective disorder. Depression 1:29–37, 1993

Oren DA, Moul DE, Schwartz PJ, et al: A controlled trial of levodopa plus carbidopa in the treatment of winter seasonal affective disorder: a test of the dopamine hypothesis. J Clin Psychopharmacol 14:196–200, 1994

O'Rourke D, Wurtman JJ, Wurtman RJ, et al: Treatment of seasonal depression with d-fenfluramine. J Clin Psychiatry 50: 343–347, 1989

Ozaki N, Rosenthal NE, Moul DE, et al: Effects of phototherapy on electrooculographic ratio in winter seasonal affective disorder. Psychiatry Res 49:99–107, 1993

Ozaki N, Rosenthal NE, Mazzola P, et al: Platelet [^{3}H]paroxetine binding, 5-HT-stimulated Ca^{2+} response, and 5-HT content in winter seasonal affective disorder. Biol Psychiatry 36:458–466, 1994

Reme C, Terman M, Wirz-Justice A: Are deficient retinal photoreceptor renewal mechanisms involved in the pathogenesis of winter depression? Arch Gen Psychiatry 41:72–80, 1990

Rosenthal NE, Skwerer RG, Sack DA, et al: Biological effects of morning-plus-evening bright light treatment of seasonal affective disorder. Psychopharmacol Bull 23:364–369, 1987

Rudorfer MV, Skwerer RG, Rosenthal NE: Biogenic amines in seasonal affective disorder: effects of light therapy. Psychiatry Res 46:19–28, 1993

Schaffer CE, Davidson RJ, Saron C: Frontal and parietal electroencephalogram asymmetry in depressed and nondepressed subjects. Biol Psychiatry 18:753–762, 1983

Schoeffter P, Hoyer D: How selective is GR 43175? Interactions with functional 5-HT1A, 5-HT1B, 5HT1C, 5HT1C and 5HT1D receptors. Naunyn Schmiedebergs Arch Pharmakol 340:135–138, 1989

Spitser RL, Williams JBW, Gibbon M, et al: Structured Clinical Interview for DSM-III-R-Patient Edition (with Psychotic Screen) Version 1.0. Washington, DC, American Psychiatric Press 1990

Stahl SM: Peripheral models for the study of neurotransmitter receptors in man. Psychopharmacol Bull 21:663–671, 1985

Schwartz PJ, Murphy DL, Wehr TA, et al: Effects of meta-chlorophenylpiperazine infusions in patients with seasonal affective disorders and healthy control subjects: diurnal responses and nocturnal regulatory mechanism. Arch Gen Psychiatry 54:375–385, 1997

Szadoczky E, Falus A, Arato M, et al: Phototherapy increases platelet ^{3}H-imipramine binding in patients with winter depression. J Affect Disord 16:121–125, 1989

Szadoczky E, Falus A, Nemeth A, et al: Effect of phototherapy on ^{3}H-imipramine binding sites in patients with SAD, non-SAD and in healthy controls. J Affect Disord 22:179–184, 1991

Tam EM, Lam RW, Levitt AJ: Treatment for seasonal affective disorder: a review. Can J Psychiatry 40:457–466, 1995

Teicher MH, Glod CA, Ito Y, et al: Hemispheric asymmetry of EEG and T2* relaxation time in seasonal affective disorder (SAD) pre and post-light therapy, in SLTBR: Abstracts of the Annual Meeting of the Society for Light Treatment and Biological Rhythms. Wheat Ridge, CO, Society for Light Treatment and Biological Rhythms, 1996, p 9

Terman M, Terman JS, Quitkin FM, et al: Light therapy for seasonal affective disorder. A review of efficacy. Neuropsychopharmacology 2:1–22, 1989

Wehr TA, Rosenthal NE: Seasonality and affective illness. Am J Psychiatry 146:829–839, 1989

Williams JBW, Link M, Rosenthal NE, et al: Structured Interview Guide for the Hamilton Depression Rating Scale, Seasonal Affective Disorders Version (SIGH-SAD). New York, New York Psychiatric Institute, 1991

Witkovsky P: Excitation and adaptation in the vertebrate retina. Curr Top Eye Res 2:1–66, 1980

Yatham LN, Steiner M: Neuroendocrine probes of serotonergic function—a critical review. Life Sciences 53:6:447–463, 1993

Yatham LN, Lam RW, Zis AP: Growth hormone responses to sumatriptan (5-HTID agonist) challenge in seasonal affective disorder: effects of light therapy. Biol Psychiatry 42: 24–29 1997

Young SN, Smith SE, Pihl R, et al: Tryptophan depletion causes a rapid lowering of mood in normal males. Psychopharmacology 87:173–177, 1985

Young SN, Ervin FR, Pihl RO, et al: Biochemical aspects of tryptophan depletion in primates. Psychopharmacology 98:508–511, 1989

FIVE

Dawn Simulation and Bright Light Therapy in Subsyndromal Seasonal Affective Disorder

David H. Avery, M.D.
Michael J. Norden, M.D.

Bright light therapy is a well-established treatment for seasonal affective disorder (SAD), also known as winter depression, which is defined as recurrent major depressive episodes with a seasonal pattern (Rosenthal 1993; Rosenthal, et al. 1984; Terman et al. 1989a; Wesson and Levitt, this volume). Dawn simulation is a newer form of light therapy that may be effective in SAD (Avery et al. 1993, 1994). These light therapies may also be effective in subsyndromal SAD, a milder form of SAD. In subsyndromal SAD, full criteria for a major depression may not be present, yet seasonal symptoms pose a problem for the person.

The most common form of SAD in more northern latitudes is a recurrent fall-winter depression; less common is the recurrent spring-summer pattern (Wehr and Rosenthal 1989). Fall-winter SAD is typically associated with increased sleep, increased appetite, weight gain, decreased social activity, decreased mood, and decreased energy. Subsequent references to SAD and subsyndromal SAD will refer to the fall-winter type of depression.

The Seasonal Pattern Assessment Questionnaire (SPAQ) (Rosenthal et al. 1987a) is an instrument commonly used to assess the seasonality of symptoms. The SPAQ rates the degree of seasonality by asking the subject to what degree (0 = no change, 1 = slight change, 2 = moderate change, 3 = marked change, 4 = extreme change) each of six items (mood, sleep, weight, energy, social activity, and energy) varies with the seasons. The total of the score for the six items yields a Global Seasonality score ranging from 0 to 24. The test-retest reliability of the SPAQ may be dependent on the sample tested; the intraclass correlation coefficient for a sample of patients with SAD is 0.80, for nonseasonally affected normal subjects it is 0.61, and for subsyndromal subjects with SAD it is 0.44 (Hardin et al. 1991). The SPAQ appears to have validity in that the Global Seasonality scores increase with latitude (Rosen et al. 1990) and correlate with other measures of seasonality (Marriott 1993; Rosen and Rosenthal 1991). The Global Seasonality scores are higher in subjects diagnosed with SAD compared with subjects with subsyndromal SAD; subjects with subsyndromal SAD have higher Global Seasonality scores than nonseasonally affected subjects (Terman 1988).

Seasonality is best thought of as a dimension rather than an either-or phenomenon. In an epidemiological study of the general population of Montgomery County, Maryland, Kasper et al. (1989a) found that the frequency distribution of the SPAQ scores in the random sample of the population (Figure 5–1) did not show a bimodal distribution; a continuum exists between those who are not seasonally affected at all and those who have SAD. In that study, SAD was defined as a Global Seasonality score of 10 or greater, *and* seasonality identified as a problem of moderate or greater severity. Only 8% of the sample reported no seasonality whatsoever (Global Seasonality score = 0); a minimum estimate of winter-pattern SAD using stringent criteria was 4.3%. A large proportion of the sample experienced intermediate degrees of seasonality; for 27% of the sample, seasonal symptoms were a problem.

The Kasper group defined subsyndromal SAD as non-SAD individuals who had either 1) a Global Seasonality score of 10 or above but who considered their seasonality to be only a mild problem or no problem, or 2) a Global Seasonality score of 8 or 9 but who consid-

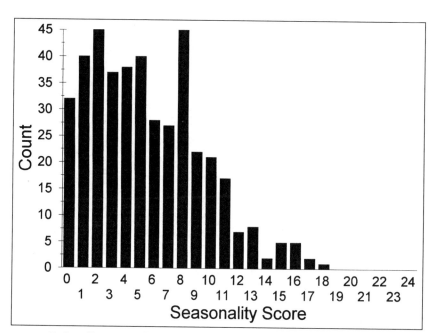

FIGURE 5–1. Frequency distribution of Seasonal Pattern Assessment Questionnaire (SPAQ) scores in a random sample of Montgomery County, Maryland, residents.

Source. Reprinted from Kasper S, Wehr T, Bartko J, et al: Epidemiological findings of seasonal changes in mood and behavior: a telephone survey of Montgomery County, Maryland. Arch Gen Psychiatry 46:823–833, 1989. Copyright 1989 American Medical Association. Used with permission.

ered their seasonal symptoms to be at least a moderate problem (Kasper et al. 1989a). Using these criteria they estimated that about 13.5% of the sample experienced subsyndromal winter SAD.

Studies using neutral multivariate statistical techniques support the concept of winter depression, both syndromal and subsyndromal SAD. Bartko and Kasper (1989) used a cluster analytic technique to examine the Montgomery County data and found a small winter-SAD cluster, as well as a large subsyndromal winter-depression cluster; interestingly, no cluster emerged with no seasonal changes. Using a factor analytic approach and a sample from multiple latitudes (Rosen et al. 1990), Rosen and Rosenthal (1991) found that seasonal dimensional factors emerged, including winter depression, winter weight gain, and winter hypersomnia, as well as mild winter depression. The correlations between factors are consistent with the view of behavioral changes being on a continuum with no seasonal changes at all. These results show that it is unlikely that the seasonal pattern of symptoms seen in SAD and subsyndromal SAD are simply the result of investigator bias or the bias of affected individuals.

Rosen et al. (1990), using the SPAQ, found the prevalence of SAD and subsyndromal SAD to increase with latitude: Alaska (64°N latitude), SAD 8.9%, subsyndromal SAD 24.9%; New Hampshire (42°) 9.7%, 11.0%); New York City (41°), 4.7%, 12.5%; Maryland (39°), 4.3%, 13.5%; and Florida (28°), 1.4%, 2.6%. Note that subsyndromal SAD is more common than SAD at all latitudes. Rosenthal (1989) estimates that, in the United States, about 6.1% of the population (10.8 million) have SAD, and about 14.3% (25.3 million) have subsyndromal SAD. Even small decrements in mood, productivity, or alertness in such a large proportion of the population in northern latitudes could have a significant impact in terms of safety, economics, and personal suffering.

Seasonality has also been explored among patients with other disorders. Hardin et al. (1991) found that patients with major depression and patients with bipolar disorder have Global Seasonality scores that are similar to those of normal populations. However, in both groups there was a tendency in the winter to sleep more, eat more, and gain weight. Patients with eating disorders tended to be more seasonally affected (see Lam and Goldner, this volume). Thompson et al. (1988) found that an unselected sample of patients with bipolar disorder reported significantly greater seasonality than control subjects, but less than patients with SAD. Hansen et al. (1987) has noted that 24% of Norwegians living at 69°N latitude complained of sleep difficulties (termed midwinter insomnia), and the most common problem was initial insomnia. In that study, sleep latency was significantly decreased with morning bright light exposure (2,000–2,500 lux for 30 minutes/day).

Bright Light Therapy of Subsyndromal SAD

In contrast to the many studies of bright light treatment of SAD, relatively few studies have involved normal controls or subjects with subsyndromal SAD. In an uncontrolled study, Wirz-Justice et al. (1986) administered 2 hours of bright light (1 hour in the morning and 1 hour in the evening) to 10 normal subjects and found significant improvement in the mornings but not the evenings, according to a visual analogue scale. In normal subjects, Saletu et al. (1986) compared 7 hours of bright light in one 24-hour period (2,800 lux, 6:00 A.M. to 9:00 A.M. and 5:00 P.M. to 9:00 P.M.) with partial sleep deprivation and found significant improvement on a general well-being scale in both conditions. In the first controlled study of normal subjects, Rosenthal et al. (1987b) found that the results of 2 hours of bright light (2,500 lux) in the morning for 1 week were no different from the results of 2 hours of a dim (300 lux) control condition, and the bright light therapy was associated with no significant improvement compared with baseline values. Among the 11 subjects receiving bright light therapy, only one reported that seasonal changes were a problem, and that subject had the only positive response to bright light therapy. In the earlier studies by Wirz-Justice et al. (1986) and Saletu et al. (1986), seasonality was not carefully assessed among the normal participants, and some with subsyndromal SAD may have been included.

Bauer et al. (1994) studied 24 normal control subjects who were randomized to receive 4 weeks of bright light exposure (2,500 lux from 6:00 A.M. to 8:00 A.M.) or 4 weeks of simply rising at 6:00 A.M. for quiet activities. The control subjects were not depressed at baseline, and no significant changes in depression ratings were noted with treatment. However, several controls subjects who received bright light developed hypomanic symptoms, and members of the light-treated group had significantly more of these symptoms than those in the no-light group. These individuals experienced symptoms including increased sex drive, a "sped up" feeling, irritability, decreased sleep, and racing thoughts. When the controls, whose scores showed varying degrees of seasonality, were combined with SAD patients who were treated with bright light treatment over 4 weeks, a stepwise logistic regression revealed that the Global Seasonality score from the SPAQ was the most powerful predictor ($P < .05$) of the emergence of hypomania.

In a controlled study, Kasper et al. (1989b) administered bright light therapy to both patients with subsydromal SAD ($n = 20$) and those who reported no seasonal difficulties ($n = 20$). Five hours of bright light therapy (2,500 lux) divided equally between morning and evening was found to be more effective in relieving the symptoms than 2 hours of bright light exposure (2,500 lux, 1 hour in the morning and 1 in the evening) for those with subsyndromal SAD. The response of the subjects with subsyndromal SAD to the 5 hours of bright light was significantly better than the response of the non-seasonally affected group to the same light regimen. Those who had no seasonal symptoms did not benefit from either bright light treatment regimen. The study demonstrates that improvement with bright light treatment was clearly associated with the presence of seasonal symptoms. Further, a higher Global Seasonality score was correlated with a greater increase in hypomania score for the 20 nonseasonally affected control subjects ($r = 0.42, P < .01$) and for the total sample of 40 participants ($r = 0.67, P < .001$).

In a controlled study using a dim light "placebo" condition, Kasper et al. (1989c, 1990) studied a random sample of the general population. Using a balanced randomization based on the Global Seasonality score, they assigned subjects to either 1 week of bright light (2,500 lux for 2 hours daily in the morning, $n = 20$) or 1 week of a dim light (300 lux for 2 hours daily in the morning, $n = 20$). In each group, nine subjects had significant seasonal symptoms (two with SAD and seven with subsyndromal SAD). For those subjects without seasonal symptoms, neither bright light nor dim light had any significant effects. In those subjects with SAD and subsyndromal SAD, bright light resulted in a significantly greater reduction in depression ratings compared with dim light. The results suggest that bright light therapy may be helpful even for those with subsyndromal SAD.

Overall, the small database for bright light therapy suggests that individuals whose symptoms lack any seasonal pattern do not respond to the therapy, and that those who have symptoms with some degree of seasonality not only are more likely to respond positively to light but also may be at risk for developing hypomania.

Dawn Simulation Treatment of SAD

Dawn simulation is a technique that simulates a summer dawn signal during the winter. Dawn simulation consists of dim light that gradually increases in illuminance to a peak of only 100–500 lux prior to awakening (Terman et al. 1989b). Commercially available dawn simulators are able to create, at a specified time, a gradually increasing voltage over a specified time (e.g., 1 minute to 3 hours) to a light source.

In an open study design, Terman and Schlager (1990) found that dawn simulation lowered the average Hamilton Rating Scale for Depression (HAM-D) (Hamilton 1967) score from 13.1 to 4.9, among eight patients with SAD. In another open study, Jacobsen et al. (1990) treated 25 patients with major depression and complaints of either oversleeping or difficulty awakening, with a 150-W floodlight that came on abruptly 10 minutes before the desired time of awakening and found that 60% had a full response and 36% had a partial response. However, concomitant medication and lack of a control group make this study difficult to interpret.

A total of five controlled studies of dawn simulation have been performed, four with SAD patients and one with subjects with subsyndromal SAD. After two pilot studies (Avery et al. 1992a, 1992b) that helped determine an optimal "dose" of dawn, two subsequent studies found dawn simulation to be superior to a "placebo" condition.

In a parallel-design study of SAD, the response to a 2-hour, 250-lux dawn was superior to a 30-minute, 0.2-lux "placebo" dawn in treating patients with winter depression (Avery et al. 1993). Prior to randomization, the subjects were told that the 2-hour, 250-lux dawn would be "gradual," and that the 30-minute, 0.2-lux dawn would be "rapid," with the final illuminances being equal. Fourteen patients were randomized to 1 week of the 2-hour, 250-lux dawn; 13 patients to 1 week of the 30-minute, 0.2-lux dawn. Among the 13 patients completing the 2-hour, 250-lux dawn, the average HAM-D decreased from 17.1 to 5.5. Among the nine patients completing the 30-minute, 0.2-lux dawn, the average HAM-D decreased from 18.6 to 11.1. The 2-hour, 250-lux dawn resulted in a significantly better response compared with the 30-minute, 0.2-lux dawn (ANCOVA with the baseline HAM-D as the covariate: $F = 7.0$, df $= 1,19$, $P <$ .05). The atypical symptoms associated with SAD, such as hypersomnia, increased appetite, and weight gain, were assessed with the Atypical Score (ATYP) of the Structured Interview Guide for the Hamilton Depression Rating Scale—Seasonal Affective Disorder version (SIGH-SAD) (Williams et al. 1988). With the 2-hour dawn, the average ATYP decreased from 13.1 to 4.3; with 30-minute dawn, from 16.1 to 8.8. The postdawn ATYP was lower following the "active" dawn, compared with the dim placebo dawn (ANCOVA with the baseline ATYP as covariate: $F = 4.38$, df = 1,19, $P = .05$).

In another dawn simulation study of SAD, we used a parallel design to compare a 1.5-hour, 250-lux white-light dawn with a 1.5-hour, 2-lux red-light dawn (Avery et al. 1994). Prior to randomization, the participants were told that a white-light dawn would be compared with a red-light dawn. Thirteen patients were randomized to the white-light dawn, and 10 patients were randomized to the dim red-light dawn. Among the 10 patients completing the white-light dawn, the average HAM-D decreased from 20.7 to 8.0. Among the nine patients completing the dim red-light dawn, the average HAM-D decreased from 20.4 to 15.5. The postdawn HAM-D was significantly lower following the white-light dawn compared with the dim red-light dawn (ANCOVA with the baseline HAM-D as the covariate: $F = 8.1$, df = 1,16, $P < .05$). The average ATYP score resulting from the white-light dawn decreased from 14.4 to 6.7; that from the dim red-light dawn, decreased from 16.1 to 11.7. The postdawn ATYP showed a nonsignificant trend to be lower following the white-light dawn compared with the dim red-light dawn (ANCOVA with the baseline ATYP as the covariate: $F = 2.9$, df = 1,16, $P = .10$). The subjective rating by the participants who experienced the white-light dawn was significantly better ($P < .01$) than that of the participants who experienced the dim red-light dawn. The change in a quality of awakening score was also significantly better with the white-light dawn.

The baseline expectations for the white-light dawn and red-light dawn were similar for our total sample. Baseline expectations for the treatment actually received were similar and did not correlate with the response to treatment. The global improvement rating after treatment was significantly better with the white, 250-lux dawn compared with the red, 2-lux dawn, using ANCOVA with baseline expectations for the treatment received as the covariate ($P < .005$).

Together, these small studies suggest that dawn simulation is effective in SAD compared with a "placebo" signal.

Dawn Simulation Treatment of Subsyndromal SAD

A small study of dawn simulation in subjects with subsyndromal SAD also suggests that dawn simulation is effective (Norden and Avery 1993). Persons with SAD symptoms such as hypersomnia, drowsiness, increased appetite, or weight gain on a seasonal basis, but who did not fulfill criteria for major depression, were selected for the study. Over 500 Washington State doctors were mailed invitations to participate in this study. Sixteen nondepressed subjects, 6 women and 10 men, with an average SPAQ Global Seasonality score of 8 were given two courses of dawn signals, a dawn simulation signal and a rapid "placebo" signal. The signals were given Monday through Thursday nights over consecutive weeks in a randomized, single-blind, balanced cross-over design study. In the dawn condition, the light achieved full intensity over 45 minutes (slow); in the placebo condition, full intensity was achieved over about 4 seconds (rapid). The lighting source was a 60-W frosted halogen bulb positioned at the bedside 4 feet from the individual's eyes in his or her usual sleeping position, 18 inches above eye level, and controlled by a dawn simulator. At peak illuminance this system delivered about 100 lux to the closed eyes. Questionnaires using analogue scales were administered by telephone, blind to treatment assignment, at baseline and after each course of treatment. Both conditions were associated with improvements over baseline functioning. However, as hypothesized, the slow dawn condition was associated with significantly greater overall improvement than the rapid, placebo condition ($P < .01$). Improvement was significantly greater for the slow condition over the rapid condition with respect to daytime drowsiness ($P < .01$), energy, mood, social interest, concentration, productivity, quality of waking, and quality of sleep (all $P < .05$). The overall quality of awakening was significantly ($P < .01$) better with the slow dawn compared with the rapid dawn.

All of the above variables improved significantly ($P < .05$) with respect to the dawn signal compared with baseline. The overall rating of awakening compared with an alarm clock (using an analogue scale rated from -100 = very much worse than an alarm clock, 0 = same as an alarm clock, 100 = very much better than an alarm clock) showed that the slow dawn was significantly better than the rapid dawn (54.9 vs. 17.7, $P < .01$). In addition, with the 45-minute dawn, the average time it took subjects to get out of bed decreased significantly ($P < .05$) from 24.5 minutes to 9.6 minutes, and the average time required to become alert decreased from 49.2 minutes to 21 minutes. The Global Seasonality score of subjects in our study had a broad range from 2 to 16, but the effect of the dawn signal appeared unrelated to the score. In the slow condition, five subjects noted early awakenings, but only one called it a problem. Overall, the dawn signal appeared to be effective in relieving symptoms bothersome to those with subsyndromal SAD, and dawn simulation had few significant side effects.

Dawn simulation offers some advantages over traditional bright light box therapy. Because dawn simulation occurs during sleep, it is very convenient, unlike bright light therapy. Oren et al. (1991) noted that up to 69% of bright light box users reported that bright light therapy is inconvenient. The convenience of the dawn simulator is likely to result in better compliance than the bright light therapy. Because dawn simulators are small (one model measures 1.5 inches × 5.25 inches × 3 inches), they are much more portable than bright light boxes. They easily can be taken on trips and used with any incandescent light source under 400 W. The degree of improvement in SAD with dawn simulation is similar to that seen in previous studies of bright light boxes, but no direct comparison has yet been made.

The mechanisms of action for both bright light therapy and dawn simulation are unclear. Light therapy probably works through the eyes, since eye exposure to bright light is more effective than skin exposure in treating SAD (Wehr et al. 1987). Even though dawn simulation takes place while the person is asleep and has his or her eyes closed, a light signal could still reach the retinas through the translucent eyelids. About 10% of red spectrum and 2% of blue-green spectrum light is transmitted through the eyelids (Moseley 1988). Furthermore, the retinas are especially sensitive to light in the early morning hours (Bassi and Powers 1986; O'Keefe and Baker 1987). Because of the change in positioning of the subject in bed, for example, rolling away from the light source, it is difficult to know the precise light exposure experienced by the subjects. However, in spite of the experimental "noise" introduced by positioning, the small controlled studies appear to support the efficacy of dawn simulation.

Whether a treatment is started depends on the benefit-to-risk ratio. Because of the milder symptoms of subsyndromal SAD compared with SAD, a careful assessment of the potential side effects of a treatment may be even more important. Bright light therapy has been associated with several side effects including eyestrain, headache, insomnia, overactivity, irritability, nausea, tingling sensation, drowsiness, constipation, and tremor (Oren et al. 1991). Dawn simulation has also been associated with several side effects including early morning awakening, headache, agitation, and increased muscle tension (Avery et al. 1992a, 1992b, 1993, 1994). Both bright light therapy and dawn simulation have been associated with the occurrence of hypomania that appears to resolve with discontinuance of the light treatment (Avery et al. 1994; Bauer et al. 1994).

Although there was some initial concern about potential ocular side effects of bright light therapy (Terman et al. 1990), subsequent studies have been negative. Ophthalmologic exams before and after bright light therapy (e.g., 10,000 lux for 30 minutes daily) show no changes even after chronic treatment (Gallin et al. 1995). Gorman et al. (1993) also found no changes in a 5-year follow-up study of 71 patients with SAD who were treated daily during the winter with 2 hours of 700-lux to 2,500-lux light administered via a light visor. The illuminance of a cloudy day may reach 10,000 lux; 10,000 lux is much dimmer than the 100,000 lux seen on a bright sunny day. Extensive ophthalmologic tests prior to bright light therapy are not routine (Waxler et al. 1992). While formal testing of the safety of dawn simulation has not been performed, the highest illumination used (<500 lux) is dimmer than the illumination of a well-lit office.

Antidepressant medication, such as fluoxetine, might be effective in treating SAD (Lam et al. 1995), but medication studies of subsyndromal SAD have not been done. Antidepressant medications are now being used for dysthymia (Hellerstein et al. 1993), a condition characterized by chronic, intermittent, low-grade depressive symptoms. Since dysthymia may overlap with subsyndromal SAD, careful diagnosis is necessary, and the relative side effects of medication and light therapies should be considered in treatment planning. Because of the possible teratogenic risks of antidepressant medications (Miller et al. 1991), research on the effectiveness of nondrug treatments is especially important for women, who compose a majority of patients with SAD and subsyndromal SAD (Kasper et al. 1989a). One study found no increase in congenital malformations among mothers on fluoxetine (Pastuszak et al. 1993). Nonetheless, there continue to be concerns about more subtle in utero effects of psychoactive drugs.

Even though convenience, compliance, portability, cost, and safety argue for the use of the dawn simulator in the treatment of not only SAD but also subsyndromal SAD, the efficacy of dawn simulation needs to be clarified relative to a placebo condition and standard bright light therapy.

References

Avery D, Bolte MA, Millet M: Bright dawn simulation compared with bright morning light in the treatment of winter depression. Acta Psychiatr Scand 85:430–434, 1992a

Avery D, Bolte MA, Cohen S, et al: Gradual versus rapid dawn simulation treatment of winter depression. J Clin Psychiatry 53:359-363, 1992b

Avery DH, Bolte MA, Dager SR, et al:Dawn simulation treatment of winter depression: A controlled study. Am J Psychiatry 150:113–117, 1993

Avery DH, Bolte MA, Wolfson JK, et al: Dawn simulation compared with a dim red signal in the treatment of winter depression. Biol Psychiatry 36:181–188, 1994

Bartko JJ, Kasper S: Seasonal changes in mood and behavior: a cluster analytic approach. Psychiatry Res 28:227–239, 1989

Bassi CJ, Powers MK: Daily fluctuations in the detectability of dim lights by humans. Physiol Behav 38:871–877, 1986

Bauer MS, Kurtz JW, Rubin LB, et al: Mood and behavioral effects of four-week light treatment in winter depressives and controls. J Psychiatr Res 28:135–45, 1994

Gallin PF, Terman M, Reme CE, et al: Ophthalmologic examination of patients with seasonal affective disorder, before and after bright light therapy. Am J Ophthalmol 119:202–210, 1995

Gorman CP, Wyse PH, Demjen S, et al: Ophthalmological profile of 71 SAD patients: a significant correlation between myopia and SAD (abstract), in SLTBR: Abstracts of the Annual Meeting of the Society for Light Treatment and Biological Rhythms, Vol 5. Wilsonville, OR, Society for Light Treatment and Biological Rhythms, 1993, p 8

Hamilton M: Development of a rating scale for primary depressive illness. Br J Soc Clin Psychol 6:278–296, 1967

Hansen T, Bratlid T, Lingjaerde O, et al: Midwinter insomnia in the subarctic region: evening levels of serum melatonin and cortisol before and after treatment with bright artificial light. Acta Psychiatr Scand 75: 428–434, 1987

Hardin TA, Wehr TA, Brewerton T, et al: Evaluation of seasonality in six clinical populations and two normal populations. J Psychiatr Res 25: 75–87, 1991

Hellerstein D-J, Yanowitch P, Rosenthal J, et al: A randomized double-blind study of fluozetine versus placebo in the treatment of dysthymia.

Jacobsen FM: Waking in a lighted room. Biol Psychiatry 27:372–374, 1990

Kasper S, Wehr T, Bartko J, et al: Epidemiological findings of seasonal changes in mood and behavior. A telephone survey of Montgomery County, Maryland. Arch Gen Psychiatry 46:823–833, 1989a

Kasper S, Rogers SLB, Yancy A, et al: Phototherapy in individuals with and without subsyndromal seasonal affective disorder. Arch Gen Psychiatry 46:837–844, 1989b

Kasper S, Rogers SLB, Yancey A, et al: Psychological effects of light therapy in normals, in Seasonal Affective Disorders and Phototherapy. Edited by Rosenthal NE, Blehar MC. New York, Guilford, 1989c, pp 260–270

Kasper S, Rogers SL, Madden PA, et al: The effects of phototherapy in the general population. J Affect Disord 18:211–219, 1990

Lam RW, Gorman C, Michalon M, et al: A multicentre, placebo-controlled study of fluoxetine in seasonal affective disorder. Am J Psychiatry 152: 1765–1770, 1995

Marriott PF: An assessment of SPAQ and SPAQ+ reliability. Light Treatment and Biological Rhythms 5(3):33–34, 1993

Miller LJ: Clinical strategies of the use of psychotropic drugs during pregnancy. Psychiatr Med 9:275–298, 1991

Moseley MJ: Light transmission through the human eyelid: in vivo measurement. Ophthalmic Physiol Opt 8:229–230, 1988

Norden MJ, Avery DH: A controlled study of dawn simulation in subsyndromal winter depression. Acta Psychiatr Scand 88:67–71, 1993

O'Keefe LP, Baker HD: Diurnal changes in human psychophysical luminance sensitivity. Physiol Behav 41:193–200, 1987

Oren DA, Shannon NJ, Carpenter CJ, et al: Usage patterns of phototherapy in seasonal affective disorder. Compr Psychiatry 32:147–152, 1991

Pastuszak A, Schick-Boschetto B, Zuber C, et al: Pregnancy outcome following first-trimester exposure to fluoxetine (Prozac). JAMA 269: 2246–2248, 1993

Rosen LN, Rosenthal NE: Seasonal variations in mood and behavior in the general population: a factor-analytic approach. Psychiatry Res 38: 271–283, 1991

Rosen LN, Targum SD, Terman M, et al: Prevalence of seasonal affective disorder at four latitudes. Psychiatry Res 31:131–144, 1990

Rosenthal NE: Seasons of the Mind. New York, Bantam, 1989

Rosenthal NE: Diagnosis and treatment of seasonal affective disorder. JAMA 270:2717–2720, 1993

Rosenthal NE, Sack DA, Gillin JC, et al: Seasonal affective disorder: a description of the syndrome and preliminary findings with light therapy. Arch Gen Psychiatry 41:72–80, 1984

Rosenthal NE, Genhardt M, Sack DA, et al: Seasonal affective disorder: relevance for treatment and research of bulimia, in Psychobiology of Bulimia. Edited by Hudson JI, Pope HG. Washington, DC, American Psychiatric Press, 1987a, pp 203–228

Rosenthal NE, Rotter A, Jacobsen FM, et al: No mood-altering effects found following treatment of subjects with bright light in the morning. Psychiatry Res 22:1–9, 1987b

Saletu B, Dietzel M, Lesch OM, et al: Effect of biologically active light and partial sleep deprivation on sleep, awakening and circadian rhythms in normals. Eur Neurol 25(suppl 2):82–92, 1986

Terman M: On the question of mechanism in phototherapy for seasonal affective disorder: questions of clinical efficacy and epidemiology. J Biol Rhythms 3:155–172, 1988

Terman M, Schlager DS: Twilight therapeutics, winter depression, melatonin and sleep, in Sleep and Biological Rhythms: Basic Mechanisms and Applications to Psychiatry. Edited by Montplaisir J, Godbout R. New York, Oxford University Press, 1990, pp 113–128

Terman M, Terman J, Quitkin F, et al: Light therapy for seasonal affective disorder. A review of efficacy. Neuropsychopharmacology 2:1–22, 1989a

Terman M, Schlager D, Fairhurst S, et al: Dawn and dusk simulation as a therapeutic intervention. Biol Psychiatry 25:966–970, 1989b

Terman M, Reme CE, Rafferty B, et al: Bright light therapy for winter depression: potential ocular effects and theoretical implications. Photochem Photobiol 51:781–792, 1990

Thompson C, Stinson D, Fernandez M, et al: A comparison of normal, bipolar, and seasonal affective disorder subjects using the Seasonal Pattern Assessment Questionnaire. J Affect Disord 14:257–264, 1988

Waxler M, James RH, Brainard GC, et al: Retinopathy and bright light therapy. Am J Psychiatry 149:1610–1611, 1992

Wehr TA, Rosenthal NE: Seasonality and affective illness. Am J Psychiatry 146:829–839, 1989

Wehr TA, Skwerer RG, Jacobsen FM, et al: Eye versus skin phototherapy of seasonal affective disorder. Am J Psychiatry 144:753–757, 1987

Williams JBW, Link MJ, Rosenthal NE, et al: Structured Interview Guide for the Hamilton Depression Rating Scale, Seasonal Affective Disorder Version (SIGH-SAD). New York, New York State Psychiatric Institute, 1988

Wirz-Justice A, Buchelli C, Graw P, et al: Light treatment of seasonal affective disorder in Switzerland. Acta Psychiatr Scand 74:193–204, 1986

SIX

Light Treatment for Nonseasonal Major Depression: Are We Ready?

Daniel F. Kripke, M.D.

In 1981, I reported that bright light had an antidepressant effect among patients with ordinary serious depression, that is, patients with nonseasonal major depressive disorders. Although within a day, a single hour of light treatment produced only about a 12% reduction in depression ratings as compared with placebo, the result was statistically significant in the first seven patients (Kripke 1981). It did not seem then that the evidence was sufficient to immediately recommend bright light to clinicians as a new treatment. Further clinical testing was needed. The question now is whether in the intervening years, sufficient testing has been completed so that this treatment should be made available to patients with nonseasonal major depression.

Clinical Trials of Bright Light for Nonseasonal Depression

After our first report, we extended our 1-hour-treatment trial (Kripke et al. 1983a), replicated it (Kripke et al. 1983b), then did a

Supported by National Institute of Health grants MH00117 (National Institute of Mental Health); HL40930 (National Heart, Lung, and Blood Institute); and AG12364 (National Institute on Aging).

5-day trial that produced equivocal results (Kripke et al. 1987), and finally completed a 1-week bright light trial that produced unequivocal evidence for an antidepressant effect (Kripke et al. 1992). In the 1-week trial, 25 drug-free patients with major depression, randomly assigned to bright light treatment, were contrasted with 26 similar patients randomly assigned to a dim red placebo light. Measured expectations of the two groups were similar. Most of the experimental patients spent 3 hours in the evening in specially designed rooms illuminated to 2,000–3,000 lux at eye level; the placebo condition provided a similar daily exposure of 50 lux. After 7 evenings of bright light, Hamilton Depression Scale (HAM-D) (Hamilton 1967) ratings dropped 18%, rebounding somewhat by 2 days posttreatment, whereas the average ratings of placebo-treated patients hardly changed after 7 evenings of dim red light. Bright light treatment produced hypomania in two patients and agitation in two more, and evidently tended to delay sleep onset. Otherwise, side effects were minimal.

Our studies were all carried out with hospitalized veterans (almost all male) who were inpatients on a research ward. These patients were *not* admitted specifically for light treatment, and, indeed, the procedures of the ward tended to select patients who were either treatment refractory or in little hurry to get well. Further, over half of the patients had comorbid substance abuse problems or other comorbid conditions (Kripke et al. 1992). Thus, the roughly 18% reduction in depressive symptoms that 7-day bright light treatment produced (as compared with placebo responses) might underestimate what could be achieved among patients with less comorbidity and greater motivation.

Another study showing an unequivocal therapeutic effect of bright light in nonseasonal depression was reported by Yamada and colleagues (Yamada et al. 1995). In that study, 27 hospitalized patients with major depressive episodes were randomized to one of four conditions for 7 days: 2,500-lux bright light for 2 hours daily (morning or evening exposure), or 500-lux dim light for 2 hours daily (morning or evening exposure). Results showed the bright light was significantly superior to the dim light, although the time of day of exposure did not make a difference. On average, patients treated with bright light had a 35% reduction in depression scores compared with only 11% reduction in the dim light group.

Quite a few other clinical trials of bright light for treatment of nonseasonal depression have been reported by other investigators, for the most part with similar positive results (Deltito et al. 1991; Dietzel et al. 1986; Heim 1988; Kjellman et al. 1993; Kusumi et al. 1995; Leibenluft et al, 1995; Levitt et al. 1991; Neumeister et al. 1996; Papatheodorou and Kutcher, 1995; Peter 1986; Prasko et al. 1988; Schuchardt and Kasper 1992; Tsujimoto et al. 1990). There have also been some abstracts suggesting that bright light benefited depressed geriatric patients in nursing homes (Hanger et al. 1992; Moffit et al. 1993). A particularly valuable trial was that of Schuchardt and Kasper (1992). In this study, although the 1-week bright light response relative to placebo was rather less than the response we had observed, by 4 weeks the relative benefit was 27%. This study confirmed that, as with other antidepressants and with bright light treatment of SAD, benefits increase as treatment is continued for several weeks. Another 3-week study reported by Prasko and colleagues showed a 67% response rate (as defined by greater than 50% reduction in HAM-D scores to a termination score of less than 8) in bright light–treated patients compared with a 33% response rate in patients treated with imipramine (Prasko et al. 1995). Apart from occasional triggering of hypomania and mania (which also occurs with antidepressant pharmacotherapy), few appreciable side effects of bright light treatment have been reported.

It is unfortunate that the literature has given too much emphasis to the minority of studies in which no significant benefits were reported. For example, in the widely quoted study of Yerevanian et al. (1986), no statistically significant benefit was reported, but the degree of benefit observed was actually rather similar to what our group has observed. Further, the statistical procedure reported by the authors was probably inappropriate. If a paired t test was applied to the light responses of nonseasonally affected patients with depression who completed the trial, the benefit observed was indeed statistically significant ($P = .04$). In the report of Mackert and colleagues, no significant benefit of bright light was observed after 1 week of 2,500 lux given for 2 hours in the morning (Mackert et al. 1991). Nevertheless, all of the final results were in the direction of greater benefit with bright light than with placebo, and the magnitude of benefit was almost as great as what we had observed. The failure of Mackert and colleagues to observe statistical significance might be attributable to a Type II error that resulted from a sample somewhat smaller than ours (Kripke et al. 1992). Of note is that several papers also published by Mackert and colleagues referred to interim reports of the same aforementioned study (Mackert et al. 1990; Volz et al. 1990). Stewart and colleagues reported that patients with SAD responded more to light treatment than did patients with nonseasonal atypical depressions (Stewart et al. 1990), but the recruitment of the groups differed, and the atypical depressives had a mean duration of depression of 142 months (incomparably more chronicity than patients with SAD have, by definition). Moreover, the atypical depressives improved after bright light treatment with respect to 9 out of 10 measures. A more troubling result was reported by Holsboer-Trachsler and colleagues, who actually obtained better results with trimipramine alone than with trimipramine plus bright light or tri-mipramine plus sleep deprivation, although patients treated with the combinations did improve significantly (Holsboer-Trachsler et al. 1994). The response to nightly bright light in the initial week of this study (a 22% improvement in HAM-D scores) was quite favorable, but the benefits progressed little after the light treatment frequency was reduced to 3 times per week. This unexpected result, in some ways an outlier among reports, may have been attributable to unexpectedly high benefit observed with trimipramine alone or to the accident that patients with significantly poorer prognostic factors were assigned to the bright light treatment.

Many observers have an exaggerated impression of the efficacy of standard therapies of nonseasonal depression. This has encouraged a misguided expectation for light treatment. The 18% relative benefit that we obtained in 1 week, and even the smaller response described by Mackert and colleagues (Mackert et al. 1991), is larger than the response that standard therapy generally produces in a similar time. For example, in the landmark NIMH Treatment of Depression Collaborative Research Program (Elkin et al. 1989), the 16-week benefit of imipramine was only 10% better than placebo. This was substantially less than the 18% 1-week benefit that bright light produced in our study (Kripke et al. 1992), the 27% 6-day benefit reported by

Prasko et al. (1988), or the 27% 4-week benefit found by Schuchardt and Kasper (1992). In the NIMH Treatment of Depression Collaborative Research Program (Elkin et al. 1989), the relative benefits of cognitive and interpersonal psychotherapies were merely 6% and 9%, respectively. To give another example, in the distinguished study of DiMascio et al. (1979), no significant benefit of amitriptyline or psychotherapy was noted after 1 week. At 16 weeks, improvements about 32% greater in the amitriptyline and psychotherapy groups than with placebo were attributable partly to the higher baseline levels of depression in the active treatment groups; the 16-week depression ratings with active treatment were only about 26% lower than the placebo ratings. Some of the most successful recent studies of antidepressants have shown a relative advantage of antidepressant over placebo of less than 20% after 4 weeks or more (Fabre et al. 1995; Schulberg et al. 1996; Thase et al. 1996). Thus, the 1- to 4-week responses to bright light in nonseasonally affected patients with depression appear roughly equivalent in magnitude to the slower responses to standard drug treatments.

In summary, available data concerning nonseasonally affected patients with depression have indicated that bright light treatment responses may be more rapid than responses to standard treatment, and perhaps of equivalent magnitude. Such conclusions can be suggested only tentatively because direct randomized comparisons between bright light and standard treatment in patients with nonseasonal depression are not yet available.

Bright Light Combined With Antidepressants

In studies from our laboratory, the first-day response to bright light was larger in our first study, in which the patients were receiving antidepressants (Kripke et al. 1983a), than in our later study of drug-free patients with nonseasonal depression (Kripke et al. 1992). Rather large bright-light responses were likewise noted by Prasko et al. (1988) and by Schuchardt and Kasper (1992), who were similarly comparing responses to bright light plus antidepressants, with responses to antidepressants alone. Quite dramatic bright light augmentation among those who did not respond to antidepressants was reported by Levitt et al. (1991). Such studies may indicate that the incremental benefit of bright light is particularly favorable when light is combined with an antidepressant drug. Possibly, the benefits of both treatments are synergistic when combined, that is, better than additive in combination. A particularly dramatic speed and magnitude of response was obtained by Neumeister and colleagues, who combined bright light (2,000–3,000 lux vs. a 300-lux placebo condition for 6 days), a half-night of sleep deprivation, and antidepressant pharmacotherapy (Neumeister et al. 1996), which, in a fashion, extended the 1-hour treatment combination of our early study (Kripke et al. 1983a). Further studies of this very promising triple combination are needed because it may provide substantial and lasting relief within a single day.

Whether bright light alone works better than antidepressants alone may be of clinical interest only for those patients who tolerate the antidepressant drugs poorly. The clinician need not choose between the known benefits of standard antidepressant drugs and the benefits of bright light, but rather, the clinician can consider the potential benefits of combining bright light with antidepressant drugs. Perhaps a half-night of sleep deprivation, with its well-described benefits, should also be added.

Several investigators have also suggested that light therapy may be particularly useful for patients with nonseasonal bipolar depression. Deltito et al. (1991) found that patients who were medication free and had bipolar II depression showed significantly better response to light treatment than patients with unipolar depression. Bauer (1993) reported that light therapy was beneficial in treating episodes of major depression in patients (maintained on thymoleptic medications) who had bipolar I depression during the summertime. A recent study showed that breakthrough depressive symptoms in nonseasonally affected patients with bipolar depression were helped by light treatment (Papatheodorou and Kutcher 1995). Seven patients with bipolar I depression, kept on their mood-stabilizing medications, were treated with 10,000 lux for 45–60 minutes during the morning and the evening for 1 week; three patients showed a marked response, two patients had moderate response, and two had a mild or no response. Two studies have also reported that bright light may have a beneficial influence on rapid-cycling bipolar disorder (Kusumi et al. 1995; Leibenluft et al. 1995). Although these studies are case series and thus limited because they were not placebo controlled, to date, no negative results have been reported for light treatment of patients with nonseasonal bipolar depression.

Bright Light Treatment for SAD

The reputation of bright light treatment of seasonal affective disorder (SAD), also known as winter depression, was initially stimulated by two extremely enthusiastic reports. In the first modern report, the single volunteer studied had very positive expectations for light treatment (Lewy et al. 1982); moreover, he had previously experienced spontaneous remissions at about the same time of year (Rosenthal et al. 1983). This was an uncontrolled study. In the second enthusiastic report, bright light treatment produced 52% greater reduction in symptoms than a dim light placebo, but there were several limitations to the study design (Rosenthal et al. 1984). This landmark study had recruited subjects with newspaper stories that created high expectations for bright light, and the expectations for placebo were not equivalent. The strongly positive results may have been related to the high spontaneous remission rate in SAD, and important order effects in SAD cross-over studies (Terman 1993).

Subsequent studies of treatment of SAD have shown average advantages of bright light over placebo that are considerably lower than those in the landmark reports (Terman et al. 1989). Further, those subjects with HAM-D ratings of less than 15 have the best responses (Terman et al. 1989), and the early studies summarized by Terman showed a bias favoring bright light, because the bright light–treated patients had significantly lower scores at baseline than those who received the placebo (Terman et al. 1989). Most clinical trials of SAD have continued to recruit volunteers through newspapers and advertising, which produces risks of strong suggestion and placebo effects. It has even been suggested that most of the benefit of bright light in SAD patients can be attributed to placebo effects. In one of the comparisons that contrasted bright light and placebo most meticulously, the advantage of bright light was only 10%, which was not significant (Eastman et al. 1993). Growing evidence does confirm that bright light is significantly better than placebo for treatment of SAD, but the benefit might be of the same order of magnitude as with the patients who are nonseasonally depressed.

There remain serious limitations to our knowledge of bright light treatment of SAD. First, although SAD by definition lasts at least several weeks and is chronically recurrent, no light treatment studies have extended randomized trials over even one entire winter. Second, there have been no adequate contrasts of light treatment with standard treatments such as antidepressants and psychotherapy. A particularly important problem is the relative lack of consensus on diagnostic criteria for SAD. Further, the majority of patients with identified SAD who continue to show symptoms eventually manifest nonwinter depression, and they often require antidepressants as well as light treatment (Schwartz et al. 1996). Although this condition has been described as "complicated SAD," the diagnosis of patients displaying nonwinter symptoms may become major depression but *not* SAD under current definitions. It is ironic that even the archetypal SAD patient did display nonwinter depression (Rosenthal et al. 1983). These data and a particularly detailed case study (Summers et al. 1992) raise the question of whether SAD can be fully distinguished from nonseasonal major depressive disorders on a year-to-year basis.

Likewise, it is doubtful whether the light response of patients with seasonal and nonseasonal depression can be reliably distinguished. Magnitudes of treatment benefits obtained in seasonal and nonseasonal patient groups are overlapping. As has been mentioned, the outpatients with SAD, recruited by advertisement, often with HAM-D scores of less than 15, have been quite different from the inpatients used in many studies of light treatment of nonseasonal depression, and the induced expectations were different. Perhaps the benefits would be similar if the biases were similar.

Although the initial enthusiasm for bright light treatment of SAD may have been excessive, bright light treatment restricted to SAD has been accepted in various national and governmental guidelines (Depression Guideline Panel 1993), and bright light treatment may now be considered accepted practice in the United States.

Recommendations

In considering our current evidence, I believe we should now recommend bright light treatment for nonseasonal major depression, both in combination with antidepressant drugs and alone (for those patients who do not tolerate or accept antidepressant drugs). Initial results suggest that benefits with an initial end-of-night sleep deprivation are particularly favorable, but this needs further confirmation. It would also seem reasonable to combine bright light treatment with psychotherapy of depression, though this combination has not been formally studied in patients with either SAD or nonseasonal depression. The time has come to accept bright light treatment into our therapeutic armamentarium. Supporting this decision is a preponderance of evidence that bright light produces statistically significant benefits of an order of magnitude comparable with standard treatments. Further, the benefits of bright light and antidepressant drugs appear to be additive or even synergistic, so there is no need to deny standard treatment in order to add bright light therapy. Although there have been some small studies that have failed to show statistically significant advantages for bright light treatment, most of the weak results can be explained by problems in experimental design. With one exception (where the prospective prognoses were not balanced successfully) (Holsboer-Trachsler et al. 1994), there have been no studies in which bright light treatment risks seemingly outweighed benefits. Because bright light is in fact a very old treatment (Kellogg 1910; Wehr 1989), and human responses to sunlight are well known, it is unlikely that excessive long-term risks will be found. The cost of a suitable bright light fixture for treatment may be less than the cost of a 6-month supply of the newer patented antidepressant drugs. The cost would be much less than the cost of 12–18 psychotherapy sessions. Thus, bright light treatment will be a cost-effective addition to modern health care.

It would be desirable to have more extensive testing of long-term responses to bright light treatment. However, it does not appear in the public benefit to delay this treatment another decade while such studies are being done. Most accepted contemporary treatments have not received as much long-term efficacy testing as would be desirable. In particular, the evidence supporting bright light treatment for nonseasonal depression is rather similar to that supporting such treatment for SAD. There is little point in accepting the treatment for one condition but not the other, when the two conditions may not even be readily distinguishable.

It is time now to recommend bright light for patients with nonseasonal depression.

Recommended Treatment Method

For acute treatment of major depressions, patients should receive 2–3 hours of bright light treatment per day in addition to standard therapies such as antidepressant drugs, psychotherapy, and milieu therapy. Treatment should consist of 2,000- to 3,000-lux illumination at eye level in the direction of gaze, administered either by ceiling fixtures or by portable light fixtures providing well-diffused light. Although 10,000 lux seems preferred for treatment of SAD, some caution in exceeding 3,000 lux for treatment of major depression might be advisable when advanced age and various drugs might increase the retinal sensitivity of patients with major depressions. So-called full-spectrum lighting sometimes contains sufficient ultraviolet radiation to pose unnecessary risks for the eyes and skin, and there is no proven advantage over ordinary lighting such as cool-white fluorescents. To date, there is no convincing evidence favoring any particular time-of-day of treatment, but it is likely that patients who awaken early will be most comfortable with evening bright light treatment, whereas patients with trouble falling asleep and trouble getting up will be more comfortable with morning treatment.

Relative contraindications for bright light treatment are retinitis or other conditions that produce photophobia, and prior history of mania (unless the patient is simultaneously receiving a mood stabilizer). No serious manias have been reported resulting from bright light treatment of patients maintained on lithium.

References

Bauer MS: Summertime bright-light treatment of bipolar major depressive episodes. Biol Psychiatry 33:663–665, 1993

Deltito JA, Moline M, Pollak C, et al: Effects of phototherapy on nonseasonal unipolar and bipolar depressive spectrum disorders. J Affect Disord 23:231–237. 1991

Depression Guideline Panel: Depression in Primary Care, Vol. 2. Treatment of Major Depression (DHHS, AHCPR Publication No. 93–0551). Washington, DC, Agency for Health Care Policy and Research, U.S. Government Printing Office, 1993

Dietzel M, Saletu B, Lesch OM, et al: Light treatment in depressive illness: polysomnographic, psychometric and neuroendocrinological findings. Eur Neurol 25(suppl):93–103, 1986

DiMascio A, Weissman MM, Prusoff BA, et al: Differential symptom reduction by drugs and psychotherapy in acute depression. Arch Gen Psychiatry 36:1450–1456, 1979

Eastman CI, Young MA, Fogg LF: A comparison of two different placebo-controlled SAD light treatment studies, in Light and Biological Rhythms in Man. Edited by Wetterberg L. Stockholm, Pergamon, 1993, pp 371–383

Elkin I, Shea T, Watkins JT, et al: National Institute of Mental Health Treatment of Depression Collaborative Research Program: general effectiveness of treatment. Arch Gen Psychiatry 46:971–982, 1989

Fabre LF, Abuzzahab FS, Amin M, et al: Sertraline safety and efficacy in major depression: a double-blind, fixed-dose comparison with placebo. Biol Psychiatry 38:592–602, 1995

Hamilton M: Development of a rating scale for primary depressive illness. Br J Soc ClinPsychol 6:278–296, 1967

Hanger MA, Ancoli-Israel S, Kripke DF, et al: Effect of phototherapy on depression in nursing home residents (abstract). Sleep Res 21:88, 1992

Heim M: Zur Effizienz der Bright-Light-Therapie bei zyklothymen Achsensyndromen—eine cross-over Studie gegenuber partiellem Schlafentzug. Psychiatr Neurol Med Psychol (Leipz) 40:269–277, 1988

Holsboer-Trachsler E, Hemmeter U, Hatzinger M, et al: Sleep deprivation and bright light as potential augmenters of antidepressant drug treatment—neurobiological and psychometric assessment of course. J Psychiat Res 28:381–399, 1994

Kellogg JH: Light Therapeutics: A Practical Manual of Phototherapy for the Student and Practitioner. Battle Creek, MI, Good Health Publishing, 1910, pp 1–213

Kjellman BF, Thalen BE, Wetterberg L: Light treatment of depressive states: Swedish experiences at latitude 59 north, in Light and Biological Rhythms in Man. Edited by Wetterberg L. Stockholm, Pergamon, 1993, pp 351–370

Kripke DF: Photoperiodic mechanisms for depression and its treatment, in Biological Psychiatry. Edited by Perris C, Struwe G, Jansson B. Amsterdam, Elsevier–North Holland Biomedical, 1981, pp 1249–1252

Kripke DF, Risch SC, Janowsky DS: Bright white light alleviates depression. Psychiatry Res 10:105–112, 1983a

Kripke DF, Risch SC, Janowsky DS: Lighting up depression. Psychopharmacol Bull 19:526–530, 1983b

Kripke DF, Gillin JC, Mullaney DJ, et al: Treatment of major depressive disorders by bright white light for 5 days, in Chronobiology and Psychiatric Disorders. Edited by Halaris A. New York, Elsevier Science, 1987, pp 207–218

Kripke DF, Mullaney DJ, Klauber MR, et al: Controlled trial of bright light for non-seasonal major depressive disorders. Biol Psychiatry 31:119–134, 1992

Kusumi I, Ohmori T, Kohsaka M, et al: Chronobiological approach for treatment-resistant rapid cycling affective disorders. Biol Psychiatry 37:553–559, 1995

Leibenluft E, Turner EH, Feldman-Naim S, et al: Light therapy in patients with rapid cycling bipolar disorder: preliminary results. Psychopharmacol Bull 31:705–710, 1995

Levitt AJ, Joffe RT, Kennedy SH: Bright light augmentation in antidepressant nonresponders. J Clin Psychiatry 52:336–337, 1991

Lewy AJ, Kern HA, Rosenthal NE, et al: Bright artificial light treatment of a manic-depressive patient with a seasonal mood cycle. Am J Psychiatry 139:1496–1498, 1982

Mackert A, Volz HP, Stieglitz RD, et al: Effect of bright white light on non-seasonal depressive disorder. Pharmacopsychiatry 23:151–154, 1990.

Mackert A, Volz HP, Stieglitz RD, et al: Phototherapy in non-seasonal depression. Biol Psychiatry 30:257–268, 1991

Moffit MT, Ancoli-Israel S: Bright light treatment of late-life depression (abstract), in SLTBR: Abstracts of the Annual Meeting of the Society for Light Treatment and Biological Rhythms, Vol. 5. Wilsonville, OR, Society for Light Treatment and Biological Rhythms, 1993, p 41

Neumeister A, Goessler R, Lucht M, et al: Bright light therapy stabilizes the antidepressant effect of partial sleep deprivation. Biol Psychiatry 39: 16–21, 1996

Papatheodorou G, Kutcher S: The effect of adjunctive light therapy on ameliorating breakthrough depressive symptoms in adolescent-onset bipolar disorder. J Psychiatr Neurosci 20:226–232, 1995

Peter K: First results with bright light in affective psychosis. Psychiatr Neurol Med Psychol 38:384–390, 1986

Prasko J, Foldmann P, Praskova H, et al: Hastened onset of the effect of antidepressive drugs when using three types of timing of intensive white light. Ceskoslovenská Psychiatrie 84:373–383, 1988

Prasko J, Baudis P, Klaschka J, et al: Bright light therapy in patients with recurrent nonseasonal unipolar depressive disorder—a double blind study (abstract), in SLTBR: Abstracts of the Annual Meeting of the Society for Light Treatment and Biological Rhythms, Vol. 7. Wheat Ridge, CO, Society for Light Treatment and Biological Rhythms, 1995, p 48

Rosenthal NE, Lewy AJ, Wehr TA, et al: Seasonal cycling in a bipolar patient. Psychiatry Res 8:25–31, 1983

Rosenthal NE, Sack DA, Gillin JC, et al: Seasonal affective disorder: a description of the syndrome and preliminary findings with light therapy. Arch Gen Psychiatry 41:72–80, 1984

Schuchardt HM, Kasper S: Lichttherapie in der psychiatrischen praxis. Fortschr Neurol Psychiatr 60:193–194, 1992

Schulberg HC, Block MR, Madonia MJ, et al: Treating major depression in primary care practice. Arch Gen Psychiatry 53:913–919, 1996

Schwartz PJ, Brown C, Wehr TA, et al: Winter seasonal affective disorder: a follow-up study of the first 59 patients of the National Institute of Mental Health Seasonal Studies Program. Am J Psychiatry 153:1028–1036, 1996

Stewart JW, Quitkin FM, Terman M, et al: Is seasonal affective disorder a variant of atypical depression? Differential response to light therapy. Psychiatry Res 33:121–128, 1990

Summers L, Shur E: The relationship between onsets of depression and sudden drops in solar irradiation. Biol Psychiatry 32:1164–1172, 1992

Terman M: Problems and prospects for use of bright light as a therapeutic intervention, in Light and Biological Rhythms in Man. Edited by Wetterberg L. Stockholm, Pergamon, 1993, pp 421–436

Terman M, Terman JS, Quitkin FM, et al: Light therapy for seasonal affective disorder: a review of efficacy. Neuropsychopharmacology 2:1–22, 1989

Thase ME, Fava M, Halbreich U, et al: A placebo-controlled, randomized clinical trial comparing sertraline and imipramine for the treatment of dysthymia. Arch Gen Psychiatry 53:777–784, 1996

Tsujimoto T, Hanada K, Shioiri T, et al: Effect of phototherapy on mood disorders (abstract), in SRBR: Abstracts of the Annual Meeting of the Society for Research on Biological Rhythms, Vol. 2. New York, Society for Research on Biological Rhythms, 1990, p 39

Volz HP, Mackert A, Stieglitz RD, et al: Effect of bright white light therapy on non-seasonal depressive disorder. Preliminary results. J Affect Disord 19:15–21, 1990

Wehr TA: Seasonal affective disorders: a historical overview, in Seasonal Affective Disorder and Phototherapy. Edited by Rosenthal NE, Blehar M. New York, Guilford, 1989, pp 11–32

Yamada N, Martin-Iverson MT, Daimon K, et al: Clinical and chronobiological effects of light therapy on nonseasonal affective disorders. Biol Psychiatry 37:866–873, 1995

Yerevanian BI, Anderson JL, Grota LJ, et al: Effects of bright incandescent light on seasonal and non-seasonal major depressive disorder. Psychiatry Res 18:355–364, 1986

SEVEN

Light Therapy of Premenstrual Depression

Barbara L. Parry, M.D.

Bright light therapy has been used to treat patients with seasonal affective disorder (SAD) (Rosenthal et al. 1985), some patients with major depressive disorders (Kripke et al. 1992), patients with seasonal premenstrual syndrome (Parry et al. 1987), and, most recently, patients with nonseasonal premenstrual syndrome (Parry et al. 1989a). In a pilot study, we reported greater effectiveness of evening bright light compared with morning bright light in the treatment of six patients with prospectively documented premenstrual depression (Parry et al. 1989a). To extend our preliminary investigation, in a subsequent study we reported on effects of bright light treatment in an additional 19 patients with prospectively documented premenstrual depression (who met DSM-III-R criteria [American Psychiatric Association 1987] for late luteal phase dysphoric disorder) and in 11 normal control subjects (Parry et al. 1993). In our initial pilot study, morning bright light treatment, hypothesized to exacerbate symptoms by phase-advancing already pathologically advanced circadian rhythms in

The figures and portions of the text in Chapter 7 are adapted from Parry BL, Mahan AM, Mostofi N, et al.: "Light Therapy of Late Luteal Phase Dysphoric Disorder: An Extended Study," *Am J Psychiatry* 150: 1417–1419, 1993. Copyright 1993 American Psychiatric Association. Used with permission.

Supported in part by NIMH grant #R29MH42831, CRC grant #M01RR00827, and NIMH CRC grant #MH30914–14. D. F. Kripke, M.D., served as a consultant.

patients with premenstrual depression, was intended to serve as an internal control. In that pilot study, depression ratings, although not statistically different from ratings obtained at baseline (before treatment), did decrease after morning light treatment. Thus, morning bright light did not serve as a sufficient control condition. In the present study, we added an additional placebo control condition: dim red evening light. In the extended study, summarized in this chapter, we report the effects on mood of morning bright white, evening bright white, and evening dim red light administered in a crossover design to patients with premenstrual depression and to normal control subjects.

Method

Subjects

For purposes of familiarity and succinctness, we will use the term *PMS* to describe subjects with prospectively documented premenstrual depression who met DSM-III-R criteria for late luteal phase dysphoric disorder. The patients were referred by local professionals or were recruited by advertisement. Screening procedures consisted of a structured menstrual assessment questionnaire (adapted by B. L. Parry and N. Mostofi from D. R. Rubinow et al.; Roy-Byrne et al. 1986), a Structured Clinical Interview for DSM-III-R (SCID) (Spitzer et al. 1990), psychiatric interview, physical examination, and laboratory tests including chemistry panel, complete blood count, urinalysis, and measurements of thyroid indexes. If the subject did not have major medical, gynecologic, or psychiatric illness, had regular (26- to 32-day) menstrual cycles, appeared consistently to have premenstrual affective symptoms sufficiently severe to disrupt social or occupational functioning, and was willing to endure the rigors of a long-term research study, she was admitted for a 2- to 3-month prospective evaluation for diagnostic assessment. A past history of affective illness in PMS, but not in normal control subjects, was permissible for the study. Normal control subjects were selected only if they also met exclusion criteria for medical and psychiatric illness, and first-degree relatives were free of psychiatric illness, with the exception of alcohol abuse. (We found that requiring a negative history of this latter criterion was so strict as to prevent us from recruiting participants.)

During the evaluation, subjects completed twice-daily mood ratings (100-mm visual analogue scales of depression, anxiety, irritability, fatigue, withdrawal, physical symptoms, and appetite) and visited the clinic weekly for objective (21-item Hamilton Rating Scale for Depression, HAM-D) (Hamilton 1967) and self-report (Beck Depression Inventory, BDI) (Beck et al. 1961) depression ratings. Based on this examination, to be selected for the study, patients had to 1) meet DSM-III-R criteria for late luteal phase dysphoric disorder; 2) have mean scores of 14 or more on the HAM-D, and 10 or more on the BDI in the late luteal phase (1 week before the onset of menses); and 3) demonstrate a reduction in scores to 7 or less on the HAM-D and 5 or less on the BDI by the week after the cessation of menses. All patients had debilitating affective symptoms that occurred during the late luteal phase of each menstrual cycle throughout the year (i.e., they did not have seasonal premenstrual symptoms).

Normal control subjects also underwent a 2-month diagnostic evaluation: mean HAM-D ratings were less than 7, and BDI ratings less than 5 at all menstrual cycle phases, and daily ratings showed no important (>30%) clinical variation in association with the menstrual cycle.

Procedures

Subjects selected for the study underwent, in random order, the six possible orders of treatment in a crossover trial of morning bright white light (>2,500 lux, 6:30 A.M. to 8:30 A.M.), evening bright white light (>2,500 lux, 7:00 P.M. to 9:00 P.M.), or placebo evening dim red light (<10 lux, 7:00 P.M. to 9:00 P.M.) treatment. Each treatment was administered for 7 consecutive days during the luteal phase of a separate menstrual cycle (7–10 days before the onset of menses). We administered the dim red light placebo in the evening to contrast with the evening bright light, which our preliminary study had indicated was more effective than morning light in alleviating PMS symptoms.

Menstrual cycle phase was determined by using a colorimetric urinary immunoassay (Ovustick Company, Irvine, CA) for the midcycle luteinizing hormone surge. Patients were asked to sit 3 feet from the light source. The bright light was a portable illumination box (Apollo Light, Orem, UT) containing cool-white fluorescent light bulbs that produced 2,500 lux at 3 feet. The dim light was one fluorescent bulb behind a red filter encased in the same size box and producing 10 lux at 3 feet. Subjects were asked to keep their eyes open and to gaze every few minutes at the light. During each month of study, patients were asked to maintain their normal sleep patterns, take no naps, and document their sleep times on daily sleep logs. They also were asked to wear dark sunglasses or goggles to block out light when outdoors between 6:30 A.M. and 8:30 A.M. if they were being treated with evening light, or between 7:00 P.M. and 9:00 P.M. if they were being treated with morning light, in order to balance the amount of light exposure during both treatment conditions. Subjects also completed daily light logs, expectation forms (100-mm visual analog scales from "much better than usual" to "much worse than usual" for each light treatment condition administered at the beginning of the study), and Horne-Ostberg ratings (Horne and Ostberg 1976) to assess for morningness and eveningness.

At the end of 7 days of light treatment in the luteal phase, mood over the past several days was assessed by two raters who were blind to the treatment condition, using the HAM-D, an addendum that assessed atypical depressive symptoms such as fatigue, social withdrawal, carbohydrate craving, weight gain, and hypersomnia (ATYP, maximum of 23 points), and a mania rating scale (Rosenthal and Heffernan 1986). Criteria of Terman et al. (1989) were used to define responders to light treatment: a 50% reduction in scores on the 21-item HAM-D, to a termination score of less than 8. In addition, subjects completed the BDI after each treatment, and they were asked to continue filling out the daily ratings forms throughout the light study.

Subjects had been off psychoactive medication for at least 2 months before the initiation of the study. All gave written informed consent after the procedures had been fully explained.

After completion of the acute treatment study, PMS subjects who wished to continue with the light treatments were invited to do so in a follow-up study. Menstrual phase continued to be monitored by urinary leutinizing hormone assay, and the light treatment (morning bright white light, evening bright white light, or evening dim red light) that was found to be most effective in the acute treatment study was administered during the premenstrual phase for a subsequent 6- to 18-month period. Each month, HAM-D ratings were performed following a week of the specified light treatment. Patients continued to complete daily mood ratings, sleep and light logs, and BDI ratings during each follow-up light treatment.

Data Analysis

Baseline measures for each rating scale (HAM-D, BDI, ATYP, mania, or daily ratings) were determined by taking the mean of the ratings during the premenstrual weeks of the 2–3 month evaluation phase before treatment. Mood assessments also were made during a month of hormonal study (circadian measurements for melatonin, cortisol, prolactin, and thyroid-stimulating hormone) that was completed before light treatments were initiated. Ratings done during this month of hormonal study were not significantly different from ratings done during the evaluation phase. Thus, there was no spontaneous improvement in symptoms over a 3-month interval before the treatment protocol was begun. The ratings made during the month of hormonal assessment were not used for these data analyses because of the possible confounding effects of hospitalization and because the hormonal data will be reported separately. For each of the rating scales, normality was tested by the Shapiro-Wilk approach. Preliminary analysis showed trivial differences by order of treatment; hence, treatment order was not taken into account in the statistical model. The nonparametric tests used were those of Friedman and Wilcoxon. PMS patients and normal control subjects were analyzed separately. Since this was a small-sample exploratory study, no adjustment for multiple comparisons was used. The $P < .05$ level was used for statistical significance.

Results

Of 884 screening questionnaires that were mailed, 449 (51%) were returned, and 186 (41%) of those returned were deemed appropriate for a screening interview (21% of total questionnaires sent). Of those patients screened, 107 (58%) were admitted to the study for diagnostic evaluation (12% of questionnaires sent). Of those subjects who completed the diagnostic evaluation, 35% entered the light study (4% of questionnaires sent). Reasons for exclusion included being on oral contraceptives or other medications, not having regular, ovulatory menstrual cycles, not meeting DSM-III-R criteria for late luteal phase dysphoric disorder or our inclusion criteria for severity of symptomatology, or not being willing to meet the demands of a rigorous long-term research study.

The age distribution of the PMS patients (mean 36 years, range 28–45 years) was nearly identical to that of the normal controls (mean 36 years, range 27–43 years). Not including students (2 of whom were normal controls and 2 of whom were PMS patients), 9 of 11 (82%) control subjects, and 15 of 19 (79%) PMS patients were employed outside the home. Including students, 90% of PMS patients and 91% of normal controls were employed. Of the PMS patients, 12 (63%) were married, 5 (26%) were single, and 2 (10%) were divorced. Of the normal control subjects, 4 (36%) were married, 5 (45%) were single, and 2 (18%) were divorced ($P = .36$). As expected, PMS and control groups differed markedly on mood, behavior, and physical symptoms (Table 7–1). Over 75% of the PMS patients were rated moderate or severe for each of the following items: irritable, feel sad/cry, and loss of energy or fatigue, versus 0% for controls.

In parity the two groups were very similar. Of the PMS patients, 10 (53%) had no children, 1 (5%) had one child, 4 (21%) had two children, 3 (16%) had three children, and 1 (5%) had 4 children. Of the normal control subjects, 6 (54%) had no children, 2 (18%) had one child, 3 (27%) had two children, and none had three or more children. Normal control subjects and PMS subjects were not significantly different with regard to number of children.

There was no significant difference in menstrual cycle lengths between the PMS patients (mean ±SD: 27.5 ± 3.44 days) and the normal control subjects (mean ±SD: 28.8 ± 2.79 days).

Regarding family history of psychiatric illness, 8 of 19 (42%) of the PMS patients had a history of depression in a first-degree family relative. By the exclusion criteria, none of the normal control sub-

TABLE **7-1.**

Clinical variables in patients with premenstrual depression and normal control subjects

Mood, behavior, or physical change*	% rated moderate or severe	
	PMS patients ($n = 19$)	Normal controls ($n = 11$)
Irritable	83	0
Feel sad/cry	78	0
Crave specific foods	72	9
Difficulty concentrating/ making decisions	68	9
Loss of energy or fatigue	78	0
Appetite	67	0
Anxious or jittery	67	0
Difficult to enjoy self	65	0
Past postpartum depression	57	0
Decrease in efficiency	56	0
Feel guilty	39	0
Decrease in sexual drive	39	0
Increase in accidents	28	0
Excessive sleeping	28	0
Seasonal change in mood	26	0
Seasonal change in energy level	21	0
Thoughts of hurting self	17	0

Note. PMS, premenstrual depression.
*Comparison between patients and controls, $P < .05$ for all variables listed.

jects had a history of depression in first-degree relatives. Nine of 19 (42%) PMS patients had a family history of alcoholism compared to 1 of 11 (9%) normal control subjects.

Of the PMS patients, 19 (61%) had received counseling or had been treated by a mental health professional, whereas 3 (21%) of normal controls had received counseling, related mainly to relationship issues. Of the PMS patients, 7 (35%) had been previously treated for a mood problem, whereas none of the normal control subjects had been so treated.

Of those subjects who had SCID interviews, 14% of PMS patients had a lifetime history of major depression, 14% had anxiety disorder (simple phobia), and 14% had psychoactive substance use disorders. Twenty percent of normal control subjects had a lifetime history of psychoactive substance use disorders.

Acute Treatment Study

HAM-D ratings (Figure 7–1)

In PMS patients, a Friedman's test on the HAM-D ratings showed statistically significant effects of condition (baseline, morning bright white light, evening bright white light, evening dim red light; $P = .001$). Wilcoxon signed rank tests for pairwise comparisons showed that HAM-D baseline ratings (before treatment) were significantly

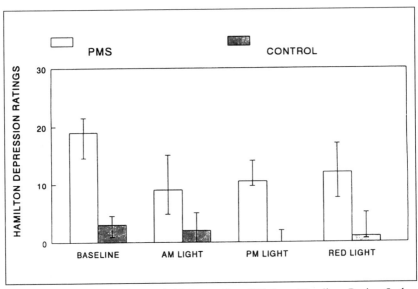

FIGURE 7–1. Median, first, and third quartiles of 21-item Hamilton Rating Scale of Depression (HAM-D) ratings in PMS ($n = 19$) and normal control ($n = 11$) subjects, by baseline and treatment values. Each of the light treatments (morning bright white, evening bright white, evening dim red) was significantly different from baseline ($P < .01$), but none of the light treatments differed significantly from each other.

greater than those ratings obtained after treatment with evening bright white light ($P < .01$), morning bright white light ($P < .01$), and evening dim red light ($P < .01$). None of the light treatments (morning bright white, evening bright white, evening dim red) differed significantly from each other ($P > .10$).

Using the response criteria of Terman et al. (1989), eight (39%) patients responded to morning bright light, four (22%) responded to evening bright light, and five (28%) responded to evening dim light.

For normal control subjects, Friedman's test showed no statistically significant effects of light treatment on HAM-D ratings ($P = .71$).

BDI ratings (Figure 7–2)

Friedman's test on BDI scores showed statistically significant effects for condition (baseline, morning bright white light, evening bright

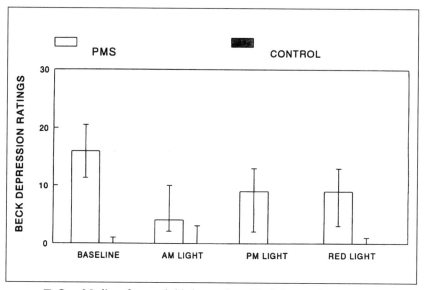

FIGURE 7–2. Median, first, and third quartiles of Beck Depression Inventory (BDI) ratings in PMS ($n = 19$) and normal control ($n = 11$) subjects, by baseline and treatment values. Each of the light treatments (morning bright white, evening bright white, evening dim red) was significantly different from baseline ($P < .01$), but none of the light treatments differed significantly from each other.

white light, evening dim red light; $P < .005$). BDI ratings obtained at baseline (before treatment) were significantly higher than ratings obtained after morning bright white ($P < .01$), evening bright white ($P < .01$), and evening dim red ($P < .01$) light treatments (by Wilcoxon tests). The three light treatments did not differ significantly from each other ($P > .10$).

Normal control subjects showed no statistically significant effects of light treatment on BDI ratings (by Friedman's test, $P = .85$).

ATYP ratings (Figure 7–3)

The ATYP ratings showed statistically significant effects of condition (baseline, morning bright, evening bright, and evening dim light treatment; Friedman's test, $P < .001$). Baseline premenstrual ATYP ratings before treatment were significantly higher than those after

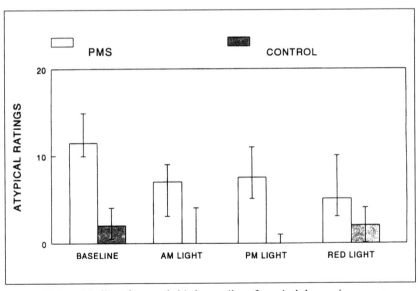

FIGURE 7–3. Median, first, and third quartiles of atypical depressive symptoms assessment (ATYP) ratings in PMS ($n = 19$) and normal control ($n = 11$) subjects, by baseline and treatment values. Each of the light treatments (morning bright white, evening bright white, evening dim red) was significantly different from baseline ($P < .01$), but none of the light treatments differed significantly from each other.

treatment with morning bright white ($P < .01$), evening bright white ($P < .01$), or evening dim red ($P < .01$) light treatment (by Wilcoxon tests). The effects of the three light treatments were not significantly different from each other ($P > .10$).

For normal control subjects, Friedman's test showed no statistically significant effects of light treatment on ATYP ratings ($P > .17$).

Mania ratings (Figure 7–4)

Treatment conditions had no statistically significant effect on mania ratings in PMS patients (Friedman's test, $P > .70$).

In normal control subjects, there were statistically significant differences of treatment condition on mania ratings (Friedman's test, $P < .02$). By Wilcoxon signed ranks tests, there were no statistically significant differences between baseline and morning bright light ($P > .10$), or baseline and evening bright light ratings ($P > .10$), but there was a statistically significant reduction in ratings between base-

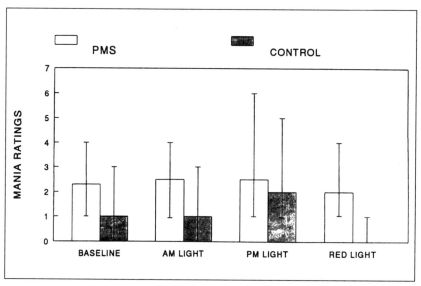

FIGURE 7–4. Median, first, and third quartiles of mania ratings in PMS ($n = 19$) and normal control ($n = 11$) subjects, by baseline and treatment values. In normal control subjects, there was a significant difference in mania ratings when baseline and evening dim red light were compared ($P < .05$).

line and evening dim red light treatment ($P < .05$). Also, there was a statistically significant increase in mania ratings after evening bright white light compared with evening dim red light treatment ($P < .05$). However, the magnitude of these effects was not considered clinically important.

Daily ratings

Only daily ratings after 4 days of light treatment were used in the analysis, because light treatment generally takes 3–4 days to produce therapeutic effects (Rosenthal et al. 1985). Friedman's tests showed statistically significant differences between conditions (baseline, morning bright white light, evening bright white light, and evening dim red light) for the daily visual analog ratings of depression ($P < .04$), irritability ($P < .001$), and physical symptoms ($P < .002$). For each of these symptoms, Wilcoxon tests showed significant ($P < .05$) improvement in reported symptoms between baseline and each of the three light treatments. There were no statistically significant differences between pairwise comparisons of the three treatments. By Friedman's test there were no statistically significant differences of condition (baseline, the three light treatments) for anxiety or appetite. Items rating fatigue ($P = .07$) and withdrawal ($P = .06$) approached statistical significance.

Subject expectations

For PMS patients, the only statistically significant correlations between expectation of improvement with each condition, and clinical response by observed ratings, were in BDI ratings for evening bright white light ($P = .015$), and in HAM-D ratings for evening dim red light ($P < .03$).

Horne-Ostberg ratings

There were no statistically significant correlations of morningness-eveningness with response to morning bright, evening bright, or evening dim light treatment based on HAM-D, BDI, ATYP, or mania ratings.

Sleep logs

In PMS patients, there was a statistically significant difference in the reported amount of sleep with treatment condition (Friedman's test, $P < .02$). By Wilcoxon tests, there was a significant reduction of sleep reported by the PMS patients during the morning bright white light treatment compared with evening dim red light treatment ($P < .01$). There were no significant differences in sleep duration during different light treatment conditions in normal control subjects.

Side-effects checklist

Only PMS patients reported significant side effects from the light treatments. The most frequently reported side effect of morning bright white light was increased activity (agitation), which was reported in 6 of 10 patients (3 reported mild symptoms, 3 moderate). Eye strain was the most frequently reported symptom from evening bright white light, and was reported in 5 of 10 patients (3 reported mild, 1 moderate, and 1 marked symptoms). Drowsiness was the most frequently reported symptom under evening dim red light, and was reported in 7 of 10 patients (1 mild, 5 moderate, 1 marked).

Follow-up study (Figure 7–5)

No patient who participated in the follow-up study did the best on evening dim red light treatment during the initial study, and, therefore, dim red light treatment was not used in the follow-up study. Four patients (two who chose to continue with morning bright light and two who chose to continue with evening bright light) completed at least 12 months, and three of them completed 18 months, of follow-up bright light treatment. The mean ±SD of HAM-D, BDI, ATYP, and mania ratings after 6 months, 12 months, and 18 months of bright light treatment (morning and evening) are illustrated in Figure 7–5.

Mean ratings for HAM-D ($P < .01$), BDI ($P < .005$), and ATYP scales ($P < .04$) at 18 months after bright light treatment continued to show statistically significant reductions in depressive symptoms compared with baseline. Mania ratings did not change during the months of light treatment. There were no statistically significant diff-

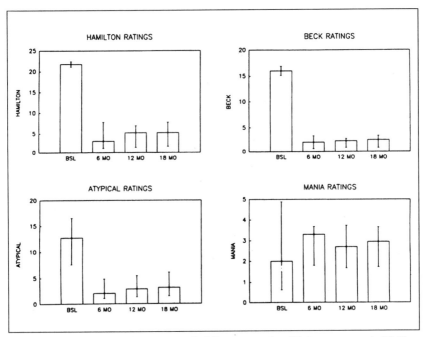

FIGURE 7–5. Results of an 18-month follow-up study of light treatment in PMS subjects, comparing baseline (before treatment) premenstrual 21-item Hamilton Rating Scale for Depression (HAM-D), Beck Depression Inventory (BDI), atypical symptoms of depression assessment (ATYP), and mania ratings with the same premenstrual ratings obtained after morning or evening bright white light treatment. Compared with baseline ratings, HAM-D, BDI, and ATYP ratings were significantly ($P < .05$) reduced during follow up months 1–6, 7–12, and 13–18. Ratings obtained during months 1–6, months 7–12, and months 13–18 did not differ from each other. Mania ratings did not significantly change during the months of light treatment compared with baseline.

erences between morning and evening bright light treatment on any of the rating scales. Furthermore, there were no statistically significant differences in any of the ratings when months 1–3 were compared with months 4–6, or when months 1–6 were compared with months 7–12 or months 13–18 in the follow-up study.

The daily ratings after 18 months of follow-up bright light treatment continued to show significant improvement from baseline in withdrawal ($P < .02$), irritability ($P < .04$), and physical discomfort ($P < .04$).

Discussion

The results of this study suggest that light treatments may have therapeutic effects in patients with prospectively diagnosed premenstrual depression. Depression ratings fell significantly from baseline after morning bright white light, evening bright white light, and evening dim red light treatments. The lack of discernible order of treatment effects is consistent with the observation that the three treatments were nearly equally effective. The fact that the three light treatments were not significantly different from each other raises several questions regarding possible mechanisms for the observed effects of light therapy in PMS.

First, a placebo effect of light therapy cannot be ruled out, as Eastman (1990) described in her discussion of the placebo response to light therapy in SAD. However, our patients' expectations showed little correlation with clinical response, which tends to argue against this possibility. Also, results of our 18-month follow up study, although they are based on a small number of subjects, show that all subjects continued to benefit from morning or evening bright light treatment over time. Thus, if bright light treatment is a placebo response, it appears to be stable over time in patients who do respond. Further controlled follow-up trials with a larger number of subjects are indicated. Such trials should include a completely untreated (i.e., negative) control group, especially to evaluate any long-term effects.

Alternatively, the various light treatments may be exerting their therapeutic effects through different biological mechanisms. We had initially hypothesized, based on preliminary data examining sleep (Parry and Wehr 1987), temperature (Parry et al. 1989b), and melatonin (Parry et al. 1990), that circadian rhythms in patients with premenstrual depression tended to be phase-advanced with respect to the sleep-wake cycle. Because morning bright light tends to advance and evening bright light to delay circadian rhythms (Lewy et al. 1987), we hypothesized that evening bright light, by delaying circadian rhythms, would correct the underlying phase-advanced disturbances in PMS patients and thereby improve mood. Alternatively, morning bright light, by advancing circadian rhythms, would be expected to exacerbate the underlying phase-advanced disturbances, thereby exacerbating symptoms and serving as an internal control. Our pilot study comparing the efficacy of morning and evening bright light treatment in PMS subjects suggested, as hypothesized, a superior efficacy of evening compared with morning bright light treatment (Parry et al. 1989a). However, although the morning bright light treatment did not significantly reduce depression ratings compared to baseline, it did not exacerbate symptoms and thus did not serve as an adequate internal control condition. Our current study suggests equal efficacy of morning and evening bright light treatment in PMS patients. It is possible that circadian phase heterogeneity, which would contribute to variable responses to morning versus evening bright light treatment, exists among PMS patients, similar to what has been reported by Lewy et al. (1991) in patients with SAD. PMS patients whose circadian rhythms are phase-advanced may respond better to evening bright light treatment, whereas PMS patients whose circadian rhythms are phase-delayed may respond more to morning bright light treatment. Indeed, variability of circadian phase responsiveness, similar to what Siever and David (1985) have hypothetically described for receptor sensitivity variability in depressive illness, may characterize PMS patients. In a previous report we described low or dampened melatonin circadian profiles in PMS patients compared with control subjects (Parry et al. 1990). Low melatonin levels may reflect a decreased strength of the underlying circadian oscillator (Pittendrigh 1981). Low amplitude rhythms, as Aschoff (1983) suggested, may contribute to phase lability. Thus, PMS patients may have a specific vulnerability to circadian phase lability or heterogeneity because of dampened circadian oscillators, and this phase heterogeneity may contribute to their variable response to morning and evening bright light. We have begun to test this hypothesis by measuring melatonin circadian profiles before and after light treatment in PMS patients and control subjects. Our early preliminary data suggest another alternative of both phase and amplitude disturbances, described later, that might explain how different light treatments may be working through different mechanisms to exert their therapeutic effects.

As Czeisler observed, bright light, depending on its timing, has the capacity to alter not only the phase but also the amplitude of circadian rhythms (Czeisler et al. 1987). Our preliminary data suggest the possibility that evening bright light may serve to delay circadian rhythms (that may be pathologically phase-advanced in PMS patients), and that morning bright light may serve to increase the amplitude of circadian rhythms (which may be pathologically blunted in PMS patients). We are currently investigating whether similar responses of circadian phase and amplitude to light treatments characterize a larger number of PMS patients.

A remaining question is how the dim red light might be working. One possibility is that because of its dimness (<10 lux), it may serve as a dark pulse. Increasing evidence suggests the importance of dark pulses in entraining human circadian rhythms (Czeisler et al. 1987; Wehr 1991). In fact, our preliminary results of the effects of different light treatments on cortisol secretion suggested that dim red evening light treatment serves to advance the acrophase of cortisol secretion in PMS patients compared with controls (Parry et al. 1991). Thus, dim red evening light, similar to morning bright white light, may exert its effects by advancing circadian rhythms in some PMS patients.

In summary, we found that morning bright light, evening bright light, and evening dim light treatments significantly reduced premenstrual symptoms. Light treatment had no significant effects on mood ratings in normal control subjects. Different psychological and biological mechanisms are proposed for the therapeutic effects of light treatment. These findings, if replicated, suggest the potential use of light therapy as an alternative to the pharmacologic management of patients with debilitating premenstrual depression.

References

American Psychiatric Association: Diagnostic and Statistical Manual of Mental Disorders, 3rd Edition, Revised. Washington, DC, American Psychiatric Association, 1987

Aschoff J: Disorders of the circadian system as discussed in psychiatric research, in Circadian Rhythms in Psychiatry. Edited by Wehr TA, Goodwin FK. Pacific Grove, CA, Boxwood Press, 1983, pp 33–39

Beck AT, Ward CH, Mendelson M, et al: Inventory for measuring depression. Arch Gen Psychiatry 4:561–571, 1961

Czeisler CA, Kronauer RE, Mooney JJ, et al: Biologic rhythm disorders, depression and phototherapy: a new hypothesis. Psychiatr Clin North Am 10:687–709, 1987

Eastman CI: What the placebo literature can tell us about phototherapy for SAD. Psychopharmacol Bull 26:495–504, 1990

Hamilton M: Development of a rating scale for primary depressive illness. Br J Soc Clin Psychol 6:278–296, 1967

Horne JA, Ostberg O: A self-assessment questionnaire to determine morningness-eveningness in human circadian rhythms. Int J Chronobiol 4: 97–110, 1976

Kripke DF, Klauber MR, Risch SC, et al: Controlled trial of bright light for nonseasonal major depressive disorders. Biol Psychiatry 31:119–134, 1992

Lewy AJ, Sack RL, Miller S, et al: Antidepressant and circadian phase-shifting effects of light. Science 235:352–354, 1987

Lewy AJ, Sack RL, Latham JM: Melatonin and the acute suppressant effect of light may help regulate circadian rhythms in humans, in Advances in Pineal Research, Volume 5. Edited by Arendt J, Pivet P. London, John Libey, 1991, pp 285–293

Parry BL, Wehr TA: Therapeutic effect of sleep deprivation in patients with premenstrual syndrome. Am J Psychiatry 144:808–810, 1987

Parry BL, Rosenthal NE, Tamarkin L, et al: Treatment of a patient with seasonal premenstrual syndrome. Am J Psychiatry 144:762–766, 1987

Parry BL, Berga SL, Mostofi N, et al: Morning versus evening bright light treatment of late luteal phase dysphoric disorder. Am J Psychiatry 146: 1215–1217, 1989a

Parry BL, Mendelson WB, Duncan W, et al: Longitudinal sleep EEG, temperature and activity measurements across the menstrual cycle in patients with premenstrual depression and in age-matched controls. Psychiatry Res 30:285–303, 1989b

Parry BL, Berga SL, Kripke DF, et al: Altered waveform of plasma nocturnal melatonin secretion in premenstrual depression. Arch Gen Psychiatry 47:1139–1146, 1990

Parry BL, Berga SL, Hauger R, et al: Melatonin and cortisol circadian rhythms in premenstrual depression (abstract). Abstracts of the 5th World Congress of Biological Psychiatry, Florence, Italy, World Congress of Biological Psychiatry 1991, p 547

Parry BL, Mahan AM, Mostofi N, et al: Light therapy of late luteal phase dysphoric disorder: an extended study. Am J Psychiatry 150: 1417–1419, 1993

Pittendrigh CS: Circadian systems: Entrainment, in Biological Rhythms: Handbook of Behavioral Neurobiology, IV. Edited by Aschoff J. New York, Plenum, 1981, pp 95–124

Rosenthal NE, Heffernan MM: Bulimia, carbohydrate craving and depression: a central connection? in Nutrition and the Brain, Vol. 7. Edited by Wurtman RJ, Wurtman JJ. New York, Raven, 1986, pp 139–166

Rosenthal NE, Sack DA, Carpenter CJ, et al: Antidepressant effects of light in seasonal affective disorder. Am J Psychiatry 142:163–170, 1985

Roy-Byrne PP, Rubinow DR, Hoban MC, et al: Premenstrual changes: a comparison of five populations. Psychiatry Res 17:77–85, 1986

Siever LJ, David KL: Overview: Toward a dysregulation hypothesis of depression. Am J Psychiatry 142:1017–1031, 1985

Spitzer RL, Williams JBW, Gibbon M, et al: Structured Clinical Interview for DSM-III-R. Patient Edition (SCID-P, Version 1.0). Washington, DC, American Psychiatric Press, 1990

Terman M, Terman JS, Quitkin FM, et al: Light therapy for seasonal affective disorder. A review of efficacy. Neuropsychopharmacology 2:1–22, 1989

Wehr TA: The durations of human melatonin secretion and sleep respond to changes in daylength (photoperiod). J Clin Endocrin Metab 73:1276–1280, 1991

EIGHT

Seasonality of Bulimia Nervosa and Treatment With Light Therapy

Raymond W. Lam, M.D.
Elliot M. Goldner, M.D.

Whoever wishes to investigate Medicine properly, should proceed thus: in the first place, to consider the seasons of the year, and what effects each of them produces for they are not all alike . . .
— *Hippocrates: On Airs, Waters and Places, circa 400 B.C.*

All diseases occur at all seasons, but certain of them are more apt to occur and be exacerbated at certain seasons.
— *Hippocrates: Aphorisms, Section III, circa 400 B.C.*

Hippocrates made important observations about the influence of the seasons on medical illnesses, that went unrecognized by subsequent generations of physicians. When seasonal affective disorder (SAD) was first systematically reported by Rosenthal and colleagues in 1984, there was initial skepticism about a subtype of depression with recurrent seasonal episodes. Some wondered how a phenomenon

Dr. Lam's research is supported by the British Columbia Health Research Foundation and the Medical Research Council of Canada. We thank Ms. Arvinder Grewal, Dr. Maria Corral, and Dr. Joseph Mador for their help in data collection and patient assessment.

193

thought to affect such a significant percentage of the mood disorders population could have been missed. Only after numerous published reports from researchers around the world did acceptance of SAD ensue. It became apparent that the old medical truism was applicable: that which is not looked for is rarely found.

The search for seasonality has extended to other psychiatric conditions such as alcohol and substance abuse, panic disorder, obsessive-compulsive disorder, and schizophrenia. This chapter focuses on seasonality and eating disorders, and our studies of seasonality in bulimia nervosa and treatment with light therapy.

Seasonality in Bulimia Nervosa

Bulimia nervosa and anorexia nervosa are disorders characterized by specific disturbances in eating behavior, mood, and cognition. Patients with bulimia nervosa have frequent binge-eating episodes, that is, rapid eating of large amounts of food over a short period of time while feeling "out of control." These binges are generally accompanied by intense feelings of depression, guilt, and self-deprecation and are often followed by compensatory behaviors such as self-induced vomiting, laxative/diuretic abuse, and overexercise (Fairburn 1993). Patients with anorexia nervosa are preoccupied with concerns about their body shape and weight and systematically starve themselves by restricting food intake. Individuals with anorexia nervosa may also binge and purge, and the DSM-IV classification (American Psychiatric Association 1994) differentiates two subtypes of anorexia nervosa based on the presence or absence of binge/purge symptoms. Table 8–1 summarizes the DSM-IV diagnostic criteria for anorexia nervosa and bulimia nervosa.

Eating disorders most commonly affect women, with an estimated prevalence for bulimia nervosa of 1%–3% in young women (Fairburn and Beglin 1990; Garfinkel et al. 1995), whereas the prevalence for anorexia nervosa is approximately 0.1% (Hsu 1989; Yates 1989). Depressive symptoms are frequently seen in both disorders, and comorbid major depression may be as high as 79% in bulimia nervosa (Levy et al. 1989). The causes of these eating disorders are unknown but likely involve multifactorial etiologies (Garfinkel and Garner 1982; Hsu 1989).

TABLE **8-1**

DSM-IV criteria for anorexia nervosa and bulimia nervosa

Anorexia nervosa

A. Refusal to maintain body weight at or above a minimally normal weight for age and height (e.g., weight loss leading to maintenance of body weight less than 85% of that expected; or failure to make expected weight gain during period of growth, leading to body weight less than 85% of that expected).

B. Intense fear of gaining weight or becoming fat, even though underweight.

C. Disturbance in the way in which one's body weight or shape is experienced; undue influence of body weight or shape on self-evaluation, or denial of the seriousness of the current low body weight.

D. In premenopausal females, amenorrhea (i.e., the absence of at least three consecutive menstrual cycles). (A woman is considered to have amenorrhea if her periods occur only following hormone, e.g., estrogen, administration.)

Specify type of symptoms

A. Restricting type: During the currect episode of anorexia nervosa, the person has not regularly engaged in binge-eating or purging behavior (i.e., self-induced vomiting or the misuse of laxatives, diuretics, or enemas).

B. Binge eating/purging type: During the current episode of anorexia nervosa, the person has regularly engaged in binge-eating or purging behavior (i.e., self-induced vomiting or the misuse of laxatives, diuretics, or enemas).

Bulimia nervosa

A. Recurrent episodes of binge eating. An episode of binge eating is characterized by both of the following:

   1. Eating, in a discrete period of times (e.g., within any 2-hour period), an amount of food that is definitely larger than most people would eat during a similar period of time and under similar circumstances.

   2. A sense of lack of control over eating during the episode (e.g., a feeling that one cannot stop eating or control what or how much one is eating).

B. Recurrent inappropriate compensatory behavior to prevent weight gain, such as self-induced vomiting; misuse of laxatives, diuretics, enemas, or other medications; fasting; or excessive exercise.

C. The binge eating and inappropriate compensatory behaviors both occur, on average, at least twice a week for 3 months.

D. Self-evaluation is unduly influenced by body shape and weight.

E. The disturbance does not occur exclusively during episodes of anorexia nervosa.

(continued)

TABLE **8-1**

DSM-IV criteria for anorexia nervosa and bulimia nervosa
Continued

Specify type of symptoms

A. Purging type: During the current episode of bulimia nervosa, the person has regularly engaged in self-induced vomiting or the misuse of laxatives, diuretics, or enemas.

B. Nonpurging type: During the current episode of bulimia nervosa, the person has used other inappropriate compensatory behaviors, such as fasting or excessive exercise, but has not regularly engaged in self-induced vomiting or the misuse of laxatives, diuretics, or enemas.

Our group began investigating seasonality in eating disorders in 1987 when a colleague, Leslie Solyom, M.D., remarked that there seemed to be a high rate of seasonal (winter) depression in his patients with bulimia. The connection between eating disorders and seasonal affective disorder (SAD) had been noted in previous reports (Rosenthal and Heffernan 1986), but no systematic studies had been done. We began by administering the Seasonal Pattern Assessment Questionnaire (SPAQ) (Rosenthal et al. 1987a) to female patients with bulimia nervosa, patients with SAD, and matched normal subjects. The SPAQ is a self-rated questionnaire that was initially designed as a screening tool for SAD and is widely used in studies of seasonality and seasonal depression. One section of the SPAQ inquires about the degree of seasonal change in six items: mood, sleep, social activity, energy, appetite, and weight. Possible responses are none, mild, moderate, marked, and disabling, scored from 0 to 6 for each item. The sum of the scores for these six items is termed the Global Seasonality score, which ranges from 0, indicating no seasonality, to 24, indicating extreme seasonality. Another section of the SPAQ asks respondents to indicate the months of the year, if any, when they feel best and feel worst, sleep most and sleep least, and so on. Finally, there is a question that asks whether these seasonal changes are a problem, with possible responses of none, mild, moderate, severe, and disabling. Epidemiologic studies using the SPAQ have defined operational criteria to classify subjects as having a diagnosis of SAD (Booker et al. 1992; Kasper et al. 1989; Magnusson and Stefansson 1993; Rosen et al. 1990). These criteria are defined as a Global Seasonality score of 10 or greater *and* a response on the seasonal problem question of moderate or greater. Using these criteria, the prevalence of SAD has been estimated at 5%–10% in random population samples. A brief report by Fornari et al. (1989), based on the SPAQ, suggested that seasonality scores were higher in patients with bulimia nervosa compared with patients with SAD and normal comparison subjects. (Table 8–2 shows results of studies in this area.)

In our initial study, we compared SPAQ data from 38 patients with bulimia nervosa, 38 patients with SAD, and 25 normal comparison subjects (Lam et al. 1991). All patients were women diagnosed using DSM-III-R criteria (American Psychiatric Association 1987). The patients with SAD did not have any eating disorder diagnoses, and the normal subjects had no previous history or family history of mood disorder or eating disorders. There was no significant difference in age between the groups. We found that, as expected, the patients with SAD had the highest Global Seasonality scores (mean score 18.7). However, the patients with bulimia also had significantly higher Global Seasonality scores than normal subjects (mean score 11.7 vs. 5.1, respectively, $P < .01$). As expected, all of the patients with SAD and none of the normal subjects met the operational SPAQ criteria for a diagnosis of SAD. However, 42% of the bulimic patients also met SPAQ criteria for winter SAD ($\chi^2 = 14.1$, df = 1, $P < .001$). This percentage is much higher than the prevalence of SAD reported in the general population (5%–10%), using the same instrument. The patients with bulimia meeting SAD criteria also reported significantly greater number of sleep hours in the winter and greater seasonal weight gain compared with the group with bulimia but not SAD, suggesting that they had winter symptoms that were similar to those found in patients with SAD.

These results were replicated by Blouin et al. (1992) using the same questionnaire for 31 women with bulimia and 31 matched comparison subjects. They found that 26% of the group with bulimia met SPAQ criteria for SAD, compared with 3% of the comparison group. In a separate study of 197 patients with bulimia, consecutively referred to their clinic, they also noted a significant correlation between the frequency of binge eating (but not purging) at initial assessment, and the scotoperiod (the daily number of hours of darkness) (Blouin et al. 1992). That is, patients binged more when they were assessed during the shorter days of winter than when assessed in summer. Hardin et al. (1991) also reported that patients with eating disorders had high seasonality scores on the SPAQ. In a comparison of six diagnostic groups (winter SAD, summer SAD, subsyndromal SAD, eating disorders, bipolar depression, and nonseasonal depression), they found that the eating disorders group, a mixed group of patients with bulimia nervosa and anorexia nervosa, had Global Seasonality scores second only to the winter SAD group.

The seasonality identified in eating disorders, however, may be specific to bulimia nervosa. In a second study, we administered the SPAQ, modified to include questions relating to seasonality of eating disorder symptoms, to a consecutive series of 91 women diagnosed with DSM-III-R eating disorders, and to a nonclinical comparison group (Lam et al. 1996a). We again found that the patients with bulimia nervosa ($n = 60$) had the highest Global Seasonality scores. Women with anorexia nervosa, independent of whether they had bulimic symptoms, had low seasonality scores not significantly different from those of the nonclinical comparison group.

In contrast to these results, Brewerton et al. (1994) found that patients with the bulimic subtype of anorexia nervosa had higher seasonality scores than those with nonbulimic anorexia nervosa and bulimia nervosa. Their study encompassed 159 patients with eating disorders, seen in three locations, including the U.S. National Institute of Mental Health, and therefore may not be generalizable to more varied clinic populations.

Other evidence also suggests that the symptoms of patients with anorexia nervosa are less likely to demonstrate seasonality. Fornari et al. (1989) found that seasonal symptom scores in restrictive anorexic patients were not significantly different from normal controls. A "bulimic group" (a mixed group of patients with bulimic anorexia nervosa and bulimia nervosa) had higher seasonality scores than both the normal comparison group and the group with anorexia nervosa. Subsequently, they compared SPAQ data from patients with anorexia nervosa ($n = 60$), bulimia nervosa ($n = 31$), and bulimic anorexia nervosa ($n = 34$) (Fornari et al. 1994). The patients with

TABLE 8–2

Studies of seasonality in eating disorders

Study	Sample and number	Instrument	Findings
Fornari et al. 1989	35 BN (18 AN-B) 27 AN-R 149 SAD 46 NC	SPAQ	Seasonality of symptoms: SAD > BN > AN-R, NC BN group had some AN-B patients
Lam et al. 1991	38 BN 38 SAD 25 NC	SPAQ	GSS: SAD > BN > NC SAD diagnosis: 46% of BN vs. 0% of NC
Hardin et al. 1991	41 ED (10 AN-R, 31 BN) 20 NC 55 NCC 5 other clinical groups	SPAQ	GSS: Winter SAD > (ED, Summer SAD, subsyndromal SAD) > (MD, NC, NCC)
Blouin et al. 1992	28 BN (3 AN-B) 31 NCC	SPAQ (modified)	SAD diagnosis: 26% of BN vs. 3% of NC
Blouin et al. 1992	197 BN (16 AN-B)	SCL-90R binge-purge ratings	Binge frequency (but not purge frequency or depression score) at time of assessment correlated with scotoperiod
Brewerton et al. 1994	109 BN 30 AN-R 20 AN-B 50 NC	SPAQ	GSS: AN-B > BN, AN-R > NC Seasonal syndromes: BN > AN-R SAD Diagnosis: 15% of total eating disorders group

(continued)

TABLE 8–2

Studies of seasonality in eating disorders
Continued

Study	Sample and number	Instrument	Findings
Levitan et al. 1994	103 BN	SPAQ (modified)	69% seasonal positive
	35 BN	Interview	10% of entire sample diagnosed as SAD by interview 18% had winter worsening of bulimia without SAD
Fornari et al. 1994	60 AN-R 31 BN 34 AN-B 29 ED-NOS	SPAQ	GSS: BN, AN-B, ED-NOS > AN-R SAD diagnosis: BN = 26%, AN-B = 18%, ED-NOS = 17%, AN-R = 10%
Lam et al. 1996a	60 BN 16 AN-B 15 AN-R 50 NCC	SPAQ (modified)	GSS: BN > all other groups AN-B, AN-R, NCC all similar SAD diagnosis: BN = 35% (28% winter, 7% summer), NCC = 8%, AN-B = 6%, AN-R = 7%
Levitan et al, 1996	51 seasonal BN 45 nonseasonal BN (defined as top 30% and bottom 30% based on GSS, some AN-B included)	SPAQ (modified) EDI binge-purge ratings	Seasonal BN had earlier age of onset of bingeing but not purging, greater current monthly binge frequency but not purge frequency, and more pathologic scores on EDI Interoceptive Awareness scale

Note. BN, bulimia nervosa; AN-R, Anorexia Nervosa, Restrictive subtype; AN-B, anorexia nervosa, bulimic subtype; SAD, seasonal affective disorder; NC, normal controls; NCC, nonclinical comparison subjects; ED, eating disorders, ED-NOS, eating disorders, not otherwise specified; SPAQ, Seasonal Pattern Assessment Questionnaire; GSS, Global Seasonality score; SCL, symptom check list; EDI, Eating Disorders Inventory.

anorexia had the lowest Global Seasonality scores, the patients with bulimia had the highest, and the patients with bulimic anorexia had intermediate scores (6.6, 9.9, and 9.4, respectively). Both groups with bulimia had significantly higher scores than the group with anorexia. The patients with anorexia also showed significantly less monthly and seasonal variability in individual symptoms than did the two groups with bulimia. A study by Levitan et al. (1996) separated 208 female patients with bulimia into groups with "seasonal" ($n = 51$) and "nonseasonal" ($n = 45$) symptoms by taking the highest and lowest 30th percentiles, respectively, based on their Global Seasonality scores from the SPAQ. Although they studied a mixed group of patients with bulimia nervosa and bulimic anorexia nervosa, they found significantly fewer patients with anorexia nervosa in the seasonal group (18%) than the nonseasonal group (33%) (Levitan et al. 1996). These data lend support to the finding that anorexia nervosa is associated with less seasonality than bulimia nervosa.

Is the seasonality found in bulimia nervosa merely due to comorbid SAD? After all, eating disturbances are common in SAD and include carbohydrate craving, increased appetite, and weight gain (Lam et al. 1989; Rosenthal et al. 1984). There is also evidence that patients with SAD have disturbances in appetite and weight regulation (Berman et al. 1993; Gruber et al. 1996; Krauchi and Wirz-Justice 1988, 1991; Krauchi et al. 1990; Rosenthal et al. 1987b, 1989). A related question is whether the seasonality of mood and eating symptoms in bulimia are similar (Kaplan and Levitan 1990). In our second study, 35% of the group with bulimia ($n = 60$) met SPAQ criteria for seasonal depression, whereas 28% endorsed marked or extreme seasonal changes in binge eating and purging behaviors. Another method of comparing the seasonal patterns of mood and binge-purging behavior is by examining the SPAQ question based on which months of the year, if any, patients identify feeling best and feeling worst, or when they binge-purge the most and the least. The relative frequency of mood change, for example, can then be calculated for each month by subtracting the percentage of respondents who feel worst in that month from the percentage feeling best (Terman 1988). A relative frequency of 0 indicates equal numbers who endorse feeling best and feeling worst for that month.

The relative frequency, if positive, gives the excess proportion of the sample that feels best during that month, whereas a negative relative frequency indicates that there is an excess of the sample that feels worst. The relative frequency distribution is considered a qualitative population measure of seasonality because it describes what percentage of the total sample feel the best or worst, but it does not rate the severity of these feelings.

Figures 8–1 and 8–2 depict the relative frequency distribution for mood (based on "feel best" and "feel worst" items) and binge-purge behavior (based on "binge-purge least" and "binge-purge most" items) for the patients with bulimia nervosa ($n = 60$). The data are double plotted to better illustrate the seasonal patterns. For mood (Figure 8–1), there is a large bipolar amplitude in the relative frequency distribution, with an excess of about 40% of the patients feeling best in the summer, the same percentage feeling worst in the

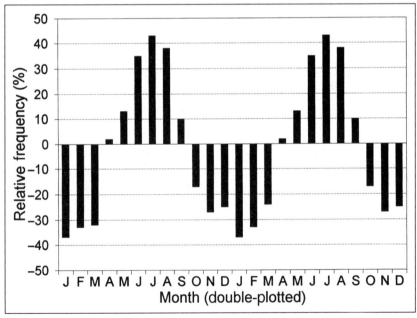

FIGURE 8–1. Relative frequency of mood change versus month. Relative frequency is the percentage of subjects who endorse feeling worse subtracted from the percentage who endorse feeling best in any given month. Data are double plotted to show pattern.

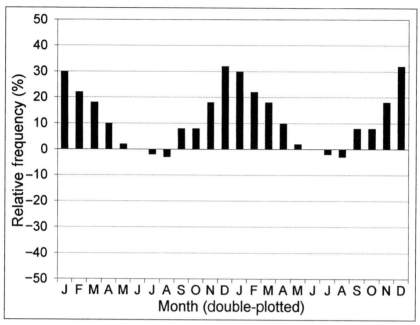

FIGURE 8-2. Relative frequency of binge eating/purging versus month. Relative frequency is the percentage of subjects who endorse binge/purging the least, subtracted from the percentage who endorse binge/purging the most in any given month. Data are double plotted to show pattern.

winter, and the switch points occurring in April and October. For binge-purge episodes (Figure 8–2), there is only a unipolar distribution, with an excess of about 30% of the patients endorsing binge-purging the most in the winter. Unlike mood, there is no equivalent positive peak indicating improvement of binge-purging during the summer months. Inspection of the raw data, however, show that this is due to the fact that whereas there is a proportion of patients with bulimia who identify binge-purging the least in summer (about 20% of the sample), there is an equal proportion who have summer worsening of their bulimia. In contrast, there are very few patients (about 2%) who endorsed binge-purging the least in the winter. This suggests that there are differences in the seasonal patterns of mood and eating for at least a proportion of these patients with bulimia.

Consistent with the relative frequency distribution results, we identified both summer and winter SAD patterns in the patients with bulimia (Lam et al. 1996a). However, of the patients who were identified as having SAD on the SPAQ, only 71% of those with winter SAD (12 of 17) and 50% of those with summer SAD (2 of 4) also had worsening of their binge eating and purging in the same season. Thus, some bulimic patients have a dissociation of seasonal worsening of mood and eating symptoms. Similarly, Blouin et al. (1992) found that only half of the patients with bulimia who were identified as having SAD, based on SPAQ criteria, actually had a lifetime diagnosis of major depression as determined by structured interview. Levitan et al. (1994) identified patients with bulimia as "seasonally positive" using a combination of SPAQ criteria and seasonal changes in eating symptoms; 71 of 103 patients (69%) expressed significant seasonality. They subsequently interviewed about half of these patients and found a heterogenous mix of seasonality diagnoses. Only 10% of the interviewed sample had comorbid winter SAD. Another 18% did not meet criteria for SAD but had greater than 100% increase in binges and purges between summer and winter, although one-third of these patients attributed their seasonal pattern to psychosocial factors (e.g., the school year). Thus, not all patients with bulimia who had seasonal worsening of their binge-purge symptoms had a seasonal depression.

In summary, accumulated evidence from several research groups has shown that many patients with bulimia nervosa have marked seasonal patterns in mood and eating symptoms that are similar to those found in patients with SAD. There are suggestions that the seasonality is more related to binge eating symptoms and less to purging or starvation. This may lead to less prominent seasonality in anorexia nervosa if restrictive symptoms are more prominent. Finally, there may be separate mechanisms for the mood symptoms and the eating symptoms in the proportion of patients (25%–50%) who express seasonality and in whom there is dissociation between seasonal depression and seasonal binge-purging.

Importance of Seasonality in Bulimia Nervosa

From a clinical perspective, it may be very important to recognize seasonality in patients with bulimia nervosa. Recognizing that up to one-third of patients with bulimia have seasonal worsening of symptoms has implications for evaluating outcomes of both treatment studies and individual patient care. Most treatment studies involve treatments (pharmacologic or psychotherapeutic) conducted over a period of several weeks to several months. Seasonal patients are more likely to present during the winter when they are most symptomatic. If, for example, a 16-week treatment program is started in December or January, patients may experience natural improvement of symptoms by April or May, at a time when the treatment is completed. Clinical improvement may be incorrectly ascribed to the treatment rather than to the natural seasonal improvement of these patients. Similarly, if a patient worsens again in October as a result of his or her usual seasonal pattern, it may be misinterpreted as a relapse caused by treatment discontinuation. Therefore outcome studies of bulimia nervosa need to consider confounding influences of season on clinical effects. For an individual patient, identifying a regular pattern of seasonal worsening may help target more intensive therapeutic interventions during the season (e.g., winter) when worsening is expected (Del Medico et al. 1991).

Studying seasonality may also provide clues as to the pathophysiology of bulimia nervosa. Several possible mechanisms may explain the winter worsening in bulimia nervosa. Cognitive factors may play a role because the winter months in the Northern Hemisphere are associated with many holidays (e.g. Halloween, Thanksgiving, Christmas, Valentine's Day) that have a prominent societal focus on food and interpersonal relationships. These stressful holidays may worsen the cognitive distortions in bulimic patients that are associated with binge-eating and purging behaviors. Levitan's study suggests that, at least for some patients, the winter worsening in bulimia may be attributed to these seasonal psychosocial stressors (Levitan et al. 1994). Also, binge eating and purging are secretive activities usually done indoors and in the evening. Because more time is usually spent indoors in winter, and the winter evenings are longer, there may be greater opportunity to engage in binge eating and purging. Many patients with bulimia use exercise, sometimes compulsively, as another means of controlling their weight. If there is less chance to exercise in the winter, they may be more likely instead to use purging as a weight-control measure. On the other hand, one might expect the body image disturbance seen in patients with bulimia to be worse in the summer because summer clothing tends to focus more attention on body shape and weight. Levitan et al. (1996) have also suggested that patients with seasonal bulimia are less aware of their bodily sensations than those with nonseasonal bulimia. Thus they may misinterpret the normal, mild physiologic changes that occur with winter in a catastrophic manner, leading them to increase binge eating and purging to correct their distorted cognitions.

We have suggested that those patients with summer worsening of bulimia may be more prone to a cognitive body image disturbance, whereas those with winter worsening may have a more neurophysiologic mechanism similar to that of winter SAD (Lam et al. 1996a). Serotonin mechanisms have become a likely candidate to mediate changes in both disorders because serotonin is involved in regulation of mood, appetite, and sleep (Wallin and Rissanen 1994). There is a significant seasonal rhythm in central serotonin metabolism in normal subjects, with highest levels in the summer and autumn, and lowest levels in the winter and spring (for review, see Lacoste and Wirz-Justice 1989). Serotonergic disturbances have been found in bulimia (Brewerton et al. 1992; Jimerson et al. 1990) and SAD (Garcia-Borreguero et al. 1995; Jacobsen et al. 1987, 1994; Joseph-Vanderpool et al. 1993; Tam et al., this volume). Thus, examining serotonergic measures in seasonal bulimic patients may increase homogeneity of the sample and lead to greater insights into the role of serotonin in bulimia.

A Controlled Study of Light Therapy for Bulimia Nervosa

One of the most intriguing clinical implications of seasonality in bulimia is whether light therapy may be useful, as it is in SAD and subsyndromal SAD. A preliminary report by us (Lam, 1989) showed that a patient with comorbid SAD and bulimia experienced improvement in both depression and bulimic symptoms after a course of light therapy. We now summarize our controlled study that confirmed this preliminary report.

Subjects and Methods

We studied 17 female patients who met DSM-III-R criteria for bulimia nervosa (Lam et al. 1994). Patients were seen at eating disorders clinics and were not selected on the basis of any seasonal patterns. After a baseline monitoring period of 2 weeks, patients underwent two weeks of either bright white light (10,000-lux cool-white fluorescent light box for 30 minutes in the early morning between 7:00 A.M. and 8:00 A.M.) or dim red light (500 lux for the same time). After 2 weeks, patients were immediately crossed over to the other condition. Deception was used to enhance the plausibility of the control condition, by telling patients that we were studying the wavelength (color) of the light, without mentioning the differences in intensity. The human ethics committee of the University of British Columbia approved the study, and patients were debriefed about the deception at study completion. Pretreatment expectation ratings did not demonstrate significantly different expectations between the red light and white light conditions. We measured outcome using the 29-item modified Hamilton Rating Scale for Depression (HAM-D) (Williams et al. 1988), Beck Depression Inventory (BDI) (Beck 1978), Clinical Global Impression (CGI) scale (Guy 1976), daily binge-purge diaries, self-rated visual analog scales (VAS), and the Eating Attitudes Test (EAT) (Garner et al. 1982).

Results

The average number of binges and purges per week during the baseline period was 7.4 (SD = 5.9) and 7.5 (SD = 6.8), respectively. Many patients were clinically depressed, and the average baseline 29-item HAM-D and BDI scores for the group were 27.1 (SD = 9.6) and 20.7 (SD = 9.6), respectively. After treatment, the bright white light was significantly superior to the dim red light for all outcome measures. As shown in Figures 8–3 and 8–4, the average improvement for bright white light versus dim red light in HAM-D scores was 53% versus 21%, in binges and purges per week it was 50% versus 13%, and in the EAT scores it was 24% versus 0%. The CGI showed clear superiority of the bright white light condition. There were no significant effects of order or pretreatment expectation ratings. However, those patients who were identified as being seasonally affected (6 patients had concurrent SAD, and 1 patient had greater than 100% worsening of binges/purges between winter and summer) did best on the continuous and global measures. For example, all of these seasonally affected patients showed marked global responses (7 of 7, 100%), but only 4 of 10 (40%) of the nonseasonally affected patients showed similar responses.

The light therapy was well tolerated by the patients. Side effects during the bright white light condition included only headaches (18%) and feeling "speedy" (12%). Headaches were also noted in 18% of patients during the dim red light condition, along with nausea (12%), eye fatigue (6%), and nightmares (6%).

This study clearly shows that light therapy produces an acute and rapid effect on both the mood and eating symptoms found in patients with bulimia nervosa. Despite the robust results, however, we consider these to be preliminary findings because of the small sample

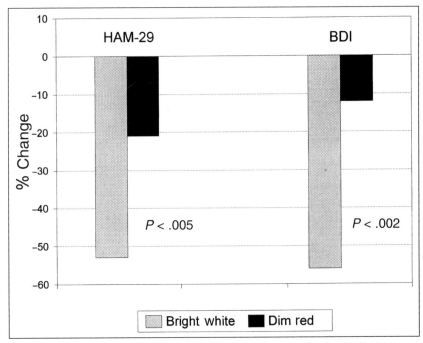

FIGURE 8–3. Percent change in modified Hamilton Depression Rating Scale scores (HAM-29) and Beck Depression Inventory scores (BDI) after light therapy ($n = 17$).

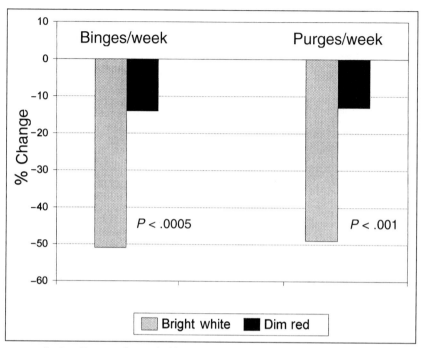

FIGURE 8–4. Percent change in bingeing and purging episodes per week after light therapy (*n* = 17).

size and the brief duration of treatment. Further controlled studies must be done to replicate these results and to ensure that the therapeutic effects of light are sustained over time.

Blouin and colleagues have recently published another controlled study of light therapy in bulimia nervosa (Blouin et al. 1996). They studied 18 female patients with DSM-III-R diagnoses of bulimia nervosa, using a randomized, double-blind, placebo-controlled parallel study design. Light therapy was administered using fluorescent light boxes. The active treatment was a large full-spectrum fluorescent light box rated at 2,500 lux. The placebo condition was a similar light box that emitted less than 500 lux. Patients used the light box for 2 hours/day for 7 days. There was a baseline week without light treatment, and a withdrawal week following light exposure. Outcome measures included daily binge/purge logs, the BDI, and the 29-item HAM-D.

Expectation testing both before and after light exposure found that patients were not able to guess which condition was "active," that is, the blinding of conditions was preserved. The results showed that, even with only 1 week of treatment, there were significant improvements in the depression ratings (both BDI and HAM-D) during the bright light treatment, but not during the dim light treatment. The depression ratings also worsened during the following week when light treatment was withdrawn. There were, however, no significant differences between the effects of bright and dim light on the mean weekly bingeing or vomiting episodes. The bright light therapy appeared effective on depressive symptoms, but not on the bulimic symptoms, of these patients.

The advantage of the parallel study design, compared to a crossover study, is that it avoids any expectation effect of patients experiencing both active and placebo treatments. However, the disadvantage of the parallel design is that it reduces the statistical power of a study, especially one already limited by small sample size, to detect significant differences between conditions. Thus, the low statistical power of this study may have resulted in a Type II error, namely, that significant clinical effects of bright light therapy on bulimic symptoms were not found. An intriguing finding in support of this hypothesis was that the daily patient ratings of binge eating consistently decreased on the last 2 days of the bright light treatment week; this finding was not found in any of the other study weeks. The investigators pointed out that this finding, together with the results of our study (Lam et al. 1994), suggests that bulimic symptoms may require higher intensity or longer duration of light treatment to show the therapeutic effects of light therapy than do mood symptoms.

Also of interest is that, in their group of patients with bulimia nervosa who were not especially selected for seasonality, 10 of 18 were found to be seasonally affected, based on the SPAQ, 13 of 18 met DSM-III-R criteria for major depression, and 3 of 18 met DSM-III-R criteria for seasonal pattern. These findings emphasize the high rate of seasonality and mood disorders associated with bulimia nervosa. However, Blouin et al. found no differences between the groups with and without SAD in their responses to the bright light therapy. Again, the different results found in our study may simply reflect selection differences resulting from the small sample sizes.

Open Studies of Light Therapy in Bulimia Nervosa

We have continued to study light therapy in bulimia in a case series of patients with bulimia who also had comorbid SAD. Patients were diagnosed with DSM-III-R criteria and were seen in winter. Entry criteria for the study included a score on the 21-item HAM-D of 15 or greater, *or* a score on the 29-item modified HAM-D of 28 or greater. All patients entered a standard protocol consisting of a 1-week baseline monitoring period when they arose at the scheduled time daily. If their depression scores did not drop by more than 20% at the end of the week, they took home a 10,000-lux cool-white fluorescent light box to use for 30 minutes between 7:00 A.M. and 8:00 A.M. daily. Patients were assessed by psychiatrists at 2-week intervals for 1 month, and BDI and HAM-D ratings were obtained. In addition, patients used a daily diary to keep track of binges and purges.

Fifteen patients have undergone this open-design, 4-week study. Demographic information on the patients is included in Table 8–3. The clinical features seen in the patients with bulimia and SAD are similar to those seen in patients with SAD but without bulimia (e.g., Lam et al. 1989). The patients had an average of 6.7 (SD = 2.6) winter depressive episodes, and an average duration of bulimia of 7.8 (SD = 3.6) years.

Results of the 4-week open study of bright light therapy are shown in Table 8–4. The 29-item modified HAM-D scores improved significantly after 2 weeks and continued to stay low at the 4-week mark, with mean scores falling from 34.7 pretreatment to 14.5 post-treatment ($t = 7.2$, df = 14, $P < .001$). There were significant reductions at 4 weeks in the number of weekly binges (from 9.7 binges/week to 5.1 binges/week, $t = 4.6$, df = 14, $P < .001$), and weekly purges (from 9.1 purges/week to 5.2 purges/week; $t = 3.6$, df = 14, $P < .005$). Again, these results were clinically significant as well as statistically significant, with average reductions of 56%, 50%, and

TABLE 8–3

Characteristics of winter depressive episodes for patients with bulimia and seasonal affective disorder ($n = 15$)

Symptom	Number	Percentage
Diagnosis		
Unipolar	13	87
Bipolar, type II	2	13
Onset of depression		
August/September	3	20
October/November	11	73
January	1	7
Offset of depression		
March	2	12
April	6	40
May	6	40
June	1	7
Sleep		
Hypersomnia	13	87
Insomnia	2	13
Appetite		
Increased	9	60
Decreased	5	33
Carbohydrate craving	12	80
Weight change		
Increased	11	73
Decreased	3	20
Low energy	14	93
Suicidal thoughts	13	87
Diurnal variation		
Morning worse	5	33
Evening worse	3	20
Past psychiatric treatment		
Outpatient contact	8	53
Hospitalization	4	29
Family history of mood disorder	9	60

TABLE 8-4

Outcome measures in seasonal affective disorder–bulimia patients before and after 4-week treatment with light therapy

Patient	Age	29-item HAM-D			Binges per week			Purges per week		
		Pre	Post	% change	Pre	Post	% change	Pre	Post	% change
1	29	44	3	93	13	2	85	13	2	85
2	23	43	3	93	9	0	100	9	0	100
3	18	33	6	82	3	0	100	3	0	100
4	29	29	7	76	14	4	71	14	4	71
5	26	35	12	66	6	2	67	5	4	20
6	33	34	12	65	14	7	50	14	5	64
7	31	43	16	63	7	2	71	7	4	43
8	30	30	12	60	7	1	86	7	1	86
9	31	37	16	57	6	3	50	6	3	50
10	24	36	19	47	13	7	46	11	9	18
11	21	35	22	37	10	11	−10	10	11	−10
12	27	31	20	35	9	8	11	7	7	0
13	34	32	21	34	15	10	33	14	10	29
14	27	34	28	18	9	10	−11	8	10	−25
15	37	24	21	13	10	10	0	8	8	00
Mean	28	34.7	14.5	56	9.7	5.1	50	9.1	5.2	42

Note. HAM-D, Hamilton Depression Rating Scale.

42% in the depression scores, binges per week, and purges per week, respectively. As shown in Table 8–4, 9 of 15 patients (60%) showed greater than 50% reduction in both depressive and eating measures. However, only 2 of 15 patients (13%) abstained from binges and purges following the 4 weeks of light therapy, whereas 7 of 15 (47%) became depression free (termination HAM-D score of 12 or less).

These data must be interpreted with caution because of the open nature of the light therapy method. Nonspecific or placebo effects of the treatment cannot be excluded. However, the case series does show that beneficial effects of light are sustained over a longer, 4-week period, as suggested by our 2-week controlled study. The mood and bulimic symptoms improved, but we still cannot tease out whether eating behaviors improve as a result of mood improvement, or whether there is a specific effect of light on the bulimic behaviors. One way to address this issue is to treat patients with seasonal bulimia (those who have greater than 100% increase in bulimic symptoms in the winter) who do not have comorbid SAD. Levitan's work (Levitan et al. 1994) suggests that this group is a sizeable sample, and thus it is plausible to seek out these patients.

Mechanism of Action of Light Therapy

How does light work to treat bulimia? There are several possible explanations. Circadian rhythm abnormalities have been suggested in SAD, and timed bright light exposure does have predictable effects in shifting circadian rhythms. It is also possible that an underlying circadian rhythm disturbance may account for both the eating and depressive symptoms in bulimia nervosa, and for the pronounced seasonality. There are as yet few studies of circadian rhythm abnormalities in bulimia. Some studies have suggested disturbances of circadian rhythms, whereas others have not found such abnormalities (Kennedy 1994; Mortola et al. 1993; Schreiber et al. 1991; Weltzin et al. 1991). Of interest is that while light is the strongest *zeitgeber*, or synchronizer, of circadian rhythms, other synchronizers include food timing and exercise. Studies have shown that increased feeding frequency or exercise can also shift rhythms (Mistlberger 1991; Reilly 1990; Van Cauter et al. 1993; Van Reeth et al. 1994). Thus, it is possible that the behavioral symptoms of bulimia nervosa (increased feeding frequency via binge eating and purging, excessive exercising for weight control) may lead to perturbation of circadian rhythms, which in turn can result in the exaggerated seasonal patterns. Light therapy may therefore correct the abnormal circadian rhythms. Further study of circadian rhythms in bulimia nervosa appear warranted.

Another major hypothesis for the mechanisms of SAD and bulimia involves serotonergic disturbances. As reviewed by Tam et al. (this volume), there is increasing evidence of serotonergic dysregulation in SAD that is corrected by light therapy. We have recently shown that light-remitted SAD patients show relapse of their depression when they undergo rapid tryptophan depletion (Lam et al. 1996b). This suggests that bright light may have direct serotonin-enhancing effects that account for or contribute to its therapeutic effect in bulimia nervosa.

Conclusions

There is converging evidence that seasonality is an important clinical dimension in bulimia nervosa. Hippocrates himself may have first recognized that eating disorders can be associated with significant seasonality, as he wrote in his *Aphorisms: "Lean persons who are easily made to vomit should be purged upwards, avoiding the winter season."* Modern studies have shown that winter worsening of bulimic and mood symptoms may be found in up to half of patients with bulimia nervosa. The use of bright light therapy has shown promising effect in preliminary studies in bulimia nervosa, although the clinical effect may be greatest in those with preexisting or concurrent seasonal patterns. Obviously, longer term controlled studies need to be done to confirm the clinical utility of light therapy. In the meantime, light therapy should be considered for patients with seasonal bulimia as an adjunctive treatment for their eating disorder.

References

American Psychiatric Association: Diagnostic and Statistical Manual of Mental Disorders, 3rd Edition, Revised. Washington, DC, American Psychiatric Association, 1987

American Psychiatric Association: Diagnostic and Statistical Manual of Mental Disorders, 4th Edition. Washington, DC, American Psychiatric Association, 1994

Beck AT: Depression Inventory. Philadelphia, PA, Philadelphia Center for Cognitive Therapy, 1978

Berman K, Lam RW, Goldner EM: Eating attitudes in seasonal affective disorder and bulimia nervosa. J Affect Disord 29:219–225, 1993

Blouin A, Blouin J, Aubin P, et al: Seasonal patterns of bulimia nervosa. Am J Psychiatry 149:73–81, 1992

Blouin AG, Blouin JH, Iversen H, et al: Light therapy in bulimia nervosa: a double-blind, placebo-controlled study. Psychiatry Res 60:1–9, 1996

Booker JM, Hellekson CJ: Prevalence of seasonal affective disorder in Alaska. Am J Psychiatry 149:1176–1182, 1992

Brewerton TD, Mueller EA, Lesem MD, et al: Neuroendocrine responses to m-chlorophenylpiperazine and L-tryptophan in bulimia. Arch Gen Psychiatry 49:852–861, 1992

Brewerton TD, Krahn DD, Hardin TA, et al: Findings from the Seasonal Pattern Assessment Questionnaire in patients with eating disorders and control subjects: effects of diagnosis and location. Psychiatry Res 52:71–84, 1994

Del Medico VJ, Qamar AB, Dilsaver SC: Seasonal worsening of bulimia nervosa (letter). Am J Psychiatry 148:1753, 1991

Fairburn CG: Binge Eating: Nature, Assessment, and Treatment. New York, Guilford, 1993

Fairburn CG, Beglin SJ: Studies of the epidemiology of bulimia nervosa. Am J Psychiatry 147:401–408, 1990

Fornari VM, Sandberg DE, Lachenmeyer J, et al: Seasonal variation in bulimia nervosa. Ann N Y Acad Sci 575:509–511, 1989

Fornari VM, Braun DL, Sunday SR, et al: Seasonal patterns in eating disorder subgroups. Compr Psychiatry 35:450–456, 1994

Garcia-Borreguero D, Jacobsen FM, Murphy DL, et al: Hormonal responses to the administration of m-chlorophenylpiperazine in patients with seasonal affective disorder and controls. Biol Psychiatry 37:740–749, 1995

Garfinkel PE, Garner DM: Anorexia Nervosa: A Multidimensional Perspective. New York, Brunner/Mazel, 1982

Garfinkel PE, Lin E, Goering P, et al: Bulimia nervosa in a Canadian community sample: prevalence and comparison of subgroups. Am J Psychiatry 152:1052–1058, 1995

Garner DM, Olmsted MP, Bohr Y, et al: The Eating Attitudes Test: psychometric features and clinical correlates. Psychol Med 12:871–878, 1982

Gruber NP, Dilsaver SC: Bulimia and anorexia nervosa in winter depression: lifetime rates in a clinical sample. J Psychiatr Neurosci 21:9–12, 1996

Guy W (ed): ECDEU Assessment Manual for Psychopharmacology, Revised (DHEW Publ No ADM-76-338). Rockvile, MD, 1976.

Hardin TA, Wehr TA, Brewerton T, et al: Evaluation of seasonality in six clinical populations and two normal populations. J Psychiatr Res 25: 75–87, 1991

Hsu LG: The gender gap in eating disorders: why are the eating disorders more common among women? Clin Psychol Rev 9:393–407, 1989

Jacobsen FM, Sack DA, Wehr TA, et al: Neuroendocrine response to 5-hydroxytryptophan in seasonal affective disorder. Arch Gen Psychiatry 44: 1086–1091, 1987

Jacobsen FM, Mueller EA, Rosenthal NE, et al: Behavioral responses to intravenous *meta*-chlorophenylpiperazine in patients with seasonal affective disorder and control subjects before and after phototherapy. Psychiatry Res 52:181–197, 1994

Jimerson DC, Lesem MD, Kaye WH, et al: Eating disorders and depression: is there a serotonin connection? Biol Psychiatry 28:443–454, 1990

Joseph-Vanderpool JR, Jacobsen FM, Murphy DL, et al: Seasonal variation in behavioral responses to m-CPP in patients with seasonal affective disorder and controls. Biol Psychiatry 33:496–504, 1993

Kaplan AS, Levitan RD: Seasonal variation in bulimic symptoms. Am J Psychiatry 147:1579–1580, 1990

Kasper S, Wehr TA, Bartko JJ, et al: Epidemiological findings of seasonal changes in mood and behavior. A telephone survey of Montgomery County, Maryland. Arch Gen Psychiatry 46:823–833, 1989

Kennedy SH: Melatonin disturbances in anorexia nervosa and bulimia nervosa. Int J Eat Disord 16:257–265, 1994

Krauchi K, Wirz-Justice A: The four seasons: food intake frequency in seasonal affective disorder during the course of a year. Psychiatry Res 25: 323–338, 1988

Krauchi K, Wirz-Justice A, Graw P: The relationship of affective state to dietary preference: winter depression and light therapy as a model. J Affect Disord 20:43–53, 1990

Lacoste V, Wirz-Justice A: Seasonal variation in normal subjects: an update of variables current in depression research, in Seasonal Affective Disorders and Phototherapy. Edited by Rosenthal NE, Blehar MC. New York, Guilford, 1989; pp 167–229

Lam RW: Light therapy for seasonal bulimia. Am J Psychiatry 146: 1640–1641, 1989

Lam RW, Buchanan A, Remick RA: Seasonal affective disorder—a Canadian sample. Ann Clin Psychiatry 1:241–245, 1989

Lam RW, Solyom L, Tompkins A: Seasonal mood symptoms in bulimia nervosa and seasonal affective disorder. Compr Psychiatry 32:552–558, 1991

Lam RW, Goldner EM, Solyom L, et al: A controlled study of light therapy for bulimia nervosa. Am J Psychiatry 151:744–750, 1994

Lam RW, Goldner EM, Grewal A: Seasonality of symptoms in anorexia and bulimia nervosa. Int J Eat Disord 19:35–44, 1996a

Lam RW, Zis AP, Grewal AK, et al: Effects of tryptophan depletion in patients with seasonal affective disorder in remission with light therapy. Arch Gen Psychiatry 53:41–44, 1996b

Levitan RD, Kaplan AS, Levitt AJ, et al: Seasonal fluctuations in mood and eating behavior in bulimia nervosa. Int J Eat Disord 16:295–299, 1994

Levitan RD, Kaplan AS, Rockert W: Characterization of the "seasonal" bulimic patient. Int J Eat Disord 19:187–192, 1996

Levy AB, Dixon KN, Stern SL: How are depression and bulimia related? Am J Psychiatry 146:162–169, 1989

Magnusson A, Stefansson JG: Prevalence of seasonal affective disorder in Iceland. Arch Gen Psychiatry 50:941–946, 1993

Mistlberger RE: Scheduled daily exercise or feeding alters the phase of photic entrainment in Syrian hamsters. Physiol Behav 50:1257–1260, 1991

Mortola JF, Laughlin GA, Yen SS: Melatonin rhythms in women with anorexia nervosa and bulimia nervosa. J Clin Endocrinol Metab 77: 1540–1544, 1993

Reilly T: Human circadian rhythms and exercise. Crit Rev Biomed Eng 18: 165–180, 1990

Rosen LN, Targum SD, Terman M, et al: Prevalence of seasonal affective disorder at four latitudes. Psychiatry Res 31:131–144, 1990

Rosenthal NE, Heffernan MM: Bulimia, carbohydrate craving, and depression: a central connection? in Nutrition and the Brain, Vol.7. Edited by Wurtman RJ, Wurtman JJ. New York, Raven, 1986, pp 139–166

Rosenthal NE, Sack DA, Gillin JC, et al: Seasonal affective disorder: a description of the syndrome and preliminary findings with light therapy. Arch Gen Psychiatry 41:72–80, 1984

Rosenthal NE, Bradt GH, Wehr TA: Seasonal Pattern Assessment Questionnaire. Bethesda, MD, National Institute of Mental Health, 1987a

Rosenthal NE, Genhart M, Jacobsen FM, et al: Disturbances of appetite and weight regulation in seasonal affective disorder. Ann N Y Acad Sc 499:216–230, 1987b

Rosenthal NE, Genhart MJ, Caballero B, et al: Psychobiological effects of carbohydrate- and protein-rich meals in patients with seasonal affective disorder and normal controls. Biol Psychiatry 25:1029–1040, 1989

Schreiber W, Schweiger U, Werner D, et al: Circadian pattern of large neutral amino acids, glucose, insulin, and food intake in anorexia nervosa and bulimia nervosa. Metabolism 40:503–507, 1991

Terman M: On the question of mechanism in phototherapy for seasonal affective disorder: consideration of clinical efficacy and epidemiology. J Biol Rhythms 3:155–172, 1988

Van Cauter E, Sturis J, Byrne MM, et al: Preliminary studies on the immediate phase-shifting effects of light and exercise on the human circadian clock. J Biol Rhythms 8(suppl):99–108, 1993

Van Reeth O, Sturis J, Byrne MM, et al: Nocturnal exercise phase delays circadian rhythms of melatonin and thyrotropin secretion in normal men. Am J Physiol 266:964–974, 1994

Wallin MS, Rissanen AM: Food and mood: relationship between food, serotonin and affective disorders. Acta Psychiatr Scand 377(suppl): 36–40, 1994

Weltzin TE, McConaha C, McKee M, et al: Circadian patterns of cortisol, prolactin, and growth hormonal secretion during bingeing and vomiting in normal weight bulimic patients. Biol Psychiatry 30:37–48, 1991

Williams JBW, Link MJ, Rosenthal NE, et al: Structured Interview Guide for the Hamilton Depression Rating Scale—Seasonal Affective Disorder Version. New York, New York State Psychiatric Unit, 1988

Yates A: Current perspectives on the eating disorders, I: history, psychological and biological aspects. J Am Acad Child Adol Psychiatry 6:813–828, 1989

NINE

Light and Melatonin Treatment of Circadian Phase Sleep Disorders

Rod J. Hughes, Ph.D.
Alfred J. Lewy, M.D., Ph.D.

Until the early 1980s, there was uniform agreement among chrono-biologists that light had a relatively minor role in regulating mela-tonin production and in entraining human biological rhythms (Vaughan et al. 1979; Wever 1979). It was generally thought that humans had evolved beyond the need for light-dark cycle entrain-ment. This thinking was based upon several failed attempts to sup-press nocturnal melatonin production and to entrain human circa-dian rhythms with light (Akerstedt et al. 1979; Jimerson et al. 1977; Vaughan et al. 1979; Weitzman et al. 1978; Wetterberg 1978; Wever 1979). There was a fundamental change after publication of the re-port that bright light (2,500 lux) could suppress nocturnal mela-tonin production in humans (Figure 9–1) (Lewy et al. 1980), which

We wish to thank the nursing staff of the Oregon Health Sciences University (OHSU) Gen-eral Clinical Research Center (GCRC) and to acknowledge the assistance of Robert Sack, Clifford Singer, Saeeduddin Ahmed, Katherine Thomas, Vance Bauer, Angela McArthur, Mary Blood, Jeannie Latham Jackson, Richard Boney, Neil Cutler, Lynette Currie, Mary Cardoza, Neil Anderson, Aaron Clemons, Joanne Otto, and Katherine Pratt. Supported by Public Health Service research grants MH40161, MH00703, MH47089, MH01005, PO1 AG10794, and M01 RR00334 (OHSU GCRC), and a grant from the National Alliance for Research on Schiz-ophrenia and Depression.

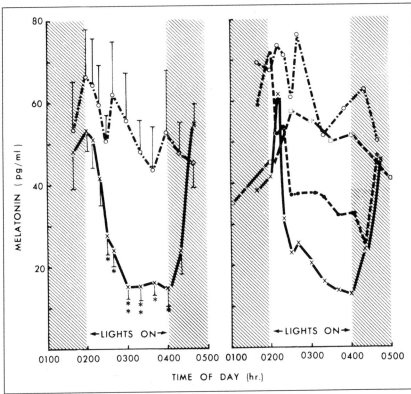

FIGURE 9–1. Effect of light on melatonin secretion. Each point represents the mean concentration of melatonin (± standard error) for six subjects. Left: A paired *t* test, comparing exposure to 500 lux with exposure to 2,500 lux, was performed for each data point. A two-way analysis of variance with repeated measures and the Newman-Keuls statistic for the comparison of means showed significant differences between 2:50 A.M. and 4:00 A.M. (*, $P < 0.05$; **, $P < 0.01$). Right: Effect of different light intensities on melatonin secretion. The averaged values for two subjects are shown. Symbols: (open circle) 500 lux; (×) 2,500 lux; (filled circle) 1,500 lux; and (open square) asleep in the dark.

Source. Reprinted with permission from Lewy AJ, Wehr TA, Goodwin FK, et al.: "Light suppresses melatonin secretion in humans." *Science* 210:1267–1269 1980. Copyright 1980 American Association for the Advancement of Science.

suggested that previous research had failed to demonstrate the importance of light in the regulation of human biological rhythms because ordinary indoor light was not sufficiently intense.

The finding that bright light but not ordinary room light could suppress nocturnal melatonin production in humans caused a "paradigm shift" in the fields of human chronobiology and human melatonin physiology. The new paradigm included the following implications 1) humans might have circadian and seasonal rhythms that respond to sunlight; 2) ordinary indoor light, which is less intense than sunlight, may not necessarily interfere with the response to sunlight; and 3) bright artificial light could be used experimentally and therapeutically to manipulate human biological rhythms. Thus the research on the suppressant effects of light was the catalyst for assessing treatment effects of bright light in psychiatric populations (Kripke 1981; Lewy et al. 1982). Shortly thereafter, Wever and co-workers (1983) showed that bright artificial light could increase the range of entrainment of the human temperature and rest-activity rhythms, and Lewy proposed that humans had a phase-response curve (PRC) to bright light (Figure 9–2) (Lewy et al. 1983).

In attempts to define the parameters of the effects of light on melatonin physiology and circadian rhythms, work done in collaboration with Brainard demonstrated that the peak wavelengths for melatonin suppression appeared to be around 509 nm (Brainard et al. 1985). Lewy suggested a relationship between the intensity of light and the degree of melatonin suppression (Lewy et al. 1980, 1985c), which was more conclusively demonstrated by Brainard and co-workers (Brainard et al. 1988). The minimum intensity required

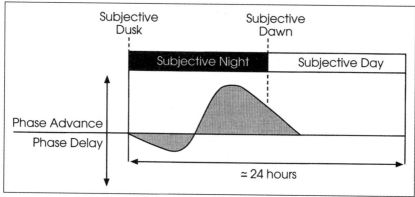

FIGURE 9–2. Schematic diagram of the hypothesized light phase-response curve (PRC) for humans.
Source. Adapted from Lewy et al. 1983.

for melatonin suppression was demonstrated to be as low as 200 lux (McIntyre et al. 1989), 300 lux (Bojkowski et al. 1987), and 500 lux (Lewy et al. 1981, 1985a). Furthermore, light suppression studies have consistently demonstrated a dose-response or fluence-response relationship (Bojkowski et al. 1987; Brainard et al. 1988; Lewy et al. 1980, 1981, 1985a; McIntyre et al. 1989).

As mentioned above, a light PRC for humans was proposed (Lewy et al. 1983), with features similar to those of other animals (Aschoff 1979; Binkley et al. 1981; DeCoursey 1964; Pittendrigh 1981; Pittendrigh and Daan 1976b). Lewy and co-workers found that, while holding the sleep-wake cycle constant, advancing dusk advanced the timing of human melatonin production, and delaying dawn delayed melatonin production, (Lewy 1985; Lewy et al. 1984, 1985b). They then demonstrated that bright artificial light given in the morning could advance circadian rhythms, and that bright light in the evening could delay them (Lewy et al. 1983, 1985d, 1987). In support of these effects, Czeisler and colleagues (1986a) demonstrated that very bright light given in the evening produced a large phase delay of the body temperature minimum (T_{min}), assessed in a constant routine protocol. To date, four complete PRCs to bright light have been described (Czeisler et al. 1989; Honma and Honma 1988; Minors et al. 1991; Wever 1989). These PRCs are similar to the human bright light PRC originally proposed in 1983 (Lewy et al. 1983).

Chronobiologic Sleep Disorders

Some sleep and mood disorders appear to be associated with underlying circadian rhythm disturbances and can be treated by interventions designed to shift the patient's endogenous circadian pacemaker (ECP), for example, appropriately timed bright light and melatonin administration. One type of desynchrony can be caused by behavioral choices to sleep out of phase with intrinsic circadian rhythms, as in shift work or rapid travel across multiple time zones. Other circadian rhythm–related sleep disorders, however, are not caused by voluntary displacement of behavioral sleep times. Rather, these circadian phase sleep disorders are characterized by an inappropriate phase relationship between habitual sleep times and the normal sleep-wake schedule.

Circadian phase sleep disorders include delayed sleep phase syndrome (International Classification of Sleep Disorders [ICSD] 780.55–0), sleep onset insomnia with normal awakening times, advanced sleep phase syndrome (ICSD 780.55–1), early morning awakening with normal sleep onset, and non-24-hour sleep-wake syndrome (ICSD 780.55–2). These chronobiologic disorders have been responsive to treatment designed to phase shift the ECP using appropriately timed bright light and, more recently, melatonin administration. Another type of chronobiologic sleep disorder is associated with hypersomnia continuing into the day, leading to excessive daytime somnolence. This disorder of sleep duration often accompanies winter depression or seasonal affective disorder (SAD), in which sleep as well as mood symptoms respond to light treatment (Lewy 1982; Lewy et al. 1987; Rosenthal et al. 1984; Sack et al. 1990).

Circadian Phase Sleep Disorders

Delayed sleep phase syndrome (DSPS) is a sleep disorder in which an individual's sleep times are delayed in relation to normal sleep time (for a recent review of DSPS, see Regestein and Monk 1995). DSPS symptoms include difficulty initiating sleep and difficulty awakening in the morning. Although delayed sleep is prevalent in the young (Thorpy et al. 1988), especially in students (Lack 1986), a DSPS diagnosis is based on the relationship between one's habitual sleep time and normal sleep time. This diagnosis is typically made only after attempts to conform to the normal sleep schedule have been attempted and failed. Thus, DSPS is different from insufficient nocturnal sleep caused by voluntarily staying up late (ICSD 307.49–4).

As noted, DSPS is characterized by difficulty initiating sleep prior to 1:00 A.M. to 3:00 A.M.; a typical sleep pattern may be from 4:00 A.M. until 12:00 noon. When assessed during habitual sleep times, polysomnographic (PSG) evaluations of patients with DSPS yield long (greater than 30 minutes) sleep latencies and delayed final awakenings, with no consistent abnormalities in either sleep duration (Czeisler et al. 1981; Shirakawa et al. 1993; Weitzman et al. 1981) or sleep architecture (Okawa et al. 1993; Uchiyama et al. 1992).

Advanced sleep phase syndrome (ASPS) is a sleep disorder in which one's sleep times are advanced in relation to normal clock time. ASPS symptoms are characterized by excessive evening somnolence, early sleep onset and early morning awakening. As with patients who have DSPS, patients with ASPS cannot, by normal means, shift their sleep times to be in phase with normal sleep time. Although both disorders can be chronic conditions, ASPS is more prevalent in older people and DSPS is more prevalent in the young (Lack 1986; Pelayo et al. 1988; Thorpy et al. 1988; Weitzman et al. 1981).

The exact circadian rhythm disturbance associated with each of the circadian phase sleep disorders is not completely defined. However, the specific insomnia characterizing each of these sleep phase disorders is often associated with altered circadian timing. For patients with DSPS, significant phase delays (about 4 hours) of T_{min} have been reported (Okawa et al. 1993). Phase delays of T_{min} have also been reported in a group of patients with sleep-onset insomnia with normal sleep duration (Morris et al. 1990). Patients with ASPS have demonstrated phase advances of T_{min} (Lack and Wright 1993). Thus, DSPS and sleep onset insomnia are generally associated with a phase delay of the ECP, and ASPS and early morning awakening are associated with a phase advance of the ECP.

These generalizations, however, do not hold for all cases of ASPS and DSPS (Singer and Lewy 1989). To examine circadian phase changes in subjects, the dim light melatonin onset (DLMO) has been used as a marker of the ECP (discussed in more detail in later sections). In normal subjects, using the time of morning bright light exposure as circadian time 0 (CT 0), the circadian time of the DLMO is typically CT 14 (about 14 hours after first bright light exposure) (Lewy and Sack 1989). Regardless of the specific clock time at which bright light is first perceived, a DLMO near CT 14 would suggest that the ECP is in normal phase. In a case report of a patient with ASPS, Singer and Lewy (1989) reported that the phase of the

DLMO was in the normal range (1950) and, when
cadian time, this subject's DLMO was at CT 14, sugg
tively normal circadian system.

Theoretical Explanations of Circadian Phase Sleep Disorders

Several explanations for these circadian phase abnormalities have
been proposed. First, in animal models, because the phase angle of
entrainment is dependent on the endogenous circadian period or τ
(e.g., Pittendrigh et al. 1976b), Czeisler and colleagues (1981) proposed that patients with ASPS may have short intrinsic periods, and
patients with DSPS may have long intrinsic periods. The only investigation of a free-running τ in a patient with ASPS did reveal a
shorter τ (Kamei et al. 1979). Other support for this explanation is
suggested by findings that elderly individuals (who are more susceptible to ASPS) tested in temporal isolation appear to have short intrinsic periods (Czeisler et al. 1986a, 1986b; Monk 1989; Monk and
Moline 1988; Weitzman et al. 1982). This work in humans was pre-
dated by similar findings in animals (Pittendrigh and Daan 1974,
1976a). It should be noted, however, that Campbell and co-workers
demonstrated that, when tested in temporal isolation, individuals
who nap during the day yield significantly shorter free-running periods of rest-activity and temperature rhythms (Campbell et al.
1993b). The tendency to nap during the day increases with increasing age (Lewis 1969; Tune 1969; Webb and Swinburne 1971).
Given this potential methodological confound in temporal isolation
testing, previous reports of shorter endogenous periods with increasing age may be the result of differential napping strategies in young
and older subjects and not to differences in the endogenous τ of the
ECP. Furthermore, using a forced desynchrony protocol to assess τ,
Duffy and Czeisler (1994) recently reported an individual with a delayed temperature rhythm but a normal τ of 24.2 hours.

An alternative explanation for DSPS suggests that these patients
are, for some reason, missing the daily corrective phase advance from
light. There are at least three ways in which this could occur: 1) patients with DSPS may have a diminished phase-advance portion of

1; Weitzman et al. 1981); 2) at the
~ may be subsensitive to light; and
obscure the phase-advance portion
1994). That bright light is able to
PS so effectively makes a diminished
ht PRC unlikely. The same argument
explanation; however, the efficacy of
) in treating DSPS alone (Ohta et al.
nd in combination with bright light
(Okawa et al. 1996, lt from vitamin B_{12}'s ability to increase
sensitivity to light (Honma et al. 1992). On the other hand, given
that some patients with ASPS and DSPS appear to have normal circadian systems (see later), Okawa's explanation has intuitive appeal.
By masking the phase-advance portion of the light PRC, more sleep
after T_{min} would likely result in delaying both the ECP and sleep.
There are some diary data to support that patients with DSPS may
sleep longer than controls, with more sleep after T_{min} (Okawa et al.
1994). However, these data are contrary to more sensitive measurements (e.g., PSG evaluations) of sleep in patients with DSPS, which
show that they do not sleep longer than normal control subjects
(Czeisler et al. 1981; Shirakawa et al. 1993; Weitzman et al. 1981).
Therefore, for these patients with DSPS, in order for sleep to cover
up the phase-advance portion of the light PRC, sleep must be shifted
more than the ECP.

Phase Typing Circadian Sleep Phase Disorders

Given that not all patients with a particular sleep phase disorder
(ASPS or DSPS) have the same phase relationship between sleep and
endogenous circadian rhythms, Lewy and Sack proposed an approach to treating chronobiologic sleep and mood disorders based
on a unified theory called *phase typing* (Lewy et al. 1984, 1985d).
What is meant by *phase typing* is that before treating an individual
one should ascertain the patient's circadian phase position. The term
sleep phase is often used clinically for *phase typing*, based on the observation that, relative to real time, all circadian rhythms, including
sleep, are shifted in the same direction, even though sleep may be

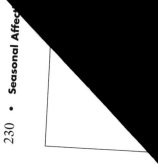

shifted to a greater or lesser extent t[...]
Phase typing becomes more difficult [...]
and awakens late, or falls asleep late [...]
we usually use sleep-offset time rath[...]
circadian phase, because it is less in[...]
such as anxiety and boredom. If a [...]
phase markers for the ECP is melat[...]
as sleep and the endogenous circad[...]
perature, are influenced by extran[...]
tivity). Melatonin is not affected by stress and activity (Lewy 1983),
only by bright light (Lewy et al. 1980). We use the DLMO as a
clearly demarcated marker for circadian phase (Lewy and Sack
1989).

Using melatonin as a marker for circadian phase, we can more
precisely classify chronobiologic sleep and mood disorders into three
subtypes (see Figure 9–3 for a graphic depiction of the various logical phase types and subtypes). In the classification of circadian phase
sleep disorders, by definition, sleep must be phase shifted with respect to real time. Many patients with ASPS and DSPS have sleep
and other circadian rhythms phase shifted to the same extent (subtype I). There is no internal phase angle abnormality in this subtype
(Figure 9–3b,c). In a recent case study of a 17-year-old male with
DSPS, Ihara and associates (1994) assessed sleep propensity using
Lavie's ultrashort sleep-wake schedule (Lavie 1986). These authors
report phase delays of approximately 5 hours for DLMO, T_{min}, and
the sleep propensity rhythm. Oren and co-workers have also recently
reported a patient with DSPS who had the circadian rhythms of
melatonin, temperature, and sleep all delayed to the same extent
(Oren et al. 1995). Subtype I patients may have general difficulty in
using *zeitgebers* (external synchronizers) to shift in one or both directions. Alternatively, social or psychological reasons may account for
why these patients have difficulty shifting sleep. Shifted sleep will
cause a corresponding shift in the other circadian rhythms of the
ECP because of the shift in the *perceived* light-dark cycle. Thus, in a
sense, subtype I patients might not actually be chronobiologically
disturbed, rather they may be sleeping at abnormal times for social
or psychological reasons.

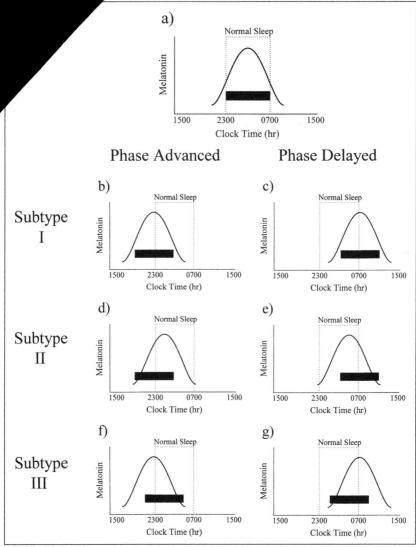

FIGURE 9–3. Proposed classification of logical subtypes of circadian phase sleep disorders. For each of the types (advanced or delayed) and subtypes, the phase relationships between melatonin and habitual sleep (solid bars) are depicted relative to normal sleep. See text for explanation of subtypes I, II, and III.

Source. Adapted from Lewy 1990.

Subtype II circadian sleep phase disorders are c having sleep phase shifted more than the other ci (Figure 9–3d,e). Thus, with respect to sleep, patients have a relatively phase-advanced ECP, and patients wiui ו…ו … ..… have a relatively phase-delayed ECP (that is, relative to sleep, but not necessarily relative to clock time). Okawa and co-workers (1994) described patients with DSPS who had this phase relationship (Figure 9–3e). For these patients, sleep was delayed more than the temperature rhythm, resulting in more sleep following T_{min} than normal control subjects. This same phase relationship was demonstrated by Dahlitz and colleagues (Alvarez et al. 1992; Dahlitz et al. 1991), who reported that for patients with DSPS, sleep was significantly phase-delayed, but when these patients were tested in a fixed light-dark cycle, melatonin was only slightly phase-delayed. As with subtype I patients, subtype II patients may not necessarily be chronobiologically disturbed. These patients may have a disturbance in the homeostatic process of sleep. Patients with DSPS may simply need to feel more tired before they can fall asleep, whereas these patients with ASPS may simply have a very low fatigue threshold. The phase of the ECP of subtype II patients may not necessarily be shifted in the expected direction (or in either direction) with respect to real time. For example, Singer, as mentioned above, reported a patient with ASPS whose DLMO was slightly advanced but still at CT 14 (Singer and Lewy 1989). Because patients with subtype II ASPS wake up into dim light (CT 0 is solar dawn not sleep offset), the ECP may not be phase-advanced relative to the light-dark cycle. In other words, using solar dawn as CT 0, these patients may have a DLMO at CT 14, reflecting a "normal" phase relationship with the light-dark cycle. This particular subtype is likely more common in ASPS because these patients are waking up into dim light, perhaps several hours before solar dawn.

The third subtype of chronobiologic sleep disorders (subtype III) occurs when sleep is not as phase shifted as the other circadian rhythms (Figure 9–3f,g). Morris and colleagues (1990) present an example of this subtype (Figure 9–3g). Compared to control subjects, individuals with sleep-onset insomnia initiated sleep more than 2 hours earlier, relative to T_{min}, despite the fact that T_{min} was delayed by 4 hours. This situation places the time of attempted sleep during the wake-maintenance zone of the sleep propensity rhythm (Strogatz et al. 1987), before the opening of Lavie's "sleep gate." It should be noted that not all individuals with this particular phase relationship between their ECP and sleep have difficulty sleeping (Duffy and Czeisler 1994). Subtype III patients likely have the most convincing circadian rhythms disturbance.

Although the three subtypes may be of interest scientifically, treatment is based on the patient's overall phase type, whether the patient is phase-delayed or phase-advanced. Once the patient is phase typed, an appropriate phase-shifting treatment strategy can be undertaken to bring the individual's sleep into normal phase and, if necessary, correct the underlying circadian rhythm disturbance. Before presenting some treatment strategies, we will first review some of the historical context behind the treatment of circadian phase sleep disorders.

Treatment of Circadian Phase Sleep Disorders

Chronotherapy

In chronotherapy, the objective is to reset the pacemaker to the normal clock time by shifting sleep (e.g., in the case of DSPS, 3 hours later each day, for about a week) until the normal sleep phase is reached (Czeisler et al. 1981). Although chronotherapy is typically done for DSPS, systematic advances have also been used to treat ASPS (Billiard et al. 1993a; Moldofsky et al. 1986; Ohta et al. 1983). Once in phase, the patients must strictly conform to the new sleep-wake schedule. This treatment strategy was, in part, based upon the presumed importance of the sleep-wake cycle in the entrainment of human circadian rhythms (Czeisler et al. 1981; Kronauer et al. 1982). It has since been shown that the sleep-wake cycle entrains the ECP only by modulation of the perceived light-dark cycle.

For individuals with DSPS, chronotherapy was originally proposed to correct a presumed decreased range of entrainment, thought

to be caused by a "mismatch" between
phase-advancing capacity of the ECP. Thi:
of either a reduction in the amplitude of
light PRC or to an increased τ that is n
creased phase-advance portion of the PRC

Chronotherapy for DSPS has been u
morning bright light exposure (Terman 1
logical hypnotic treatment (Ohta et al. 1, Uami-rascual et al.
1988). Because chronotherapy can cause a considerable sleep debt
and requires about a week of "free" time to complete, its clinical application has been limited. In short, a given patient may not have a
schedule (e.g., time off) that will allow successful completion of the
treatment (e.g., Rosenberg 1991). As shown by Ohta and colleagues
(1992) and others, there is a significant risk of relapse, which may be
associated with the degree of secondary psychiatric pathology (Billiard et al. 1993b). Furthermore, some DSPS patients have become
hypernychthemeral (non-24-hour sleep-wake syndrome [see later])
following unsuccessful chronotherapy treatment (Oren and Wehr
1992). In summary, for some patients, chronotherapy can successfully
reset the phase of sleep patterns and the ECP. However, sustaining
this effect is difficult (e.g. Ohta et al. 1992), and some patients may
actually get worse (Oren and Wehr 1992). Chronotherapy may work
by shifting the patient's light-dark cycle, exposing previously ob-
scured portions of the light PRC, so that light can achieve its corrective phase shift (evening light for DSPS and morning light for ASPS).

Bright Light Treatment

Lewy and colleagues originally proposed using appropriately timed
bright artificial light exposure to alleviate DSPS and ASPS (Lewy et
al. 1983). Initially, a patient with DSPS was successfully treated with
morning light (Lewy et al. 1983), and ASPS was treated with
evening light (Lewy et al. 1985c). Subsequent studies confirmed the
ability of bright light to treat circadian phase sleep disorders
(Czeisler et al. 1989; Joseph-Vanderpool et al. 1988, 1989; Singer
and Lewy 1989).

light to treat patients with DSPS, Rosenthal and co-
s (1990) administered 2 hours of 2,500-lux light between
0 A.M. and 9:00 A.M. and reported a more than 1-hour phase advance of T_{min}. Although sleep was not recorded, patients reported
improved sleep, and multiple sleep latency tests revealed increased
daytime alertness. In a group of patients with early morning awakening but normal sleep onset, Lack and Wright (1993) reported that 2
nights of 2,500-lux light exposure from 8:00 P.M. to 12:00 midnight delayed T_{min} and the DLMO about 2 hours and 10 minutes. In
addition, morning awakening was phase delayed by about 1 hour,
with a similar increase in sleep duration and no change in sleep-onset
time. In a study of ASPS in elderly patients, Campbell and colleagues
(1993a) delayed T_{min} by more than 3 hours with light of 4,000 lux
for 2 hours between 8:00 P.M. and 11:00 P.M. Treatment also increased sleep efficiency, stage 2 sleep, slow-wave sleep, and REM-
sleep.

Parameters of light treatment have varied. Light duration has
ranged from 15 minutes to 4 hours, illuminance levels from 2,500
lux to 10,000 lux. It appears that, holding the duration of exposure
constant, increasing light intensity can increase the magnitude of the
phase shift (e.g., Lack and Wright 1993). Of course, assuming patients awaken after solar dawn, natural sunlight is also effective (Dagan et al. 1991). As a result of the immediate alerting effects of
bright light at night (Badia et al. 1991; Campbell and Dawson
1990), some patients may complain of an energizing effect after light
treatment (Lewy and Sack 1986), causing sleep-onset insomnia, in
which case light exposure should be scheduled to end at least 1–2
hours before scheduled bedtime. In order to minimize sleep disruption, the timing of light administration can be gradually advanced to
treat DSPS. In ASPS, sleep onset may be gradually delayed.

In clinical application, scheduling of light treatment for DSPS is
usually based on the patient's sleep pattern, with no assessment of
circadian phase (e.g., T_{min} or DLMO). However, given that sleep
can occur out of phase with the subjective night, there is a risk of
obtaining phase shifts in the opposite direction to that predicted by
light exposure at a specific clock time. For example, Dr. Robert Sack

in our group treated a patien.
A.M. to 8:00 A.M. Not only did
melatonin showed a phase delay
ulation of the delay portion of
advance crossover point were mark
markers such as melatonin and tempe
able in clinical practice, the clinician
progress of sleep-phase treatment to ensu
correct direction.

Melatonin Treatment

Melatonin administration provides another option for treating circadian phase sleep disorders. As with bright light, melatonin is able to
phase shift circadian rhythms, including the sleep-wake cycle. Melatonin is particularly useful in patients who do not or cannot respond
to light treatment. About 15% of all blind people are totally blind.
That is, besides being visually blind, they have no functioning circadian photic pathway. Despite attempts to adhere to normal sleep
times, most, if not all, of these people have free-running endogenous
circadian rhythms (Lewy and Newsome 1983; Sack et al. 1992).
Many of these individuals also have sleep disturbances, typically characterized by a free-running sleep-wake cycle (Martens et al. 1990;
Miles et al. 1977; Okawa et al. 1987; Tzischinsky et al. 1991).

Because light treatment is not an option for this population, these
individuals were treated with melatonin administration. This strategy was based upon animal research that showed that daily injections
of melatonin could entrain free-running rhythms in rats that were
kept in constant darkness (Redman et al. 1983). In the first two attempts to entrain blind subjects with melatonin (5 mg), Sack and co-
workers were able to phase advance patients' free-running melatonin
rhythms (Sack et al. 1987). The initial work in blind patients eventually led to the assessment of the phase-shifting effects of exogenous
melatonin in sighted people.

In a group of sighted individuals, Lewy and co-workers (Lewy et
al. 1992) described a PRC for melatonin administration. Doses of

ed in the morning delayed the onset of endoge-
in production, whereas doses administered in the late
on and early evening advanced the onset of endogenous mela-
in production. These data demonstrate that melatonin administration shifts human circadian rhythms according to a well-defined
PRC (Figure 9–4) that is about 12 hours out of phase with the light
PRC (Lewy et al. 1992). The shape of the melatonin PRC has recently been confirmed by Zaidan and co-workers using 1-day admin-

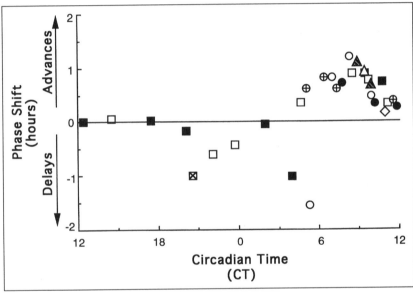

FIGURE 9–4. Phase shifts of the dim light melatonin onset (DLMO) as a function
of circadian time (CT) for nine subjects (a total of 30 trials), providing the first
evidence for a human melatonin phase response curve (PRC). Each of the nine
subjects has a separate symbol. Exogenous melatonin was administered at various
times with respect to the time of endogenous melatonin production (CT 14 =
baseline DLMO for each trial). The time of administration appears as CT by
convention and because of interindividual variability in sleep-wake cycles, perceived
light-dark cycles, and internal circadian time. On average, CT 0 = 7:00 A.M. clock
time. Two subjects (J.H. [open squares] and S.E. [closed squares]) each participated
in seven trials: when internal CT is referenced to the baseline DLMO, plots of the
data for these two subjects nearly superimpose.

Source. Lewy AJ, Ahmed S, Jackson JML, et al.: "Melatonin shifts circadian
rhythms according to a phase-response curve." *Chronobiol Int* 9:380–392, 1992.
Used with permission.

istration (Zaidan et al. 1994). This work in huma with animal studies that have demonstrated melat phase shifts at both the behavioral and cellular levels (Arm Chesworth 1987; Cassone et al. 1986; McArthur et al. 199 phase-shifting effects of melatonin are likely mediated by the tonin receptors that are found in high density in the suprachiasm nuclei (Reppert et al. 1988).

Using the melatonin PRC as a guide, melatonin administered in the late afternoon and early evening may effectively treat DSPS and sleep-onset insomnia, and melatonin administered in the late night and early morning may effectively treat ASPS and early morning awakening. Although there are no reported tests of melatonin administration to delay the advanced clocks of patients suffering from ASPS and early morning awakening, melatonin has been shown to effectively treat patients with DSPS. Dahlitz and colleagues (1991) were the first to successfully treat DSPS with melatonin administration. In a double-blind placebo-controlled clinical trial, patients were given 5 mg or placebo daily for 4 weeks. Melatonin was administered at 10:00 P.M., 5 hours prior to mean time of habitual sleep onset. Sleep was recorded by sleep logs in a fixed light-dark cycle (darkness from 11:00 P.M. to 8:00 A.M.). Melatonin treatment phase advanced the time of sleep onset by 82 minutes. Adding five patients with DSPS and one with non-24-hour sleep-wake syndrome to their original eight, these same investigators extended their findings (Alvarez et al. 1992). After having successfully advanced the time of sleep onset and sleep offset during melatonin administration, all subjects reverted back to their original sleep-wake schedule within 2–3 days of discontinuing melatonin treatment.

In an open-label trial of melatonin treatment of DSPS, Tzischinsky and co-workers (1993) administered 5 mg melatonin at 7:30 P.M. (approximately 2 hours prior to the desired time of sleep onset and 7 hours prior to mean habitual sleep onset time). Melatonin treatment continued until subjects were satisfied with their sleep phase (4–11 weeks). Melatonin treatment successfully advanced the time of sleep onset 1.98 hours, with no change in sleep duration. Contrary to earlier research, only two of the eight subjects had relapsed by the 6-month follow-up.

) reported another open-label trial
. Melatonin (5 mg) was adminis-
:00 P.M. (8.5–10.5 hours prior to
Sleep (PSG) recorded on days 28
was compared with 3 days of
prior to treatment (baseline).
onset by 115 minutes and ad-
106 minutes, with no change
the six subjects followed, all relapsed within
or discontinuation of treatment.

In a case report of melatonin treatment in a 12-year-old with DSPS, melatonin (5 mg) or placebo was administered 2 hours prior to the desired time of sleep onset (Nagtegaal et al. 1994). Melatonin was alternated with placebo in 2- to 5-day runs over a 30-day period, and the latency to sleep following pill administration was recorded in 30-minute intervals by the boy's mother. Using this observational measure of sleep, melatonin nights yielded shorter sleep latencies by an average 1.25 hours

Melatonin treatment of patients suffering from DSPS has the added advantage of utilizing the sleep-promoting effects of mela-tonin, much the same way as morning bright light treatment of DSPS has the advantage of capitalizing on the immediate alerting effects of bright lights. When administered out of phase with en-dogenous melatonin, exogenous melatonin has sleep-promoting effects in some people (Antón-Tay et al. 1971; Cramer et al. 1974; Dollins et al. 1994; Hughes et al. 1994). Whereas typical hypnotic drugs such as benzodiazepine and triazolam do help patients comply with bright light treatment for DSPS (Joseph-Vanderpool et al. 1988), triazolam alone is less effective for long-term treatment of DSPS (Uruha et al. 1987). All of the studies to date include adminis-tration of 5 mg of melatonin at approximately the same circadian time. Doses at this level given at this circadian time have been shown to consistently reduce latency to sleep via what may be an acute sleep-promoting effect (Dollins et al. 1994; Nave et al. 1995; Tzischinsky and Lavie 1994; Zhdanova et al. 1994, 1995). On the other hand, the magnitudes of the reported phase advances of the sleep-wake cycle are in the range of what is predicted by the melatonin PRC (Lewy et al. 1992). Given that melatonin can cause an immediate phase shift of as much as 90 minutes (Krauchi et al. 1995; Zaidan et al. 1994), one cannot exclude the alternative explanation that reported sleep-promoting effects from melatonin administration at this circadian time are the result of an immediate phase advance of the temperature and sleep propensity rhythms. Therefore, whether the success of melatonin treatment of DSPS is primarily the result of an acute sleep-promoting effect or a phase-shifting effect is unknown.

Non-24-Hour Sleep-Wake Syndrome

As previously mentioned, another form of sleep phase disorder is often found in individuals with total blindness. In totally blind people, endogenous melatonin and temperature rhythms can run free, independent of both the solar light-dark cycle and the behavioral sleep-wake rhythm (Klein et al. 1993; Lewy and Newsome, 1983; Miles et al. 1977; Sack et al. 1991; Tzischinsky et al. 1991). Because these individuals often attempt to keep a consistent behavioral sleep-wake cycle, despite the fact that their sleep propensity rhythm remains in phase with the free-running melatonin rhythm (Nakagawa et al. 1992), sleep disturbances in the blind are quite prevalent (Martens et al. 1990; Miles and Wilson 1977; Okawa et al. 1987; Tzischinsky et al. 1991).

This sleep disorder, which is associated with free-running sleep-wake rhythms, is classified as non-24-hour sleep-wake syndrome, or hypernychthemeral syndrome, and is primarily characterized by progressive delays of the sleep-wake cycle of 1–2 hours. Given that some patients with DSPS undergo episodes of progressive phase delays (Weitzman et al. 1981), this disorder is likely an extreme case of DSPS. Unlike patients with DSPS, who are entrained to an abnormal phase, patients with hypernychthemeral syndrome are free-running. Hypernychthemeral syndrome has also been reported in sighted people living in the presence of apparently normal social and light-dark time cues (Elliott et al. 1971; Kokkoris et al. 1978; Weber et al. 1980). These individuals also have a free-running ECP for which the sleep propensity rhythm and the melatonin rhythm remain in phase (McArthur et al. 1995).

The mechanism underlying this specific sleep phase disorder appears to be the same as for DSPS. Emens and co-workers (1994) reported a patient with free-running sleep-wake cycle (τ = 25.17 hours) who, when tested in a forced desynchrony protocol, revealed a normal period (τ = 24.51 hours). Some have suggested that these patients are subsensitive to light (McArthur et al. 1995), which again may account for the apparent success of vitamin B_{12} treatment both alone and in combination with bright light (see later). On the other hand, Okawa and co-workers (1993) report an individual with non-24-hour sleep-wake syndrome who appears to have an extreme case of DSPS subtype II. The T_{min} of this individual typically fell in the early part of his sleep episode, completely obscuring the phase-advance portion of his light PRC. McArthur and co-workers (1995) recently presented a case study of a similar patient. This individual's DLMO was significantly less than CT 14, thus indicating another case of DSPS subtype II. A close look at other case reports reveals similar phase relationships (Hoban et al. 1989; Okawa et al. 1990; Tomoda et al. 1994). It appears that most patients with non-24-hour sleep-wake syndrome have extreme cases of Lewy's DSPS subtype II, and that masking of the phase-advance portion of the light PRC is likely responsible for the progressive phase delays of the ECP (Emens et al. 1994).

These patients have been treated with light (Eastman et al. 1988; Hoban et al. 1989), vitamin B_{12} (Kamgar-Parsi et al. 1983; Okawa et al. 1990), light plus vitamin B_{12} (Ohta et al. 1991; Okawa et al. 1993), melatonin (McArthur et al. 1995), and melatonin plus vitamin B_{12} (Tomoda et al. 1994). All of these treatments have been reported to alleviate sleep disorders, although, to date, the evidence suggests that light can sometimes (Hoban et al. 1989), but not always (Eastman et al. 1988), entrain the ECP to a 24-hour day. In melatonin treatment of blind people, entrainment of endogenous circadian rhythms has been reported in only one person (Sack et al.

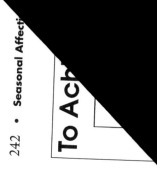

1991). However, Sack and co-work
successful treatment of sleep-wake
tonin administration (Arendt et
Lapierre and Dumont 1995; Palm
Rather than complete entrainm
shorten τ to close to 24 hours. Wh
may make it easier for the patient t
schedule (McArthur et al. 1995), c
wake cycles with a period closer to
The clinical significance of free running with a shorter τ is not yet
known. However, one can assume that free running with a shorter τ
is not necessarily better than free running with a longer τ, because
one remains out of phase for several weeks at a time rather than several days.

Conclusions

Circadian phase sleep disorders may or may not be associated with a
specific breakdown in the circadian system. Some patients may have
a normal phase relationship between their ECP and sleep, and even
though both may be out of phase with "normal" sleep times, they
may be in phase with the light-dark cycle. Other patients, however,
have endogenous circadian rhythms that are, to some degree, out of
phase with their habitual sleep times (which are out of phase with
normal sleep times). Once a patient is phase typed, an optimal treatment strategy can be initiated to phase shift the patient's sleep to normal sleep time. These treatment strategies could make use of the
phase-shifting effects of bright light or melatonin administration
(Figure 9–5). Evening bright light or morning melatonin administration is recommended for treating ASPS and early morning awakening. Morning bright light or afternoon melatonin administration
is recommended for treating DSPS and sleep-onset insomnia. Combined melatonin–bright light treatment strategies may be most effective, although melatonin administration appears to be less intrusive
than bright light exposure.

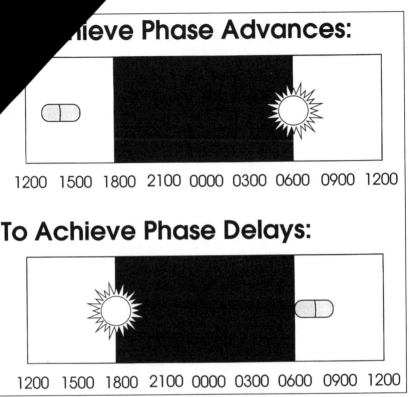

FIGURE 9–5. Phase-shifting effects of light and exogenous melatonin, assuming a normal circadian phase. To cause a phase advance, light should be administered in the morning and melatonin in the afternoon. To cause a phase delay, light should be given in the evening and melatonin should be taken in the morning. Of course, the timing of light and melatonin administration is best done with reference to circadian time rather than clock time.

References

Akerstedt T, Fröberg JE, Friberg Y, et al: Melatonin excretion, body temperature, and subjective arousal during 64 hours of sleep deprivation. Psychoneuroendocrinology 4:219–225, 1979

Alvarez B, Dahlitz MJ, Vignau J, et al: The delayed sleep phase syndrome: clinical and investigative findings in 14 subjects. J Neurol Neurosurg Psychiatry 55:665–670, 1992

Antón-Tay F, Díaz JL, Fernández-Guardiola A: On the effect of melatonin upon the human brain: it's possible therapeutic implications. Life Sci 10:841–850, 1971

Arendt J, Aldhous M, Wright J: Synchronisation of a disturbed sleep-wake cycle in a blind man by melatonin treatment. Lancet i:772–773, 1988

Armstrong SM, Chesworth MJ: Melatonin phase shifts a mammalian circadian clock, in Fundamentals and Clinics in Pineal Research. Edited by Trentini GP, de Gaetani C, Pévet P. . New York, Raven Press, 1987, pp 195–198

Aschoff J: Circadian rhythms: general features and endocrinological aspects, in Endocrine Rhythms. Edited by Krieger D. New York, Raven Press, 1979, pp 1–61

Badia P, Myers B, Boecker M, et al: Bright light effects on body temperature, alertness, EEG, and behavior. Physiol Behav 50:583–588, 1991

Billiard M, Verge M, Aldaz C, et al: A case of advanced-sleep phase syndrome. Sleep Res 22:109, 1993a

Billiard M, Verge M, Touchon J, et al: Delayed sleep phase syndrome: subjective and objective data chronotherapy and follow-up. Sleep Res 22:172, 1993b

Binkley S, Muller G, Hernandez R: Circadian rhythm in pineal N-acetyltransferase activity: phase shifting by light pulses (I). J Neurochem 37:789–800, 1981

Bojkowski CJ, Aldhous ME, English J, et al: Suppression of nocturnal plasma melatonin and 6-sulphatoxymelatonin by bright and dim light in man. Horm Metab Res 19:437–440, 1987

Brainard GC, Lewy AJ, Menaker M, et al: Effect of light wavelength on the suppression of nocturnal plasma melatonin in normal volunteers. Ann N Y Acad Sci 453:376–378, 1985

Brainard GC, Lewy AJ, Menaker M, et al: Dose-response relationship between light irradiance and the suppression of plasma melatonin in human volunteers. Brain Res 454:212–218, 1988

Campbell SS, Dawson D: Enhancement of nighttime alertness and performance with bright ambient light. Physiol Behav 48:317–20, 1990

Campbell SS, Dawson D, Anderson MW: Alleviation of sleep maintenance insomnia with timed exposure to bright light. J Am Geriatr Soc 41:829–836, 1993a

Campbell SS, Dawson D, Zulley J: When the human circadian system is caught napping: evidence for endogenous rhythms close to 24 hours. Sleep 16:638–640, 1993b

Cassone VM, Chesworth MJ, Armstrong SM: Dose dependent entrainment of rat circadian rhythms by daily injection of melatonin. J Biol Rhythms 1:219–229, 1986

Cramer H, Rudolph J, Consbruch U, et al: On the effects of melatonin on sleep and behavior in man, in Serotonin—New Vistas: Biochemistry and Behavioral and Clinical Studies (Advances in Biochemical Psychopharmacology Series). Edited by Costa E, Gessa GL, Sandler M.. New York, Raven Press, 1974, pp 187–191

Czeisler C, Richardson G, Coleman R, et al: Chronotherapy: resetting the circadian clocks of patients with delayed sleep phase insomnia. Sleep 4: 1–21, 1981

Czeisler CA, Allan JS, Strogatz SH, et al: Bright light resets the human circadian pacemaker independent of the timing of the sleep-wake cycle. Science 233:667–671, 1986a

Czeisler CA, Kronauer RE, Rios CD, et al: Attenuated output of the endogenous circadian oscillator (x) in an 85 year old man: A case study. Sleep Res 15:267, 1986b

Czeisler CA, Kronauer RE, Allan JS, et al: Bright light induction of strong (Type O) resetting of the human circadian pacemaker. Science 244: 1328–1333, 1989

Czeisler CA, Kronauer E, Johnson MP, et al: Action of light on the human circadian pacemaker: treatment of patients with circadian rhythm sleep disorders, in Sleep, Vol 88. Edited by Horne J. Stuttgart, Fisher Verlag, 1989, pp 42–47

Dagan Y, Tzischinsky O, Lavie P: Sunlight treatment for delayed sleep-phase syndrome: case report. Sleep Res 20:451, 1991

Dahlitz M, Alvarez B, Vignau J, et al: Delayed sleep phase syndrome response to melatonin. Lancet 337:1121–1123, 1991

DeCoursey PJ: Function of a light response rhythm in hamsters. J Cell Comp Physiol 63:189–196, 1964

Dollins AB, Zhdanova IV, Wurtman RJ, et al: Effect of inducing nocturnal serum melatonin concentrations in daytime on sleep, mood, body temperature, and performance. Proc Natl Acad Sci U S A 91:1824–1828, 1994

Duffy JF, Czeisler CA: Assessment of endogenous circadian period in an individual whose temperature phase is delayed with respect to his habitual sleep-wake schedule. Sleep Res 23:490, 1994

Eastman CI, Anagnopoulus CA, Cartwright RD: Can bright light entrain a free-runner? Sleep Res 17:372, 1988

Elliott AL, Mills JN, Waterhouse JM: A man with too long a day. J Physiol 212:30–31, 1971

Emens JS, Brotman DJ, Czeisler CA: Evaluation of the intrinsic period of the circadian pacemaker in a patient with a non-24-hour sleep-wake schedule disorder. Sleep Res 23:256, 1994

Folkard S, Arendt J, Aldhous M, et al: Melatonin stabilises sleep onset time in a blind man without entrainment of cortisol or temperature rhythms. Neurosci Lett 113:193–198, 1990

Hoban TM, Sack RL, Lewy AJ, et al: Entrainment of a free-running human with bright light? Chronobiol Int 6:347–353, 1989

Honma K, Honma S: A human phase response curve for bright light pulses. Jpn J Psychiatr Neurol 42:167–168, 1988

Honma K, Kohsaka M, Fukuda N, et al: Effects of vitamin B12 on plasma melatonin rhythm in humans: increased light sensitivity phase-advances the circadian clock? Experientia 48:716–20, 1992

Hughes RJ, Badia P, French J, et al: Melatonin induced changes in body temperature and daytime sleep. Sleep Res 23:496, 1994

Ihara H, Madokoro S, Nakagawa, H., et al: A case of delayed sleep phase syndrome: chronobiological study. Jpn J Psychiatr Neurol 48:451–452, 1994

Jimerson DC, Lynch HJ, Post RM, et al: Urinary melatonin rhythms during sleep deprivation in depressed patients and normals. Life Sci 20:1501–1508, 1977

Joseph-Vanderpool JR, Kelly K, Schulz PM, et al: Delayed sleep phase syndrome revisited: preliminary effects of light and triazolam. Sleep Res 17:381, 1988

Joseph-Vanderpool JR, Rosenthal NE, Levendosky AA, et al: Phase-shifting effects of bright morning light as treatment for delayed sleep phase syndrome. Sleep Res 18:422, 1989

Kamei R, Hughes L, Miles L, et al: Advanced-sleep phase syndrome studied in a time isolation facility. Chronobiologia 6:115, 1979

Kamgar-Parsi B, Wehr TA, Gillin JC: Successful treatment of human non-24-hour sleep wake syndrome. Sleep 6:257–264, 1983

Klein T, Martens H, Dijk DJ, et al: Circadian sleep regulation in the absence of light perception: chronic non-24-hour circadian rhythm sleep disorder in a blind man with a regular 24-hour sleep-wake schedule. Sleep 16:333–343, 1993

Kokkoris CP, Weitzman ED, Pollak CP, et al: Long-term ambulatory temperature monitoring in a subject with a hypernychthemeral sleep-wake cycle disturbance. Sleep 1:177–190, 1978

Krauchi K, Cajochen C, Mori D, et al: Evidence for a phase advance in circadian temperature regulation after acute melatonin and a melatonin agonist (S-20098). Sleep Res 24:526, 1995

Kripke DF: Photoperiodic mechanisms for depression and its treatment, in Biological Psychiatry. Edited by Perris C, Struwe G, Jansson B.. Amsterdam, Elsevier, 1981, pp 1249–1252

Kronauer RE, Czeisler CA, Pilato SF, et al: Mathematical model of the human circadian system with two interacting oscillators. Am J Physiology 242:R3–R17, 1982

Lack LC: Delayed sleep and sleep loss in university students. J Am Coll Health 35:105–110, 1986

Lack L, Wright H: The effect of evening bright light in delaying circadian rhythms and lengthening the sleep of early morning awakening insomniacs. Sleep 16:436–443, 1993

Lapierre O, Dumont M: Melatonin treatment of a non-24-hour sleep-wake cycle in a blind retarded child. Biol Psychiatry 38:119–122, 1995

Lavie P: Ultrashort sleep-waking schedule. III. 'Gates' and 'forbidden zones' for sleep. Electroencephalography and Clinical Neurophysiology 63:414–425, 1986

Lewis SA: Sleep patterns during afternoon naps in the young and elderly. Br J Psychiatry 115:107–108, 1969

Lewy AJ: Melatonin secretion as a neurobiological "marker" and effects of light in humans. Psychopharmacol Bull 18:127–129, 1982

Lewy AJ: Biochemistry and regulation of mammalian melatonin production, in The Pineal Gland. Edited by Relkin RM. New York, Elsevier North-Holland, 1983, pp 77–128

Lewy AJ: Regulation of melatonin production in humans by bright artificial light: evidence for a clock-gate model and a phase response curve, in The Pineal Gland: Endocrine Aspects (Advances in the Biosciences Series). Edited by Brown GM, Wainwright SD. Oxford, Pergamon Press, 1985, pp 203–208

Lewy AJ: Chronobiologic disorders, social cues and the light-dark cycle. Chronobiol Int 7:15–21, 1990

Lewy AJ, Newsome DA: Different types of melatonin circadian secretory rhythms in some blind subjects. J Clin Endocrinol Metab 56: 1103–1107, 1983

Lewy AJ, Sack RL: Minireview: light therapy and psychiatry. Proc Soc Exp Biol Med 183:11–18, 1986

Lewy AJ, Sack RL: The dim light melatonin onset (DLMO) as a marker for circadian phase position. Chronobiol Int 6:93–102, 1989

Lewy AJ, Wehr TA, Goodwin FK, et al: Light suppresses melatonin secretion in humans. Science 210:1267–1269, 1980

Lewy AJ, Wehr TA, Goodwin FK, et al: Manic-depressive patients may be supersensitive to light. Lancet 1:383–384, 1981

Lewy AJ, Kern HA, Rosenthal NE, et al: Bright artificial light treatment of a manic-depressive patient with a seasonal mood cycle. Am J Psychiatry 139:1496–1498, 1982

Lewy AJ, Sack RL, Fredrickson RH, et al: The use of bright light in the treatment of chronobiologic sleep and mood disorders: the phase-response curve. Psychopharmacol Bull 19:523–525, 1983

Lewy AJ, Sack RL, Singer CM: Assessment and treatment of chronobiologic disorders using plasma melatonin levels and bright light exposure: the clock-gate model and the phase response curve. Psychopharmacol Bull 20:561–565, 1984

Lewy AJ, Nurnberger JI, Wehr TA, et al: Supersensitivity to light: possible trait marker for manic-depressive illness. Am J Psychiatry 142:725–727, 1985a

Lewy AJ, Sack RL, Singer CM: Immediate and delayed effects of bright light on human melatonin production: shifting "dawn" and "dusk" shifts the dim light melatonin onset (DLMO). Ann NY Acad Sci 453: 253–259, 1985b

Lewy AJ, Sack RL, Singer CM: Melatonin, light and chronobiological disorders, in Photoperiodism, Melatonin and the Pineal. Edited by Evered D, Clark S. London, Pitman, 1985c, pp 231–252

Lewy AJ, Sack RL, Singer CM: Treating phase typed chronobiologic sleep and mood disorders using appropriately timed bright artificial light. Psychopharmacol Bull 21:368–372, 1985d

Lewy AJ, Sack RL, Miller S, et al: Antidepressant and circadian phase-shifting effects of light. Science 235:352–354, 1987

Lewy AJ, Ahmed S, Jackson JML, et al: Melatonin shifts circadian rhythms according to a phase-response curve. Chronobiol Int 9:380–392, 1992

Martens H, Endlich H, Hildebrandt G, et al: Sleep/wake distribution in blind subjects with and without sleep complaints. Sleep Res 19:398, 1990

McArthur AJ, Gillette MU, Prosser RA: Melatonin directly resets the rat suprachiasmatic circadian clock in vitro. Brain Res 565:158–161, 1991

McArthur AJ, Sack RL, Hughes RJ, et al: Melatonin, a stronger zeitgeber than light in some sighted individuals? Sleep Res 24a:527, 1995

McIntyre IM, Norman TR, Burrows GD, et al: Human melatonin suppression by light is intensity dependent. J Pineal Res 6:149–156, 1989

Miles LEM, Wilson MA: High incidence of cyclic sleep/wake disorders in the blind. Sleep Res 6:192, 1977

Miles LEM, Raynal DM, Wilson MA: Blind man living in normal society has circadian rhythms of 24.9 hours. Science 198:421–423, 1977

Minors DS, Waterhouse JM, Wirz-Justice A: A human phase-response curve to light. Neurosci Lett 133:36–40, 1991

Moldofsky H, Musisi S, Phillipson EA: Treatment of a case of advanced sleep phase syndrome by phase advance chronotherapy. Sleep 9:61–65, 1986

Monk TH: Circadian rhythm. Clin Geriatr Med 5:331–345, 1989

Monk TH, Moline ML: Removal of temporal constraints in the middle-aged and elderly: effects on sleep and sleepiness. Sleep 11:513–520, 1988

Morris M, Lack L, Dawson D: Sleep-onset insomniacs have delayed temperature rhythms. Sleep 13:1–14, 1990

Nagtegaal JE, Smits MG, Hemmes AM: Effects of melatonin in a child with delayed sleep phase syndrome. Sleep-Wake Research in The Netherlands 5:117–118, 1994

Nakagawa H, Sack RL, Lewy AJ: Sleep propensity free-runs with the temperature, cortisol and melatonin rhythms in a totally blind person. Sleep 15:330–336, 1992

Nave R, Shlitner A, Peled R, et al: Melatonin improves evening napping. Sleep Res 24:47, 1995

Ohta T, Iwata T, Terashima M, et al: Chronobiological study of delayed sleep phase syndrome. Sleep Res 12:270, 1983

Ohta T, Ando K, Iwata T, et al: Treatment of persistent sleep-wake schedule disorders in adolescents with methylcobalamin (vitamin B_{12}). Sleep 14: 414–418, 1991

Ohta T, Iwata T, Kayukawa Y, et al: Daily activity and persistent sleep-wake schedule disorders. Prog Neuropsychopharmacol Biol Psychiatry 16: 529–537, 1992

Okawa M, Nanami T, Wada S, et al: Four congenitally blind children with circadian sleep-wake rhythm disorder. Sleep 10:101–110, 1987

Okawa M, Mishima K, Nanami T, et al: Vitamin B12 treatment for sleep-wake rhythm disorders. Sleep 13:15–23, 1990

Okawa M, Uchiyama M, Shirakawa S, et al: Favourable effects of combined treatment with vitamin B_{12} and bright light for sleep-wake rhythm disorders, in Sleep-Wakefulness. Edited by Kumar VM, Mallick HN, Nayar U. New Delhi, Wiley Eastern Ltd., 1993, pp 71–77

Okawa M, Uchiyama M, Ozaki S, et al: The relationship between sleep-wake rhythm and body temperature rhythm in delayed sleep phase syndrome (DSPS) and non-24-hour sleep-wake rhythm. Society for Treatment of Biological Rhythms Abstract 6:19, 1994

Oldani A, Ferini-Strambi L, Zucconi M, et al: Melatonin and delayed sleep phase syndrome: ambulatory polygraphic evaluation. NeuroReport 6: 132–134, 1994

Oren DA, Wehr TA: Hypernychthemeral syndrome after chronotherapy for delayed sleep phase syndrome. N Engl J Med 327; 1762, 1992

Oren DA, Turner EH, Wehr TA: Abnormal circadian rhythms of plasma melatonin and body temperature in the delayed sleep phase syndrome [letter]. J Neurol Neurosurg Psychiatry 58:379, 1995

Palm L, Blennow G, Wetterberg L: Correction of non-24-hour sleep/wake cycle by melatonin in a blind retarded boy. Ann Neurology 29: 336–339, 1991

Pelayo RP, Thorpy MJ, Glovinsky P: Prevalence of delayed sleep phase syndrome in adolescents. Sleep Res 12:239, 1988

Pittendrigh CS: Circadian systems: entrainment, in Handbook of Behavioral Neurobiology: Biological Rhythms. Edited by Aschoff J. New York, Plenum Press, 1981, pp 95–124

Pittendrigh CS, Daan S: Circadian oscillations in rodents: A systematic increase in their frequency with age. Science 186:548–550, 1974

Pittendrigh CS, Daan S: A functional analysis of circadian pacemakers in nocturnal rodents: I. The stability and lability of spontaneous frequency. J Comp Physiology 106:291–331, 1976a

Pittendrigh CS, Daan S: A functional analysis of circadian pacemakers in nocturnal rodents: IV. Entrainment: pacemaker as a clock. J Comp Physiology 106:291–331, 1976b

Redman J, Armstrong S, Ng KT: Free-running activity rhythms in the rat: entrainment by melatonin. Science 219:1089–1091, 1983

Regestein QR, Monk TH: Delayed sleep phase syndrome: a review of its clinical aspects. Am J Psychiatry 152:602–608, 1995

Reppert SM, Weaver DR, Rivkees SA, et al: Putative melatonin receptors are located in a human biological clock. Science 242:78–81, 1988

Rosenberg R: Assessment and treatment of delayed sleep phase syndrome, in Case Studies in Insomnia. Edited by Hauri PJ. New York, Plenum, 1991, pp 193–205

Rosenthal NE, Sack DA, Gillin JC, et al: Seasonal affective disorder: a description of the syndrome and preliminary findings with light therapy. Arch Gen Psychiatry 41:72–80, 1984

Rosenthal NE, Joseph-Vanderpool JR, Levendosky AA, et al: Phase-shifting effects of bright morning light as treatment for delayed sleep phase syndrome. Sleep 13:354–361, 1990

Sack RL, Lewy AJ, Hoban TM: Free-running melatonin rhythms in blind people: phase shifts with melatonin and triazolam administration, in Temporal Disorder in Human Oscillatory Systems. Edited by Rensing L, an der Heiden U, Mackey MC. Heidelberg, Springer, 1987, pp 219–224

Sack RL, Lewy AJ, White DM, et al: Morning versus evening light treatment for winter depression; evidence that the therapeutic effects of light are mediated by circadian phase shifts. Arch Gen Psychiatry 47:343–351, 1990

Sack RL, Lewy AJ, Blood ML, et al: Melatonin administration to blind people: phase advances and entrainment. J Biol Rhythms 6:249–261, 1991

Sack RL, Lewy AJ, Blood ML, et al: Circadian rhythm abnormalities in totally blind people: incidence and clinical significance. J Clin Endocrin Metab 75:127–134, 1992

Salín-Pascual RJ, Fuentes DG, Caraveo AN: Delayed sleep phase syndrome: report of three patients. Rev Invest Clin 40:405–412, 1988

Shirakawa S, Uchiyama M, Okawa M, et al: Characteristics of sleep parameters of sleep logs on the circadian rhythm sleep disorders. Jpn J Psychiatr Neurol 47:445–446, 1993

Singer CM, Lewy AJ: Case report: use of the dim light melatonin onset in the treatment of ASPS with bright light. Sleep Res 18:445, 1989

Strogatz SH, Kronauer RE, Czeisler CA: Circadian pacemaker interferes with sleep onset at specific times each day: role in insomnia. Am J Physiology 253:R172–R178, 1987

Terman M: Light treatment, in Principles and Practice of Sleep Medicine. Edited by Kryger M, Roth T, Dement W. Philadelphia, WB Saunders, 1993, pp 1012–1029

Thorpy MJ, Korman E, Spielman AJ, et al: Delayed sleep phase syndrome in adolescents. J Adolesc Health Care 9:22–27, 1988

Tomoda A, Miike T, Uezono K, et al: A school refusal case with biological rhythm disturbance and melatonin therapy. Brain Dev 16:71–76, 1994

Tune G: The influence of age and temperament on the adult human sleep-wakefulness pattern. Br J Psychology 60:431–441, 1969

Tzischinsky O, Lavie P: Melatonin possesses time-dependent hypnotic effects. Sleep 17:638–645, 1994

Tzischinsky O, Skene D, Epstein R, et al: Circadian rhythms in 6-sulphatoxymelatonin and nocturnal sleep in blind children. Chronobiol Int 8: 168–175, 1991

Tzischinsky O, Dagan Y, Lavie P: The effects of melatonin on the timing of sleep in patients with delayed sleep phase syndrome, in Melatonin and the Pineal Gland—from Basic Science to Clinical Application. Edited by Touitou Y, Arendt J, Pévet P. New York, Elsevier, 1993, pp 351–354

Uchiyama M, Okawa M, Shirakawa S, et al: A polysomnographic study on patients with delayed sleep phase syndrome (DSPS). Jpn J Psychiatr Neurol 46:219–221, 1992

Uruha S, Mikami A, Teshima Y, et al: Effect of triazolam for delayed sleep phase syndrome. Sleep Res 16:650, 1987

Vaughan GM, Bell R, de la Peña A: Nocturnal plasma melatonin in humans: episodic pattern and influence of light. Neurosci Lett 14:81–84, 1979

Webb WB, Swinburne H: An observational study of sleep in the aged. Perception and Motor Skills 32:895–898, 1971

Weber AL, Cary MS, Connor N, et al: Human non-24-hour sleep-wake cycles in an everyday environment. Sleep 2:347–354, 1980

Weitzman ED, Weinberg V, D'Eletto R, et al: Studies of the 24-hour rhythms of melatonin in man. J Neural Trans Suppl 13:325–337, 1978

Weitzman ED, Czeisler CA, Coleman RM, et al: Delayed sleep phase syndrome: a chronobiological disorder with sleep-onset insomnia. Arch Gen Psychiatry 38:737–746, 1981

Weitzman ED, Moline ML, Czeisler CA, et al: Chronobiology of aging: temperature, sleep-wake rhythms and entrainment. Neurobiol Aging 3: 299–309, 1982

Wetterberg L: Melatonin in humans: physiological and clinical studies [review]. J Neural Trans Suppl 13:289–294, 1978

Wever RA: The Circadian System of Man. New York, Springer-Verlag, 1979

Wever RA: Light effects on human circadian rhythms. A review of recent Andechs experiments. J Biol Rhythms 4:161–186, 1989

Wever R, Polasek J, Wildgruber C: Bright light affects human circadian rhythms. Eur J Physiology 396:85–87, 1983

Zaidan R, Geoffrian M, Brun J, et al: Melatonin is able to influence its secretion in humans: description of a phase-response curve. Neuroendocrinology 60:105–112, 1994

Zhdanova IV, Wurtman RJ, Lynch HJ, et al: Evening administration of melatonin promotes sleep in humans. Society of Neuroscience Abstracts 20:1440, 1994

Zhdanova IV, Wurtman RJ, Lynch HJ, et al: Sleep-inducing effects of low melatonin doses. Sleep Res 24:66, 1995

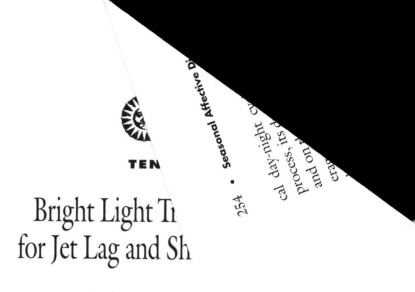

TEN

Bright Light T1
for Jet Lag and Sh

Ziad Boulos, Ph.D.

The daily cycle of rest and activity is perhaps the most visible manifestation of a species-characteristic temporal program involving virtually all aspects of animal physiology and behavior. This program is generated and coordinated by an endogenous circadian timing system that provides an internal match to the daily periodicity in the external environment (Hastings et al. 1991).

The human circadian system facilitates the initiation and maintenance of sleep at night and promotes wakefulness and activity during the day. Rapid travel across multiple time zones, and shift schedules involving night work both entail a displacement of sleep toward the activity phase of the circadian rest-activity cycle, and of wakefulness toward the rest phase. As a result, sleep quality and duration are adversely affected, as are wake-time alertness and mood and performance, the latter being caused by the combined effects of altered phase relations and prior sleep loss (Åkerstedt 1984; Comperatore and Krueger 1990; Graeber 1994; Tepas et al. 1985, 1993; U.S. Congress, Office of Technology Assessment 1991; Winget et al. 1984).

Following transmeridian travel, the symptoms of jet lag are transient, lasting until the circadian system is reentrained to the new, locle. Reentrainment, however, is a relatively slow uration depending on the number of time zones crossed he direction of travel; for flights across 5–11 time zones, average reentrainment rates of about 1.5 hours/day were obtained following westward flights, and about 1 hour/day following eastward flights (Aschoff et al. 1975; K. E. Klein and Wegmann 1980).

In contrast, circadian rhythms of shift workers show, in most cases, little or no reentrainment to the shifted sleep-work schedule, even in workers on permanent night shifts (Åkerstedt 1985; Eastman 1994; Knauth et al. 1981). Available evidence indicates limited adaptation of sleep patterns as well; self-reported sleep durations following the night shift are generally longest during permanent or prolonged shifts, followed by weekly rotating and more rapidly rotating shifts, in that order. Even during permanent night work, however, sleep duration remains shorter than during day work (Wilkinson 1992).

Phase Shifting and Entrainment of Circadian Rhythms by Light

Role of Light in Circadian Entrainment

Pittendrigh (1981) has noted that the daily light-dark (LD) cycle shows less day-to-day variability than any other daily cycle in the geophysical environment and therefore provides the most reliable index of local time. This would account for the fact that light is the primary entraining agent, or *zeitgeber*, for virtually all circadian rhythms. Indeed, most circadian pacemakers identified to date have been found to be closely associated with a photoreceptive system. Known pacemaker sites include the optic lobes of cockroaches; the eyes of molluscs and vertebrates, including mammals (Tosini and Menaker 1996); the pineal gland of nonmammalian vertebrates, which contains the photoreceptive cells involved in the regulation of melatonin secretion; and the suprachiasmatic nuclei (SCN) of mammals (and, probably, homologous hypothalamic sites in other vertebrates), which receive direct, monosynaptic input from retinal ganglion cells (for review, see Hastings et al. 1991).

Prior to 1980, the human circadian system was believed to be largely insensitive to light, and social cues were thought to be primarily responsible for human entrainment (Aschoff et al. 1971). This view was challenged by the discovery that human nighttime melatonin secretion could be suppressed by exposure to light, provided that the light was sufficiently bright: complete suppression was observed at 2,500 lux, and partial suppression at 1,500 lux. Light at 500 lux was ineffective (Lewy et al. 1980). A series of studies soon followed, clearly demonstrating that human circadian rhythms could also be phase shifted by scheduled exposure to bright light, and that this effect was not mediated by changes in the timing of the sleep-wake cycle, as originally believed (Czeisler et al. 1986; 1989; Dijk et al. 1987; Eastman 1987; Drennan et al. 1989; Duffy et al. 1996; Lewy et al. 1985; Wever et al. 1983). These and other data, including the documentation of free-running rhythms in many blind individuals, despite strict adherence to a 24-hour sleep-wake schedule (T. Klein et al. 1993; Lewy and Newsome 1983; Miles 1977; Nakagawa et al. 1992; Sack et al. 1991), increasingly indicate a primary role for light in human phase shifting and entrainment.

Human Phase-Response Curves for Light

The size and direction of light-induced phase shifts depend on the phase of the circadian cycle at which light is presented. Light exposure during the early part of an organism's subjective night causes phase delays, while light exposure during late subjective night causes phase advances. In many species, light presented during much of the subjective day is ineffective, at least for short light-exposure durations (Pittendrigh 1981). This relationship, depicted graphically in the form of a phase-response curve (PRC), has been confirmed in humans. Human PRCs have been obtained using two general procedures, one involving exposure to single bright light pulses (3–6 hours at 5,000–12,000 lux) on a dim light background (Honma and Honma 1988; Minors et al. 1991; Van Cauter et al. 1994) or following inversion of the daily sleep-wake and light-dark schedule (Jewett et al. 1994), the other consisting of 5-hour bright light pulses (7,000–12,000 lux) presented on three consecutive days following sleep-wake and light-dark schedule inversion (Czeisler et al. 1989; Jewett et al. 1997).

The PRCs derived from these two procedures are not identical and may involve different mechanisms. All single-pulse PRCs obtained thus far belong to the category of weak or type 1 PRCs, in which the maximum phase shifts are typically of the order of a few hours, and there is a more or less gradual transition between the delay and advance regions of the curve. In contrast, the triple-pulse PRC shows phase shifts of up to 12 hours, and there is an apparent discontinuity in the curve, with a sudden jump from maximum phase delays to maximum phase advances. Similar PRCs, known as strong or type 0 PRCs, have been obtained in some organisms as a result of single light pulses, but at higher light intensities and/or longer exposure durations than those that cause weak or type 1 resetting (Pittendrigh 1981). The two types of human PRC, however, share an important feature: in both cases, the transition between phase delays and phase advances occurs at or a little after the time of the minimum of the body temperature rhythm (T_{min}).

Circadian Phase Assessment

Masking Effects and the Use of Constant Routines

Accurate assessment of circadian phase is a critical requirement in studies of the circadian effects of bright light, both for determining optimal light exposure times, and for evaluating the efficacy of the treatment by measuring the size and direction of light-induced phase shifts. This is frequently based on the daily rhythm of body temperature, which provides a good index of endogenous circadian phase. However, body temperature is also directly influenced by various environmental factors, as well as by the subject's behavior, particularly motor activity, sleep, and meal intake. Such masking effects can be minimized by the use of constant routine protocols, during which subjects are required to remain awake in a resting position under constant dim illumination for at least 24 hours and are provided with small meals at frequent, regular intervals (Czeisler et al. 1985; Mills et al. 1978a).

Mathematical Demasking Procedures

Constant routines, however, are very demanding, particularly because they require prolonged sleep deprivation. A more practical alternative is provided by mathematical demasking procedures for estimating and removing the direct effects of behavior on body temperature in subjects living on a normal routine (Minors and Waterhouse 1992). The simplest of these consists of adding a constant demasking factor to temperature values recorded during sleep. The demasking factor is often derived from normative data—a mean sleep-induced lowering of rectal temperature of about 0.3°C has been reported in several studies (Barrett et al. 1993; Folkard 1989; Wever 1985a)—but may also be adjusted to individual temperature profiles. An additional step involves a negative factor that is added to wake-time temperatures and may be proportional to the type (determined from daily activity logs) or amount (measured by wrist actigraphy) of activity engaged in by the subject at different times of the day.

In a further refinement, with several variants, the diurnal temperature rhythm is modeled as the arithmetic sum of two continuous curves, representing the endogenous and exogenous components of the rhythm, respectively. One or both components may be derived from previously published normative data or from baseline recordings under normal or constant routines (Folkard 1989; Folkard et al. 1991; Minors and Waterhouse 1988). Two-component models assume that abrupt shifts of the sleep-wake schedule are accompanied immediately by an equal shift of the exogenous component. Accordingly, the phase of the endogenous rhythm is calculated after subtracting the shifted exogenous component from the overt temperature rhythm.

Validity of Mathematical Demasking

In human bright light studies, the transition between delays and advances has been found to occur at the same phase of the temperature rhythm (near the time of T_{min}), regardless of whether phase is determined from constant routine data (Czeisler et al. 1989; Van Cauter et al. 1994) or from partially demasked data (corrected for sleep-induced masking) obtained during normal routines (Eastman 1992; Minors et al. 1991). This suggests that in subjects on a normal, unshifted sleep-wake schedule, even the simplest demasking procedures can provide estimates of circadian phase that are accurate enough for determining appropriate light exposure times.

Following sleep-wake schedule shifts, the extent or rate of circadian reentrainment is consistently smaller when based on demasked temperature data than when based on raw data, both in laboratory simulations (Folkard 1989; Folkard et al. 1991; Macchi et al. 1995; Minors and Waterhouse 1988) and in field studies of shift work and jet lag (Folkard 1989; Härmä et al. 1994; Minors and Waterhouse 1993; Wever 1979). Furthermore, in some of the laboratory experiments, no differences were found between the phase shifts determined from demasked and constant routine data (Folkard et al. 1991; experiment 2 in Minors and Waterhouse 1988). In others, however, phase shifts derived from demasked data still exceeded those from constant routines, at least in some subjects (Macchi et al. 1995; experiment 1 in Minors and Waterhouse 1988).

The validity of demasking is more difficult to ascertain in the field studies, none of which included constant routines. However, two of these studies applied similar demasking procedures to the rectal temperature rhythms of nurses working the night shift. In one study, phase shifts of 4–5 hours were obtained on the first night shift (Minors and Waterhouse 1993), whereas in the other, the mean phase shift on the second night shift was only 1.65 hours (Härmä et al. 1994). The disparity between these results suggests that demasking may have been less effective in the first study than in the second.

In summary, mathematical demasking procedures provide circadian phase estimates that are more accurate than those obtained from raw temperature data. However, demasking procedures do not take into account possible circadian variations in the masking effects of sleep (Mills et al. 1978b; Wever 1985a) and physical activity (Knauth et al. 1981), nor do they allow for differences in sleep-induced masking as a function of sleep continuity and slow-wave sleep content, and of prior sleep and wake durations (Minors et al. 1994). These factors are more likely to influence phase assessment following sleep-wake schedule shifts, particularly in field situations. Under these conditions, demasking procedures can sometimes give inaccurate phase and phase-shift estimates.

The Timing of T_{min}

Individual phase assessments based on body temperature recordings, even recordings obtained during normal routines, remain impractical for widespread use in shift work and jet lag applications. Hormonal rhythms, particularly that of melatonin secretion, measured in plasma, urine, or saliva, can also provide good indexes of circadian phase, but they require frequent sampling and are therefore also impractical.

The most convenient solution, one adopted by several investigators, is to schedule bright light treatment at a constant clock time, based on normative data on the timing of T_{min}. The reliability of this approach must therefore depend on the variability in the time of T_{min} in the subject population. Data from several studies in which T_{min} was determined during constant routines are summarized in Table 10–1. Most of the studies were performed on young male subjects, but even within this restricted population, the results show considerable variability. Thus, mean T_{min} was found to occur around 5:00 A.M. in some studies (Czeisler et al. 1990; Dawson et al. 1992; Kraüchi and Wirz-Justice 1994; Van Cauter et al. 1994), but at 6:48 A.M. in another (Czeisler et al. 1992). In the latter study, individual T_{min} times in young male subjects spanned a 5-hour range, from about 4:00 A.M. to 9:00 A.M. (see Figure 1 in Czeisler et al. 1992). Constant routine data from women and from older men are much more limited, but they suggest earlier T_{min} times in both of these groups (Table 10–1). In women, the amplitude of the endogenous temperature rhythm varies with the phase of the menstrual cycle (Rogacz et al. 1988), whereas the phase of the rhythm is either unaffected (Lee 1988; Wagner et al. 1992) or occurs at a later hour in the luteal phase than in the follicular phase (Rogacz et al. 1988; Veith et al. 1993).

TABLE 10–1

Mean times of T_{min} obtained in male and female subjects in different age groups during constant routines

Gender	n	Age Mean	Age Range	Time of T_{min}[1] mean $\pm$ SD (minutes)	Reference
M	8	–	(22–29)	04:59	Czeisler et al. 1990
M	8	23.3	(18–29)	06:14 $\pm$ 64	Shanahan and Czeisler 1991
M	8	29.7	(25–35)	04:46[2] $\pm$ 68	Dawson et al. 1992
M	27	21.9	(18–31)	06:48 (06:21–07:16)[3]	Czeisler et al. 1992
M	17	–	(20–30)	05:00 $\pm$ 85	Van Cauter et al. 1994
M	7	31	(26–38)	05:19 $\pm$ 29	Kräuchi and Wirz-Justice 1994
M	9	24.4	(18–30)	06:29 $\pm$ 78	Boivin et al. 1994
M	32	21.7	(–)	06:14 $\pm$ 47	Duffy et al. 1996
M	11	69.6	(65–85)	05:14 (04:30–05:59)[3]	Czeisler et al. 1992
F	7	–	(21–35)	04:20[4] $\pm$ 144	Wagner et al. 1992
F	6	30	(21–39)	03:16 $\pm$ 59	Dahl et al. 1993
F	10	71.7	(65–85)	04:39 (03:15–06:03)[3]	Czeisler et al. 1992

[1] Some studies report two estimates of the time of T_{min}, obtained by fitting the data with a one-component (24-hour) and a two-component function (24-hour and 12-hour), respectively. Only the values obtained with the latter method are listed here. [2] Mean of two constant routines, performed 7 days apart. [3] 95% confidence interval. [4] Mean of four constant routines, performed at different phases of the menstrual cycle.

The extent of intraindividual variability in the time of T_{min} has been examined in young male (Dawson et al. 1992) and female subjects (Wagner et al. 1992) who underwent two and four sequential constant routines, respectively, in most cases at weekly intervals. In both groups, mean absolute phase differences between constant routines were about 1 hour, with standard deviations of about 30 minutes.

One final approach consists of scheduling light exposure times at a fixed interval relative to some readily determined phase marker, typically habitual wake onset, rather than at a fixed clock time. In young men, T_{min} was initially reported to precede habitual wake onset by 2–3 hours (Czeisler et al. 1989, 1990; Minors et al. 1991), but in a subsequent, more detailed report, T_{min}, measured in young men and in elderly men and women during constant routines, occurred about 1.5 hours before habitual wake onset in all three groups (Czeisler et al. 1992). This latter result is encouraging because it suggests that light-treatment programs based on habitual wake onset may be relatively immune to age and gender differences with regard to the timing of T_{min}. However, a recent analysis of data from several studies involving 101 young men (mean age 23.4, range 18–30) and 44 older men and women (mean age 68.3, range 64–81) showed that, on average, T_{min} fell 39 minutes earlier in the older than in the younger subjects (05:15 ± 2:00 versus 05:54 ± 1:30), but the interval between the time of T_{min} and wake onset was also 39 minutes shorter in the older group (1.73 ± 1.68 hours versus 2.38 ± 1.16 hours) (Duffy et al. 1997). Thus, scheduling light exposure in relation to habitual wake onset may not provide a more reliable approach than one in which light exposure is scheduled at a fixed clock time.

Bright Light Treatment

Laboratory Simulations

Laboratory studies intended as simulations of night work and of transmeridian travel are essentially similar, both involving abrupt shifts of the sleep-wake schedule. In general, however, the sleep-wake schedule is delayed in shift work simulations and advanced in jet lag simulations. Some shift work studies also include simulated work tasks, and the subjects follow the typical work-sleep-leisure sequence of workers on the night shift.

The choice of shift direction is based on the directional asymmetry of circadian reentrainment, which is usually faster following phase delays than following phase advances (Aschoff et al. 1975). This has led to the recommendation that shift work schedules rotate in a forward or delaying direction (morning-afternoon/evening-night) rather than in a backward direction (e.g., Knauth and Rutenfranz

1982), and most simulation studies are designed accordingly. In the case of transmeridian travel, the direction of the shift is dictated by the traveler's destination, and advance shifts (simulating eastward travel) are usually studied in the laboratory because they are more difficult to adapt to than delay shifts. The studies reviewed below are organized by direction of shift, regardless of whether they were intended to simulate shift work or jet lag.

Sleep-wake schedule delays

One of the earliest laboratory simulations compared the reentrainment of two subjects following two 6-hour delays of an artificial LD cycle, 2 weeks apart (Wever 1985b). Light intensity was kept below 1,500 lux in the first condition, and between 2,000 and 5,000 lux in the second. Mean reentrainment rates of the temperature rhythms on the first three days after the shift were 1.0 hours/day under the lower illumination and 1.4 hours/day under bright light.

Wever's study is unusual in that the participants were exposed to dim or bright light throughout the entire light portion of the LD cycle, and they were free to choose their daily sleep and wake times. In other studies, exposure to bright light was limited to a few hours per day, and sleep was allowed only during scheduled bedtimes. Thus, Dawson and Campbell (1991) compared the adaptation of two groups of young subjects during three consecutive night shifts (simulated night work from 12:00 midnight to 8:00 A.M.) that involved a delay of the sleep period of about 9 hours. One group was exposed to bright light (6,000 lux) between midnight and 4:00 A.M. on the first night shift, and dim light (<200 lux) during the remainder of scheduled waketime, whereas the other group was exposed to dim light throughout. On the third night shift, mean T_{min}, determined from partially demasked data, was delayed by 2.4 hours in the control group and by 5.9 hours in the experimental. The bright light group also slept better than the dim light group and showed higher onshift alertness. More recently, Campbell (1995) used a similar light-treatment protocol with middle-aged subjects, but the experimental group was also exposed to moderately bright light (1,000 lux) throughout the second and third night shifts. The mean phase shift observed following light treatment (6.25 hours) was comparable to that obtained in the young subjects. Suprisingly, however, neither daytime sleep nor onshift alertness and performance improved significantly relative to the dim light condition. These results suggest that the sleep of middle-aged subjects may be less phase tolerant than that of young subjects, and may improve only following complete reentrainment to the shifted sleep-wake schedule (Campbell 1995).

Dawson et al. (1995) also used a similar design with young subjects, except that bright light exposure (4,000–7,000 lux at midnight to 4:00 A.M.) was scheduled on all three night shifts, and dim light melatonin onset served as the circadian phase marker. On the day following the third night shift, the control and experimental groups showed mean phase delays of 4.2 hours and 8.8 hours, respectively.

Gander and Samel (1991) recorded rectal temperature and other physiological variables in 4 subjects undergoing 6-hour sleep-wake schedule delays on two consecutive days (total phase delay of 12 hours). The subjects were studied twice and were exposed both times to bright light (>3,500 lux) for 5 hours on the two shift days and the following day. In the experimental condition, bright light was scheduled to end at the predicted time of T_{min} on each of the three treatment days, whereas in the control condition, bright light was centered on the predicted time of the temperature maximum, a time at which light treatment was expected to have no phase-shifting effect. However, the temperature rhythms were delayed by a little over 2 hours/day regardless of the timing of bright light.

The latter results are all the more surprising because the subjects remained in bed throughout the two 11-day conditions, thereby minimizing activity-induced masking. It is possible, however, that by reducing the amplitude of the overt temperature rhythm, the continuous bedrest procedure also increased the relative contribution of sleep-induced masking. This may account for the unexpectedly high reentrainment rate observed in the control condition, higher even than in Wever's (1985b) bright light condition.

The phase-delaying effects of moderately bright light (1.200 lux) were assessed by Deacon and Arendt (1994). The light treatment was administered for 6 hours on three successive nights, starting at 8:00 P.M., 10:00 P.M., and midnight, respectively. Sleep was scheduled immediately following each light exposure. Circadian rhythms of melatonin secretion, measured on the first posttreatment day, showed phase delays of 2–3 hours relative to baseline. These results suggest that timed exposure to relatively low illuminance can cause significant phase shifts (see also Boivin et al. 1994), although in the absence of dim light controls, the extent of the phase shift attributable to the light treatment itself is difficult to estimate.

Sleep-wake schedule advances

Honma et al. (1991) compared reentrainment rates following an 8-hour advance shift in subjects exposed to either bright (5,000 lux) or dim light for 3 hours on three consecutive days. Light exposure began at 7:00 A.M. on the day of the shift and was advanced by 3 hours on each of the following two days. Faster reentrainment of the raw (masked) body temperature rhythm in bright than in dim light was observed in four of the five participants studied. Similar procedures were followed in a more recent study (Honma et al. 1995), except that daily light treatment was scheduled on 11 days. As in the earlier study, the timing of light exposure was advanced by 3 hours on the second and third treatment days, but it remained fixed on the following 8 days. In the bright light condition, 2 subjects reentrained antidromically, by phase delay rather than by phase advance. In the remaining 7 subjects, plasma melatonin onset advanced by an average of 2.44 hours, 4.28 hours, and 6.43 hours after the second, fifth, and eighth bright light treatments, respectively, whereas corresponding advances in the dim light condition were 1.17 hours, 1.86 hours, and 4.20 hours.

Two other studies proved less successful. In the first (Moline et al. 1989, 1990), subjects were exposed to 4-hour pulses of bright (2,500 lux) or dim light following a 6-hour advance shift. Light exposure began at the preshift mid-sleep time on the day of the shift, and immediately after waking on the next three days. Thus, a subject who slept from midnight-8:00 A.M. during baseline would be exposed to light starting at 4:00 A.M. on the first day, and at 2:00 A.M. on the following days. The bright light treatment, however, failed to accelerate reentrainment of the temperature rhythms, and no substantial differences were found between the sleep patterns of the two groups. In the second study (Samel et al. 1992), bright light exposure was scheduled for 4 hours on the first two days following a similar 6-hour advance shift. The light treatment began at 4:00 A.M. for the experimental group and at 1:00 P.M. for the control group, but reentrainment rates were similar in the two conditions.

The absence of a significant effect of the experimental treatment in these two studies may be attributable to the timing of the light exposure; in both cases, the initial light treatment was centered around 6:00 A.M.—a little later than the mean time of T_{min} reported by some investigators, but slightly earlier than that found by others (Table 10–1). In such close proximity to the transition point of the group PRC, light exposure may cause phase advances, phase delays, or have no effect at all (in the case of type I PRCs), depending on the specific characteristics of the individual's PRC (Jewett et al. 1994; Minors et al. 1991; Mitchell et al. 1995; Van Cauter et al. 1994).

Additionally, in the study by Moline et al. (1989, 1990), the second light exposure was 2 hours earlier than the first. This may have exceeded the advance of the subjects' rhythms that was caused by the first light exposure, because single pulses of bright light have been found to cause maximum phase advances of a little over 1 hour (Dawson et al. 1993; Jewett et al. 1994; Van Cauter et al. 1994). It is possible therefore that the second light exposure fell even earlier relative to the PRC transition point than the first. Finally, phase assessments in these studies were based on raw temperature data and may have been subject to strong masking effects.

Field Studies

Simulated shift work studies

Laboratory and field simulations of shift work both involve subjects drawn from the general, non–shift worker population. In field simulations, however, the subjects sleep in their own homes, and at least some of their wake time is spent outside the laboratory. They are therefore exposed on a daily basis to natural daylight and various social time cues.

In one such study (Czeisler et al. 1990), subjects received either bright (7,000–12,000 lux) or dim (150 lux) light throughout four consecutive simulated night shifts in the laboratory (midnight to 8:00 A.M.). All subjects returned to their homes in the morning; those in the bright light group slept between 9:00 A.M. and

5:00 P.M., in specially darkened bedrooms, whereas subjects in the dim light group were free to sleep at times of their own choosing and used only existing window shades and curtains when they slept. Body temperature rhythms, recorded during constant routines before and after the night shifts, were delayed on average by 9.6 hours following bright light treatment, but showed a small advance after dim light treatment (Figure 10–1). Similar shifts were observed in several other physiological and behavioral measures. The fact that complete reentrainment was obtained despite exposure to natural

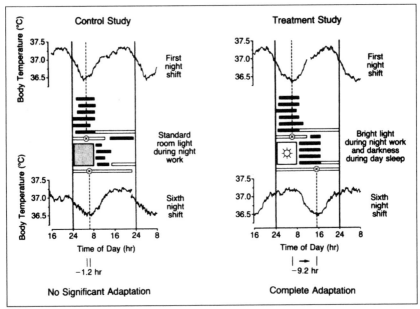

FIGURE 10–1. Body temperature data recorded from one subject during constant routines performed immediately before (top panels) and after (bottom panels) four days of exposure to dim (stippled box) or bright light (open box with solar symbol) during simulated night shifts. Solid bars in the middle panels indicate daily sleep episodes, open bars constant routines, and circled x's the calculated times of T_{min}. The temperature rhythm showed a small phase delay of 1.2 hours in the control condition, and a large delay of 9.2 hours following bright light treatment. Segments of the temperature curves are double plotted.

Source. Reprinted by permission of *The New England Journal of Medicine* from Czeisler CA, Johnson MP, Duffy JF, et al.: "Exposure to bright light and darkness to treat physiologic maladaptation to night work." *N Engl J Med* 322: 1253–1259 1990.

daylight on the way home in the morning attests to the efficacy of this light-treatment protocol.

Eastman and Miescke (1990) examined the effect of bright light exposure (2,000 or 4,000 lux) on circadian entrainment to a 26-hour sleep-wake schedule. The schedule was followed for 13 days, during which time the subjects lived at home and slept in darkened bedrooms, going to bed and getting up 2 hours later each day. Subjects in the evening-light condition were exposed to bright light for 2 hours before scheduled bedtime and to dim light for 6 hours after waking, and those in the morning-light condition were exposed to 2 hours of bright light on waking, and 6 hours of dim light before bedtime. In both conditions, the subjects wore dark goggles when they went outdoors during the scheduled dim light periods. A third, natural-light-only condition was also included. Entrainment, assessed by periodogram analysis of raw temperature recordings, was judged successful if the periodogram showed a significant peak near 26 hours but not near 24 hours. By these criteria, 74% of the subjects were entrained in the evening light condition, but only 22% in the other two conditions. In a subsequent study, the sleep-wake schedule was first delayed by 2 hours/day, then kept fixed at a 24-hour period, and finally advanced by 2 hours/day. The subjects received bright light in the evening and dim light in the morning during the first two conditions, and morning bright light and evening dim light during the third. Inspection of the partially demasked temperature rhythms, however, showed that most had not entrained to the shifting schedules, possibly because of inadequate size and placement of the bright light sources (Gallo and Eastman 1993).

Although designed for workers on rotating 2- or 3-shift systems, such gradually delaying or advancing schedules may be too inconvenient for many shift workers because they require a daily restructuring of both sleep and waketime activity, even on days off (Eastman 1994). More recently, Eastman and her colleagues have followed a different approach, combining various light-treatment protocols with abrupt, 12-hour shifts of the sleep-wake schedule. One such study (Eastman 1992) included 6-hour bright light exposures (5,000 lux) on the first four nights, and 3-hour exposures on the following 7 nights, the latter aimed at maintaining the phase position reached after the 6-hour exposures. The subjects slept in darkened bedrooms and wore goggles to avoid exposure to bright daylight. Two different temporal patterns of light exposure were studied: in the stationary pattern, all bright light exposures began at the same clock time, whereas, in the moving pattern, the 6-hour exposures were delayed by 1 hour each day (Figure 10–2). Regardless of the pattern of light exposure, the temperature rhythms shifted gradually in 21 of 24 subjects, at an initial rate of about 2 hours/day. The direction of the shift depended on the timing of bright light relative to baseline T_{min}, in a manner consistent with published PRCs.

Eastman et al. (1994) compared the relative contributions of bright light during simulated night shifts and dark goggles during daylight to the reentrainment of body temperature rhythms following a 12-hour schedule shift. A total of 50 subjects spent the first two of eight night shifts in the laboratory, and were exposed to either bright (5,000 lux) or dim light (<500 lux) for 6 hours, centered around the time of T_{min}. About half the subjects in each condition wore goggles when they went outside in the morning. Mean absolute phase shifts, calculated from demasked temperature rhythms on the last four days of the treatment, were largest with bright light and goggles (7.9 hours), and smallest with dim light and no goggles (3.2 hours). Interestingly, the mean phase shift with goggles alone (5.6 hours) was about the same as with bright light alone (6.0 hours). In addition, whereas subjects who wore goggles showed both phase advances and phase delays, those who didn't showed only phase advances. Thus, the use of goggles affected both the extent and direction of circadian reentrainment.

The phase shifting effects of 3-hour and 6-hour bright light pulses administered during simulated night shifts were compared by Eastman et al. (1995b). The design was similar to that of the preceding study, except that bright light was scheduled on all eight night shifts, and none of the subjects wore goggles. Mean absolute phase shifts were somewhat greater in the 6-hour than in the 3-hour condition (9.4 hours and 8.1 hours, respectively), but the difference was not statistically significant.

The results of a recent study (Mitchell et al. 1995) confirm the importance of the timing of bright light in determining the size and direction of the resulting phase shifts. The participants were exposed

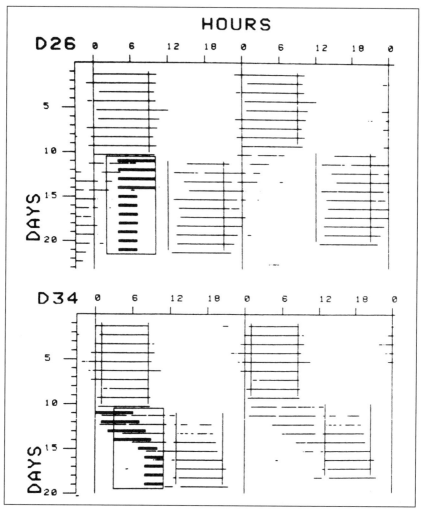

FIGURE 10–2. Double-plotted body temperature records of two subjects exposed to bright light at times indicated by thick horizontal bars. Thin horizontal lines indicate raw temperature values below the daily mean, vertical lines indicate scheduled bedtimes, and rectangles indicate times of the 8-hour simulated night shifts during which the subjects avoided exposure to daylight. The top panel shows a gradual phase advance of the temperature rhythm in a subject exposed to a stationary light pattern; the bottom panel illustrates a gradual phase delay in a subject exposed to a moving light pattern.

Source. Adapted from Eastman CI: High-intensity light for circadian adaptation to a 12-h shift of the sleep schedule. Am J Physiol 263:R428–R436, 1992. Used with permission.

to bright light (5,000 lux) for 3 hours on eight successive nights following either a 9-hour delay or a 9-hour advance of their sleep-wake schedule, with the midpoint of the bright light pulses either preceding or following the time of baseline T_{min}. Following the sleep-schedule delay, the temperature rhythms showed a larger phase delay when bright light was centered before T_{min} than when it was scheduled after (8.8 hours and 4.4 hours, respectively), whereas following the sleep-schedule advance, the rhythms advanced more when bright light was centered after T_{min} than when it was centered before (6.7 hours and 0.7 hours, respectively).

However, not all phase shifts were in the expected direction, and several individuals showed large phase delays despite bright light exposure centered after T_{min}. This may have resulted from the fact that the minimum interval between light pulse midpoint and baseline T_{min} was only 30 minutes, which left little room for inaccuracy in circadian phase estimates, or for possible individual differences in the time of T_{min} relative to the PRC delay-to-advance transition point. Indeed, in one study, the PRC transition point fell about 1 hour after, rather than exactly at, the average time of T_{min} (Van Cauter et al. 1994).

Studies on shift workers

Published studies of light treatment for real shift workers are understandably few; such treatment typically requires spending at least 2 hours/day in front of or under a bright light source, over a period of several days, and at times likely to overlap with work hours. In most cases, practical considerations have also precluded direct assessment of circadian parameters. Nevertheless, the majority of individuals who participated in such studies felt that the treatment had been helpful. This includes pilot studies involving student nurses on night duty (Ehrenstein and Weber 1990) and members of a television news crew (Powers et al. 1989), the treatment in the latter case consisting of evening exposure to only 30 minutes of bright light at 10,000 lux. In both studies, the subjects reported increased alertness during nightwork and better daytime sleep following the start of bright light treatment. Beneficial effects of bright light treatment were also reported by barge operators in the North Sea (Bougrine et al. 1995), as well as by officers on a rotating shift schedule at the Nuclear Regulatory Commission Headquarters Operations Center (Baker et al. 1995).

Härmä et al. (1993) studied a group of eight Finnish letter sorters who worked three consecutive night shifts (11:00 P.M. to 6:00 A.M.) in a shift work laboratory and were exposed to bright light (2,500 lux) from 11:00 P.M. to 3:00 A.M. on all three nights. Body temperature measurements indicated larger phase delays in most subjects during the treatment week (mean delay of 5.1 hours) than during the control week (mean delay of 2.8 hours). A decrease in subjective sleepiness and in simple reaction time was also observed, although the differences were not statistically significant. A light-treatment program was also implemented by Budnick et al. (1995) for a group of industrial workers at an Exxon Chemical Company plant in Baytown, Texas. The subjects worked rotating 12-hour shifts on a 16-day cycle consisting of 4 day shifts, 4 days off, 4 night shifts, and 4 days off. The light-treatment phase of the study lasted 3 months and consisted of an increase in ambient light intensity throughout the work shifts from 30 lux to 1,200–1,500 lux. In addition, the workers were exposed to bright light (4,000–8,000 lux) at scheduled times within the night shift. During night shifts in the baseline condition, urinary levels of 6-hydroxymelatonin sulfate, a metabolite of melatonin, were higher in late night/early morning (3:00 A.M. to 9:00 A.M.) than during the day (9:00 A.M. to 10:00 P.M.) in 9 of 10 subjects, whereas during night shifts in the light-treatment phase, nighttime levels decreased in all cases and were lower than daytime levels in 5 subjects. In general, however, self-reported sleep patterns and worktime alertness and performance levels showed little or no improvement during the light-treatment phase. Furthermore, a number of adverse effects were reported, the most common being difficulty adjusting to being off work following the night shifts (54%), as well as increased glare and the perception that the lights were too bright (38%).

The most extensive field trials, however, were carried out at NASA, with the aim of phase shifting the circadian rhythms of astronauts in preparation for night work aboard the space shuttle, as well as those of ground support personnel working the night shift. Initial trials took place in 1990 and involved four crew members of shuttle mission STS-35 (Czeisler et al. 1991). During the week preceding the scheduled launch, the subjects were exposed to 10,000 lux of light for about 9 hours on four nights, followed by maintenance light treatment (1,500–3,000 lux) on two nights. On that first occasion, cancellation of the launch provided the opportunity for measuring urinary 6-hydroxymelatonin sulfate levels. The high levels observed during daytime sleep and low levels at night indicated substantial phase shifts of the subjects' rhythms. The success of these procedures was also confirmed by the astronauts' subjective reports.

Most recently, a group of eight shuttle astronauts underwent a week-long phase resetting protocol before launch (Whitson et al. 1995). The protocol included an 11-hour delay of the sleep-wake schedule, either gradual or abrupt, combined with daily exposure to bright light (7,000–12,000 lux) for 2–6 hours on six consecutive days. The timing of bright light exposure was delayed by 1–2 hours on most treatment days. The subjects also avoided exposure to bright light at certain times of the day by remaining in a dimly lit area or by wearing dark goggles. By the end of the treatment week, melatonin and cortisol rhythms, assessed from saliva and urine samples collected during scheduled wake time, showed phase delays of 7–15 hours in seven of the eight subjects, indicating virtually complete reentrainment.

Light-treatment protocols designed for payload support crews working in control rooms at NASA's Marshall Space Flight Center have also been implemented in connection with several space shuttle missions (Eastman et al. 1995a). Results obtained during the course of two such missions were recently reported by Stewart et al. (1995). The treatment included a gradual delaying of sleep, starting several days before the first night shift and again after the end of the mission, with exposure to bright light (10,000 lux) for up to 5 hours/day before each scheduled sleep period. Some protocols also included shorter maintenance light treatments during the mission. The subjects slept in darkened bedrooms and wore dark goggles when they were outdoors at times when exposure to bright daylight would have hindered reentrainment. Control subjects received no treatment and were free to choose their own sleep schedules. Subjects in the treatment group reported better daytime sleep, less mental and physical fatigue, and improved alertness, concentration, and speed of work while on night duty.

Field studies of jet lag

An early pilot study by Daan and Lewy (1984) involved scheduled exposure to natural daylight following eastward flights across nine time zones. Two subjects participated in that study and were exposed to daylight for 3 hours on the first postflight day and on the following six days. Light exposure times, derived from animal PRCs, were intended to phase delay one subject's rhythms and advance the other's. The results were consistent with the authors' predictions, although, as discussed elsewhere (Boulos et al. 1995), the interpretation of these results is complicated by several factors. Nevertheless, the study is notable for being the first field attempt at using bright light for treating jet lag by phase shifting human circadian rhythms, particularly as it preceded the publication of the first human PRC by several years. It is also one of the few studies to have relied on natural rather than artificial bright light.

Czeisler and Allan (1987) applied a light treatment protocol to a single subject following his return from Tokyo to Boston. The subject was exposed to bright artificial light (7,000–12,000 lux) for several hours on three consecutive days, starting in early afternoon. Temperature phase assessments during constant routines before and after the light treatment showed a large delay of 11.25 hours.

Finally, Sasaki et al. (1989) recorded sleep EEG in four subjects before and after an eastward flight across eight time zones, from Tokyo to San Francisco. The first three days in San Francisco, the subjects were exposed to either bright (>3,000 lux) or dim light (<500 lux) for 3 hours, starting at 11:00 A.M., or 3:00 A.M. Tokyo time. On the first four nights, the two participants who received bright light showed higher sleep efficiency and less waking after sleep onset than the two participants who received dim light, particularly during the first half of the night. Although no circadian phase measures were reported, the improvement in sleep observed following bright light exposure suggests that the treatment may have accelerated reentrainment of the subjects' rhythms.

Alerting Effects of Light: Applications to Shift Work

Exposure to bright (>2,000 lux) or moderately bright light (500–2,000 lux) at night has been shown to exert direct effects on a number of physiological, endocrine, and behavioral functions. In particular, several laboratory studies have demonstrated that such exposure significantly enhances nighttime alertness and performance (Badia et al. 1991; Campbell and Dawson 1990; Daurat et al. 1993; French et al. 1990, 1991; Horne et al. 1991; Matsunaga et al. 1995; Myers and Badia 1993; but see Dollins et al. 1993).

In some of these studies, the alerting effects of bright light exposure were shown to be independent of its phase-resetting properties. For example, higher alertness and performance levels were observed during bright light sessions (5,000–10,000 lux) that alternated with dim light sessions (50 lux) every 90 minutes (Badia et al. 1991). These effects cannot therefore be attributed to any circadian phase shifts caused by the bright light treatment. In another study, participants were exposed to bright (3,000 lux) or dim light (150 lux) throughout a 24-hour constant routine protocol (Daurat et al. 1993). The bright light treatment improved alertness and performance during the night, but the phase and amplitude of the participants' temperature rhythms did not differ between the two conditions.

Horne et al. (1991) have shown that hourly 10-minute exposure to 2,000 lux green light enhances vigilance performance and reduces subjective sleepiness at night. Since performance and sleepiness were assessed between rather than during the 10-minute treatments, these findings indicate that the alerting effects of bright light can extend beyond the actual time of light exposure. A similar procedure was subsequently applied in a field study involving nurses on night shift (Costa et al. 1993). The treatment consisted of four 20-minute exposures to 2,350 lux, scheduled between 8:30 P.M. and 4:30 A.M. Modest improvements were observed in performance on a letter cancellation task, as well as in subjective measures of physical fitness, tiredness, and sleepiness.

In summary, these observations suggest that treatments that involve exposure to bright light during night work, though designed for and found capable of inducing large phase shifts (e.g., Czeisler et al. 1990), may have the added benefit of directly enhancing shift worker alertness and performance (Badia et al. 1991; French et al. 1990, 1991; Myers and Badia 1993). Other alertness-enhancing light treatments—those involving brief, intermittent exposure to bright light (Costa et al. 1993; Horne et al. 1991), or continuous exposure to more moderate intensity levels (Campbell and Dawson 1990; Myers and Badia 1993)—are likely to have only small phase-resetting effects (cf. Boivin et al. 1994; Deacon and Arendt 1994), especially if the subjects are also exposed to natural daylight on the way home in the morning. Such treatments would therefore be particularly useful in shift work applications in which large phase shifts are either unnecessary or undesirable (see later discussion).

Practical Considerations

Although bright light programs for phase-shifting human circadian rhythms rest on firm theoretical and empirical grounds (Dijk et al. 1995), their implementation within the constraints imposed by long-distance travel and especially by shift work schedules, in their endless variety, faces a number of challenges. The issues considered here involve the timing, duration, and intensity of bright light exposure, and the means of achieving it.

Treatments for Jet Lag

Bright light protocols intended as treatment for jet lag have called for daily light exposures lasting 3–4 hours, because shorter durations may not produce large enough phase shifts—even 4-hour exposures have had little or no effect in some studies—whereas longer durations are probably unrealistic for many travelers. Most of these protocols have sought to maximize the phase-resetting effects of the treatment by scheduling bright light exposure near the estimated time of T_{min}, on the first as well as on subsequent treatment days, based on data from human PRC studies indicating that maximum delays and advances are obtained with bright light exposures centered shortly before and shortly after the time of T_{min}, respectively.

But although there may be an advantage to scheduling light treatment near that phase of the circadian cycle, this advantage must be weighed against the risk of the light exposure falling on the opposite side of the PRC transition point, thereby causing phase shifts in the wrong direction. The risk is especially great in field settings, because of the difficulty in obtaining accurate, individual measures of circadian phase. Under these conditions, it may be preferable to allow a wider safety margin between the midpoint of light exposure and the estimated time of T_{min}. In fact, close proximity to T_{min} may not always be advantageous: in a recent study, for example, light exposures (5 hours at 1,260 lux), centered 1.5 hours and 4.3 hours after T_{min}, produced similar phase advances (Boivin et al. 1994).

Several transmeridian flight schedules provide the opportunity of using timed exposure to natural daylight as a means of accelerating circadian reentrainment. Following eastward flights across four to eight time zones, for example, the advance portion of the PRC falls in the late morning or afternoon hours of the new local day-night cycle, and exposure to daylight at those times would therefore be expected to facilitate reentrainment. In contrast, optimal light exposure times following westward flights often fall after sunset in the new time zone (depending on the number of time zones crossed, as well as on season and latitude). In these circumstances, portable artificial light sources, including head-mounted devices, provide a convenient means of bright light delivery, although the efficacy of such devices has yet to be established conclusively. Regardless of the method used, avoiding exposure to bright daylight at times when such exposure would be expected to cause phase shifts in the wrong direction should also contribute to faster reentrainment.

Detailed instructions about when to seek exposure to light and darkness on specific trips, depending on the direction of travel and the number of time zones crossed, are provided in a book by Oren et al. (1993) that is directed to the lay public reader. The authors assume that, in individuals who normally go to sleep between 10:00 P.M. and 12:00 midnight and who wake up between 6:00 and 8:00 A.M., the PRC transition point between delays and advances falls at 4:00 A.M. Accordingly, on the first day following a westward flight, they recommend exposure to bright light during the 3-hour period ending at 4:00 A.M. (or its equivalent in the new time zone), while on the day following an eastward flight, they recommend light exposure for 3 hours starting at 4:00 A.M. On subsequent days, the recommended light exposure times are delayed or advanced by 2 hours/day during westward and eastward trips, respectively, on the assumption that the circadian system of travelers following the recommended procedures will have shifted by this amount following flights in either direction.

A more flexible guide for determining light-exposure schedules is also available in the form of computer software recently described by Houpt et al. (1996). User-entered itineraries are depicted graphically, along with the ambient lighting conditions (including times of sunset, sunrise, and associated twilights) at the point of departure, during layovers, and at the final destination. Recommended times for exposure to light and darkness are calculated on the basis of a default PRC, with the transition between delays and advances preceding the user's habitual wake-up time by 3 hours; the program also assumes daily shifts of 3 hours, on trips in either direction, and light-exposure times are therefore delayed or advanced by 3 hours/day. However, the phase reference used, the time of the PRC transition point in relation to that phase reference, and the size of the daily shift can all be modified by the user.

Although the light-treatment schedules recommended by both guides seem reasonable, it should be kept in mind that they are based on a limited literature consisting primarily of studies in controlled laboratory settings, using specified light-exposure parameters, and that, except for anecdotal reports, there is little evidence that following either set of recommendations will help in reducing the severity or duration of jet lag.

Treatments for Shift Workers

The most effective bright light treatments have required about three days for achieving complete or near-complete reentrainment following schedule shifts from day to night work. Such treatments are therefore of little use to shift workers on rapidly rotating schedules. Furthermore, while complete adaptation to more slowly rotating schedules is certainly possible, the effects of undergoing large circadian phase shifts every week or two on worker health and well-being are still uncertain and may not all be positive. Finally, there are shift work schedules that defy any attempt at treatment through circadian resetting, one example being the 18-hour watch schedule (6 hours on, 12 hours off) followed on U.S. Navy submarines (e.g., Naitoh et al. 1983). In such cases, light treatments aimed at directly enhancing worker alertness and performance may be more beneficial than ones aimed at inducing large phase shifts.

Bright light protocols shown to facilitate adaptation to real or simulated shift work fall into two general categories. The first includes protocols aimed at phase shifting the subjects' rhythms prior to the first night shift, with, in some cases, maintenance treatments during and phase shifts after the period of night work; bright light exposure, however, is not scheduled during actual work hours (Czeisler et al. 1991; Stewart et al. 1995). As noted by Eastman (1994), these protocols are well suited to the work schedules of NASA astronauts and ground support crews because missions involving night work are infrequent and are preceded by a 1-week quarantine period (for astronauts) or by several days off (for ground crews), thus allowing time for adaptation to the sleep-wake schedule shifts before the start of night duty.

The second category consists of protocols in which light exposure is scheduled during nighttime work hours. Such protocols may be better suited to workers on permanent or slowly rotating shifts because they do not require devoting any free time to the light treatment. From a practical point of view, protocols calling for bright light exposure throughout the entire night shift (e.g., Czeisler et al. 1990) seem preferable to ones in which bright light is scheduled during only part of the shift (e.g., Dawson and Campbell 1991; Dawson et al. 1995), because the latter would necessitate working under two very different illumination levels within the same shift.

Bright light treatment in the work place, however, presents at least one major difficulty, that of achieving light intensities high enough to effectively reset human circadian rhythms without a concomitant increase in visual discomfort, which results primarily from reflected glare problems (e.g., Budnick et al. 1995). Such problems are often reported by workers using computer screens and are associated with such symptoms as visual focusing difficulty and eye strain. Although some lighting systems can reduce screen glare and have been shown to increase worker satisfaction (Hedge et al. 1995), these have been tested only at light intensity levels considerably lower than those required for producing large circadian phase shifts.

References

Åkerstedt T: Work schedules and sleep. Experientia 40:417–422, 1984

Åkerstedt T: Adjustment of physiological circadian rhythms and the sleep-wake cycle to shiftwork, in Hours of Work. Edited by Folkard S, Monk TH. New York, Wiley, 1985, pp 185–197

Aschoff J, Fatranska M, Giedke F: Human circadian rhythms in constant darkness: entrainment by social cues. Science 171:213–215, 1971

Aschoff J, Hoffmann K, Pohl H, et al: Re-entrainment of circadian rhythms after phase-shifts of the Zeitgeber. Chronobiologia 2:23–78, 1975

Badia P, Myers B, Boecker M, et al: Bright light effects on body temperature, alertness, EEG and behavior. Physiol Behav 50:583–588, 1991

Baker T, Morisseau D, Murphy N, et al: Timed exposure to bright light in the workplace improves night shift alertness and performance and daytime sleep. Shiftwork International Newsletter 12:109, 1995

Barrett J, Lack L, Morris M: The sleep-evoked decrease of body temperature. Sleep 16:93–99, 1993

Boivin DB, Duffy JF, Kronauer RE, et al: Sensitivity of the human circadian pacemaker to moderately bright light. J Biol Rhythms 9:315–331, 1994

Bougrine S, Cabon P, Ignazi G, et al: Exposure to bright light and adjustment of biological rhythms in a 2 × 12 hour fixed work schedule: a field research. Shiftwork International Newsletter 12:66, 1995

Boulos Z, Campbell SS, Lewy AJ, et al: Light treatment for sleep disorders: consensus report, VII: jet lag. J Biol Rhythms 10:167–176, 1995

Budnick LD, Lerman SE, Nicolich MJ: An evaluation of scheduled bright light and darkness on rotating shiftworkers: trials and limitations. Am J Indust Med 27:771–782, 1995

Campbell SS: Effects of timed bright-light exposure on shift-work adaptation in middle-aged subjects. Sleep 18:408–416, 1995

Campbell SS, Dawson D: Enhancement of nighttime alertness and performance with bright ambient light. Physiol Behav 48:317–320, 1990

Comperatore CA, Krueger GP: Circadian rhythm desynchronosis, jet lag, shift lag and coping strategies. Occup Med 5:323–341, 1990

Costa G, Ghirlanda G, Minors DS, et al: Effect of bright light on tolerance to night work. Scand J Work Environ Health 19:414–420, 1993

Czeisler CA, Allan JS: Acute circadian phase reversal in man via bright light exposure: application to jet-lag. Sleep Res 16:605, 1987

Czeisler CA, Brown EN, Ronda JM, et al: A clinical method to assess the endogenous circadian phase (ECP) of the deep circadian oscillator in man (abstract). Sleep Res 14:295, 1985

Czeisler CA, Allan JS, Strogatz SH, et al: Bright light resets the human circadian pacemaker independent of the timing of the sleep-wake cycle. Science 233:667–671, 1986

Czeisler CA, Kronauer RE, Allan JS, et al: Bright light induction of strong (type 0) resetting of the human circadian pacemaker. Science 244: 1328–1333, 1989

Czeisler CA, Johnson MP, Duffy JF, et al: Exposure to bright light and darkness to treat physiologic maladaptation to night work. N Engl J Med 322:1253–1259, 1990

Czeisler CA, Chiasera AJ, Duffy JF: Research on sleep, circadian rhythms and aging: applications to manned spaceflight. Exp Gerontol 26: 217–232, 1991

Czeisler CA, Dumont M, Duffy JF, et al: Association of sleep-wake habits in older people with changes in output of circadian pacemaker. Lancet 340:933–936, 1992

Daan S, Lewy AJ: Scheduled exposure to daylight: a potential strategy to reduce "jet lag" following transmeridian flight. Psychopharmacol Bull 20:566–568, 1984

Dahl K, Avery DH, Lewy AJ, et al: Dim light melatonin onset and circadian temperature during a constant routine in hypersomnic winter depression. Acta Psychiatr Scand 88:60–66, 1993

Daurat A, Aguirre A, Foret J, et al: Bright light affects alertness and performance rhythms during a 24-h constant routine. Physiol Behav 53: 929–936, 1993

Dawson D, Campbell SS: Timed exposure to bright light improves sleep and alertness during simulated night shifts. Sleep 14:511–516, 1991

Dawson D, Lushington K, Lack L, et al: The variability in circadian phase and amplitude estimates derived from sequential constant routines. Chronobiol Int 5:362–370, 1992

Dawson D, Lack L, Morris M: Phase resetting of the human circadian pacemaker with use of a single pulse of bright light. Chronobiol Int 10:94–102, 1993

Dawson D, Encel N, Lushington K: Improving adaptation to simulated night shift: timed exposure to bright light versus daytime melatonin administration. Sleep 18:11–21, 1995

Deacon SJ, Arendt J: Phase-shifts in melatonin, 6-sulphatoxymelatonin and alertness rhythms after treatment with moderately bright light at night. Clin Endocrinol 40:413–420, 1994

Dijk D-J, Visscher CA, Bloem GM, et al: Reduction of human sleep duration after bright light exposure in the morning. Neurosci Lett 73:181–186, 1987

Dijk D-J, Boulos Z, Eastman CI, et al: Light treatment for sleep disorders: concensus report, II: basic properties of circadian physiology and sleep regulation. J Biol Rhythms 10:113–125, 1995

Dollins AB, Lynch HJ, Wurtman RJ, et al: Effects of illumination on human nocturnal serum melatonin levels and performance. Physiol Behav 53:153–160, 1993

Drennan M, Kripke DF, Gillin JC: Bright light can delay human temperature rhythm independent of sleep. Am J Physiol 257:R136–R141, 1989

Duffy JF, Kronauer RE, Czeisler CA: Phase-shifting human circadian rhythms: influence of sleep timing, social contact and light exposure. J Physiol (Lond) 495:289–297, 1996

Duffy JF, Dijk D-J, Klerman EB, et al: Altered phase relationship between body temperature cycle and habitual awakening in older subjects. Sleep Res 26:711, 1997

Eastman CI: Bright light in work-sleep schedules for shift workers: application of circadian rhythm principles, in Temporal Disorders in Human Oscillatory Systems. Edited by Rensing L, Van der Heiden U, Mackey MC. New York, Springer-Verlag, 1987, pp 176–185

Eastman CI: High-intensity light for circadian adaptation to a 12-h shift of the sleep schedule. Am J Physiol 263:R428–R436, 1992

Eastman CI: Light treatment for circadian and sleep disturbances of shift work. Light Treatment and Biological Rhythms 6:55–62, 1994

Eastman CI, Miescke K-J: Entrainment of circadian rhythms with 26-h bright light and sleep-wake schedules. Am J Physiol 259: R1189–R1197, 1990

Eastman CI, Stewart KT, Mahoney MP, et al: Dark goggles and bright light improve circadian rhythm adaptation to night-shift work. Sleep 17: 535–543, 1994

Eastman CI, Boulos Z, Terman M, et al: Light treatment for sleep disorders: concensus report. VI. Shift work. J Biol Rhythms 10:157–164, 1995a

Eastman CI, Liu L, Fogg LF: Circadian rhythm adaptation to simulated night shift work: effect of nocturnal bright-light duration. Sleep 18: 399–407, 1995b

Ehrenstein W, Weber F: Psychophysiological field experiments into the effects of bright light on shiftworkers during prolonged shift periods, in Shiftwork: Health, Sleep and Performance. Edited by Costa G, Cesana G, Kogi K, et al. Frankfurt am Main, Lang, 1990, pp 247–252

Folkard S: The pragmatic approach to masking. Chronobiol Int 6:55–64, 1989

Folkard S, Minors DS, Waterhouse JM: "Demasking" the temperature rhythm after simulated time zone transitions. J Biol Rhythms 6:81–91, 1991

French J, Hannon P, Brainard GC: Effects of bright illuminance on body temperature and human performance. Ann Rev Chronopharmacol 7: 37–40, 1990

French J, Whitmore J, Hannon PJ, et al: Photic effects on sustained performance, in Fifth Annual Workshop on Space Operations, Applications and Research, NASA Conference Publication 3127, Vol. 2. 1991, pp 482–486

Gallo LC, Eastman CI: Circadian rhythms during gradually delaying and advancing sleep and light schedules. Physiol Behav 53:119–126, 1993

Gander PH, Samel A: Shiftwork in space: bright light as a chronobiologic countermeasure. Technical paper #911496 presented at the 21st International Conference on Environmental Systems, Society of Automotive Engineers. Warrendale, PA, 1991

Graeber RC: Jet lag and sleep disruption, . in Principles and Practice of Sleep Medicine, 2nd Edition. Edited by Kryger MH, Roth T, Dement WC, Philadelphia, WB Saunders, 1994, pp 463–470 Härmä M,

Hakola T, Åkerstadt T, et al: The effect of bright light on adaptation to night work. Ergonomics 36:314, 1993

Härmä M, Waterhouse J, Minors D, et al: Effect of masking on circadian adjustment and interindividual differences on a rapidly rotating shift schedule. Scand J Work Environ Health 20:55–61, 1994

Hastings JW, Rusak B, Boulos Z: Circadian rhythms: The physiology of biological timing, in Comparative Animal Physiology, 4th Edition. Edited by Prosser CL. New York, Wiley-Liss, 1991, pp 435–546

Hedge A, Sims WR Jr, Becker FD: Effects of lensed-indirect and parabolic lighting on the satisfaction, visual health, and productivity of office workers. Ergonomics 38:260–280, 1995

Honma KI, Honma S: A human phase response curve for bright light pulses. Jpn J Physiol 42:167–168, 1988

Honma K, Honma S, Sasaki M, et al: Bright lights accelerate the re-entrainment of circadian clock to 8-hour phase-advance shift of sleep-wake schedule, 1: circadian rhythms in rectal temperature and plasma melatonin level. Jpn J Psychiatry Neurol 45:153–154, 1991

Honma KI, Honma S, Nakamura K, et al: Differential effects of bight light and social cues on reentrainment of human circadian rhythms. Am J Physiol 268:R528–R535, 1995

Horne JA, Donlon J, Arendt J: Green light attenuates melatonin output and sleepiness during sleep deprivation. Sleep 14:233–240, 1991

Houpt TA, Boulos Z, Moore-Ede MC: MidnightSun: software for determining light exposure and phase-shifting schedules during global travel. Physiol Behav 59:561–568, 1996

Jewett ME, Kronauer RE, Czeisler CA: Phase-amplitude resetting of the human circadian pacemaker via bright light: a further analysis. J Biol Rhythms 9:295–314, 1994

Jewett ME, Rimmer DW, Duffy JF, et al: Human circadian pacemaker is sensitive to light thoughout subjective day without evidence of transients. Am J Physiol 273:R1800–R1809, 1997

Klein KE, Wegmann HM: Significance of circadian rhythms in aerospace operations, in NATO: AGARDograph No. 247, Advisory Group for Aerospace Research and Development. London, Technical Editing and Reproduction, 1980, pp 1–60

Klein T, Martens H, Dijk DJ, et al: Circadian sleep regulation in the absence of light perception: chronic non-24-hour circadian rhythm sleep disorder in a blind man with a regular 24-h sleep-wake schedule. Sleep 16:333–343, 1993

Knauth P, Rutenfranz J: Development of criteria for the design of shiftwork systems. J Hum Ergol 11(suppl):337–367, 1982

Knauth P, Emde E, Rutenfranz J, et al: Re-entrainment of body temperature in field studies of shiftwork. Int Arch Occup Environ Health 49: 137–149, 1981

Kraüchi K, Wirz-Justice A: Circadian rhythm of heat production, heart rate, and skin and core temperature under unmasking conditions in men. Am J Physiol 267:R819–R829, 1994

Lee KA: Circadian temperature rhythms in relation to menstrual cycle phase. J Biol Rhythms 3:255–263, 1988

Lewy AJ, Newsome DA: Different types of melatonin circadian secretory rhythms in some blind subjects. J Clin Endocrinol Metab 56: 1103–1107, 1983

Lewy AJ, Wehr TA, Goodwin FK, et al: Light suppresses melatonin secretion in humans. Science 210:267–269, 1980

Lewy AJ, Sack RL, Singer CM: Immediate and delayed effects of bright light on human melatonin production: shifting "dawn" and "dusk" shifts the dim light melatonin onset (DLMO). Ann N Y Acad Sci 453: 253–259, 1985

Macchi M, Aguirre A, Heitmann A, et al: Partial demasking of temperature rhythms before and after a sleep-wake schedule shift: comparison with constant routines (abstract). Sleep Res 24A:524, 1995

Matsunaga N, Itoh H, Takahashi T, et al: Effects of bright light on sleepiness at night (abstract). Sleep Res 24A:526, 1995

Miles LEM, Raynal DM, Wilson MA: Blind man living in normal society has circadian rhythms of 24.9 hours. Science 198:421–423, 1977

Mills JN, Minors DS, Waterhouse JM: Adaptation to abrupt time shifts of the oscillator(s) controlling human circadian rhythms. J Physiol 285: 455–470, 1978a

Mills JN, Minors DS, Waterhouse JM: The effect of sleep upon human circadian rhythms. Chronobiologia 5:14–27, 1978b

Minors DS, Waterhouse JM: Effects upon circadian rhythmicity of an alteration to the sleep-wake cycle: problems of assessment resulting from measurement in the presence of sleep and analysis in terms of a single shifted component. J Biol Rhythms 3:23–40, 1988

Minors DS, Waterhouse JM: Investigating the endogenous component of human circadian rhythms: a review of some simple alternatives to constant routines. Chronobiol Int 9:55–78, 1992

Minors DS, Waterhouse JM: Separating the endogenous and exogenous components of the circadian rhythm of body temperature during night work using some "purification" methods. Ergonomics 36:497–507, 1993

Minors DS, Waterhouse JM, Wirz-Justice A: A human phase response curve to light. Neurosci Lett 133:36–40, 1991

Minors DS, Waterhouse JM, Åkerstedt T: The effect of the timing, quality and quantity of sleep upon the depression (masking) of body temperature on an irregular sleep/wake schedule. J Sleep Res 3:45–51, 1994

Mitchell PJ, Hoese EK, Liu L, et al: Facilitating versus conflicting bright light exposure during night shifts for circadian adaptation to delayed and advanced sleep schedule shifts. Sleep Res 24:528, 1995

Moline ML, Pollak CP, Hirsch E: Effects of bright light on sleep following an acute phase advance. Sleep Res 18:432, 1989

Moline ML, Pollak CP, Zendell S, et al: A laboratory study of the effects of diet and bright light countermeasures to jet lag (Technical Report Natick/TR-90/024) U.S. Army Natick, Research, Development, and Engineering Center, Natick, MA, 1990, pp 1–84

Myers BL, Badia P: Immediate effects of different light intensities on body temperature and alertness. Physiol Behav 54:199–202, 1993

Naitoh P, Beare AN, Biersner RJ, et al: Altered circadian periodicities in oral temperature and mood in men on an 18-hour work/rest cycle during a nuclear submarine patrol. Int J Chronobiol 8:149–173, 1983

Nakagawa H, Sack RL, Lewy AJ: Sleep propensity free-runs with the temperature, melatonin and cortisol rhythms in a totally blind person. Sleep 15:330–336, 1992

Oren DA, Reich W, Rosenthal NE, et al: How to Beat Jet Lag: A Practical Guide for Air Travelers. New York, Henry Holt, 1993

Pittendrigh CS: Circadian systems: Entrainment, in Handbook of Behavioral Neurobiology, Volume 4: Biological Rhythms. Edited by Aschoff J. New York, Plenum, 1981, pp 95–124

Powers LM, Terman M, Link MJ: Bright light treatment of night-shift workers, in SLTBR: Abstracts of the Annual Meeting of the Society for

Light Treatment and Biological Rhythms, Vol. 1. Wilsonville, OR, Society for Light Treatment and Biological Rhythms, 1989, p 34

Rogacz S, Duffy JF, Ronda JM, et al: The increase in body temperature during the luteal phase of the menstrual cycle is only observed during the subjective night and is independent of sleep. Sleep Res 17:395, 1988

Sack RL, Lewy AJ, Blood ML, et al: Circadian rhythm abnormalities in totally blind people: phase advances and entrainment. J Biol Rhythms 6: 249–261, 1991

Samel A, Gundel A, Wegmann HM: Bright light exposure in the morning and in the afternoon after 6-h advance shift. Society for Research on Biological Rhythms Abstracts 3:25, 1992

Sasaki M, Kurosaki Y, Onda M, et al: Effects of bright light on circadian rhythmicity and sleep after transmeridian flight. Sleep Res 18:442, 1989

Shanahan TL, Czeisler CA: Light exposure induces equivalent phase shifts of the endogenous circadian rhythms of circulating plasma melatonin and core body temperature in men. J Clin Endocrinol Metab 73: 227–235, 1991

Stewart KT, Hayes BC, Eastman CI: Light treatment for NASA shiftworkers. Chronobiol Int 12:141–151, 1995

Tepas DI, Armstrong DR, Carlson ML, et al: Changing industry to continuous operations: different strokes for different plants. Behavior Research Methods, Instruments, and Computers 17:670–676, 1985

Tepas DI, Duchon JC, Gersten AH: Shiftwork and the older worker. Exp Aging Res, 9:295–320, 1993

Tosini G, Menaker M: Circadian rhythms in cultured mammalian retina. Science 272:419–421, 1996

U.S. Congress, Office of Technology Assessment: Biological Rhythms: Implications for the Worker (OTA-BA-463). Washington, DC, U.S. Government Printing Office, 1991

Van Cauter E, Sturis J, Byrne MM, et al: Demonstration of rapid light-induced advances and delays of the human circadian clock using hormonal phase markers. Am J Physiol 266:E953–E963, 1994

Veith S, Kohler WK, Fey P, et al: The influence of the menstrual cycle on the female circadian system, in SLTBR: Abstracts of the Annual Meeting of the Society for Light Treatment and Biological Rhythms, Vol. 5. Wilsonville, OR, Society for Light Treatment and Biological Rhythms, 1993, p 50

Wagner DR, Zindell S, Hurt S, et al: Circadian temperature phase variability and the menstrual cycle (abstract). Sleep Res 21:391, 1992

Wever RA: The Circadian System of Man: Results of Experiments Under Temporal Isolation. Berlin, Springer-Verlag, 1979

Wever RA: Internal interactions within the human circadian system: the masking effect. Experientia 41:332–342, 1985a

Wever RA: Use of light to treat jet lag: differential effects of normal and bright artificial light on human circadian rhythms. Ann N Y Acad Sci 453:282–304, 1985b

Wever RA, Polásek J, Wildgruber CM: Bright light affects human circadian rhythms. Pflügers Arch 396:85–87, 1983

Whitson PA, Putcha L, Chen Y-M, et al: Melatonin and cortisol assessment of circadian shifts in astronauts before flight. J Pineal Res 18:141–147, 1995

Wilkinson RT: How fast should the night shift rotate? Ergonomics 35: 1425–1446, 1992

Winget CM, DeRoshia CW, Markley CL, et al: A review of human physiological and performance changes associated with desynchronosis of biological rhythms. Aviat Space Environ Med 55:1085–1096, 1984

ELEVEN

Bright Light Treatment of Sleep Maintenance Insomnia and Behavioral Disturbance

Scott S. Campbell, Ph.D.

As much as half of the population over 65 years of age suffers from chronic sleep disturbance. Age-related sleep changes are typically expressed as fragmented nocturnal sleep, multiple and prolonged awakenings in the second half of the night, and increased daytime napping. In contrast, few elderly report difficulties getting to sleep. Thus, insomnia in people over 65 is generally regarded as a disorder of *maintaining*, rather than *initiating*, sleep.

It has been suggested by a number of researchers that such sleep disturbance is caused, in large part, to age-related changes in the circadian system, such that the temporal relationship between sleep and body temperature is altered. With aging, circadian rhythms (e.g., body core temperature) are phase-advanced, leading to an altered phase relationship between the timing of nocturnal sleep and these rhythms. It is this altered phase relationship that is hypothesized to cause, at least in part, the characteristic sleep disturbance associated with aging.

The author gratefully acknowledges the support of grants K02 MH01099, R01 MH45067, R01 AG12112, and a grant from the Tolly Vinik Trust (Cornell University Medical College).

As a consequence of such sleep disturbance, up to 40% of all hypnotic medications are prescribed to the elderly, despite an increasing body of evidence suggesting that hypnotics may be deleterious to the well-being of older individuals. The American Psychiatric Association Task Force on Benzodiazepine Dependency included high dosage and advanced age among the conditions most likely to lead to greater risks of chronic toxicity, especially cognitive impairment, and true physiological dependency (American Psychiatric Association 1990). This constellation of problems associated with pharmacological interventions to alleviate age-related sleep disturbance has led to the development of a number of nondrug strategies to treat sleep-maintenance insomnia. In this chapter, we examine one such strategy: timed exposure to bright light.

The underlying rationale for the use of light therapy to treat sleep disturbance in the elderly is based on the aforementioned changes in circadian rhythms that accompany aging. Timed exposure to bright light is used to re-set (delay) the circadian clock and thereby reinstitute the appropriate phase relationship between the circadian timing system and habitual sleep times. Although several laboratories have documented the nature of both circadian changes and sleep-wake disturbance in aging (Campbell et al. 1989; Czeisler et al. 1992; Moe et al. 1991; Weitzman et al. 1982; Zepelin and McDonald 1987), and a number of researchers have demonstrated the phase-shifting properties of timed bright light exposure (Campbell and Dawson 1992; Czeisler et al. 1986, 1989; Dawson and Campbell 1991; Dijk et al. 1989; Eastman 1986, 1991, 1992;), few investigators have employed light therapy in an effort to alleviate sleep-maintenance insomnia.

In the following section, results of one such study are presented in detail. These findings are then discussed within the general framework of other studies that have addressed this issue.

Bright Light Treatment of Age-Related Sleep Disturbance

As a first step to examine whether timed exposure to bright light would be an effective treatment for age-related sleep disturbance, we initiated a study to assess the *acute* effects of such an intervention (Campbell et al. 1993). That is, we sought to determine whether reestablishing the normal phase relationship between sleep time and the 24-hour rhythm of body core temperature would result in immediate, short-term improvement in sleep quality and consolidation measures.

Participants

Our study included 16 participants (9 females, 7 males) between the ages of 62 and 81 years (mean 70.4 years). All had experienced sleep disturbance for at least a year prior to entering the study, and none was taking hypnotic medications at the time of participation. All were in good general health and living independently in the community.

Methods

To obtain a measure of baseline sleep quality, each individual was polygraphically recorded for 4 consecutive nights in the laboratory. Nights 1 and 2 in both the baseline and the posttreatment recording intervals were treated as adaptation nights, and the data obtained on those nights were not used in the analyses. Sleep parameters from nights 3 and 4 of each laboratory session were averaged, and it is these data that were employed in all analyses. On all recording nights, bedtime and wakeup time were at the discretion of each participant. All sleep records were visually scored by trained scorers using standard criteria (Rechtschaffen and Kales 1968). Also, during this baseline phase of the study, core body temperature was recorded continuously for 36 hours, using an indwelling rectal thermistor connected to a portable data storage device. This permitted us to obtain baseline measures of the circadian phase.

Immediately following the 4 nights of baseline recording, the participants began the treatment phase of the study. During this 10-day interval, they were exposed to 2 hours of either bright white light of approximately 4,000 lux (active group, $n = 8$; 4 females, 4 males), or dim red light of approximately 50 lux (control group, $n = 8$; 5 females, 3 males). They received treatment in their homes, and they were encouraged to continue their normal daily activities during the treatment interval. Illumination was provided by a light source (Apollo Brite Lite III, Orem, UT) situated on each side of a television, at eye level when the individual was seated. Participants were instructed to watch television for the entire 2-hour treatment interval. They were specifically instructed to avoid any activities (such as reading or writing) that would cause them to divert their gaze from the light source for appreciable amounts of time, because previous research had shown that compliance with such instructions may be critical to insuring treatment efficacy (Dawson and Campbell 1990). For all participants, the 2-hour treatment interval fell within a window between 8:00 P.M. and 11:00 P.M. Based on established phase-response curves to light in humans, this interval was selected in order to delay circadian phase, without interfering with the participants' usual bedtimes.

Immediately following the 10 days of home treatment, the participants returned to the laboratory for posttreatment evaluation. This consisted of a laboratory session identical to the baseline protocol (i.e., 4 nights), with the exception that participants received light treatment on the first 2 nights in the laboratory, at the same time as during the home treatment. Thus, the entire treatment interval continued for 12 consecutive nights (10 nights at home, 2 in the lab) prior to posttreatment evaluation of sleep.

Results

At baseline, the average temperature minimum (T_{min}) for the group was at 3:53 A.M. (SD = 1.9 hours). In an earlier study (Campbell et al. 1989) we had found that older women were significantly more phase-advanced than age-matched men. In this group, however, there were no such gender differences in temperature minima, nor was there a significant relationship between age and temperature. There were, however, large individual differences in temperature measures. The range in minima was almost 8 hours (from 11:05 P.M. to 6:55 A.M.), and the amplitudes of the individual baseline temperature curve ranged by almost 1°C.

Following the 12-day treatment period, the average T_{min} for the active group was 6:44 A.M. (SD = 1.7 hours) compared with 4:23 A.M. (SD = 1.9 hours) for the control group. Thus, evening bright light exposure induced an average phase delay of just over 3 hours, compared with an average delay of only 8 minutes for the control group. Figure 11–1 shows the relationship between night-time temperature values and the timing of sleep for the active group, at baseline (Figure 11–1a) and following treatment (Figure 11–1b). Before bright light exposure, the average fitted minimum occurred about half an hour after the midpoint of sleep, whereas the minimum occurred 3 hours following midsleep after bright light exposure.

This phase shift in the circadian course of body core temperature was accompanied by several important changes in sleep electroencephalogram (EEG) measures. Table 11–1 shows group averages for a number of measures of sleep quality at baseline and following treatment. At baseline, average sleep efficiency for the active group was 77.5% (SD = 3.2%) (sleep efficiency = the ratio of total sleep time to sleep-period time). There was a strong negative correlation between sleep efficiency and age at baseline, both for the entire sample ($\rho = -0.79, P < .002$) and for each group considered separately (active: $\rho = -0.87, P < .02$); control: $\rho = -0.85, P < .02$). Following bright light treatment, average sleep efficiency increased to 90.1% (SD = 5.1%) ($F = 54.01$, df = 1,14, $P < .0001$). The overall increase in sleep efficiency for the active group was not a result of large improvements by a few individuals. Rather, the improvement was consistent across the entire group. Enhancements over baseline values ranged from 11.4% to 23.4% (mean 16.2%, SD = 3.8%; median 15.9%).

By definition, the significant improvement in sleep efficiency came as the result of a decline in the amount of wakefulness within the night. This was reflected in several measures of within-sleep waking (see Table 11–1). In response to bright light exposure, total time spent awake after initial sleep onset (WASO) declined by an average of 59.6 minutes (SD = 14.4), from 102.8 minutes to 43.2 minutes ($F = 45.1$, df = 1,14, $P < .0001$). Likewise, the proportion of stage 0 sleep within the night declined significantly in response to bright

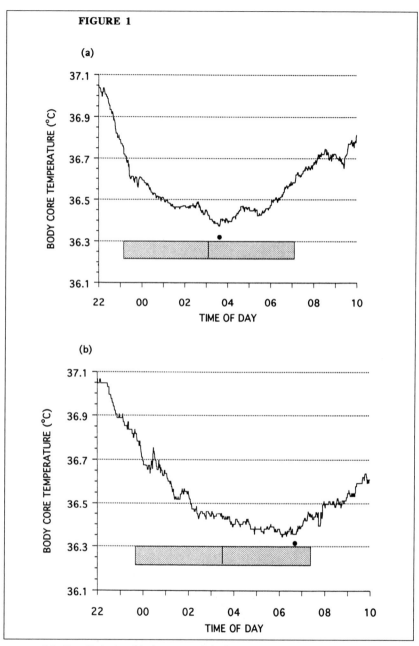

FIGURE 1

(a)

(b)

FIGURE **11-1.** Relationship between nighttime temperature values and the timing of sleep for the active group at baseline (a) and following treatment (b). Shaded bars represent average time in bed (with vertical line for midpoint), closed circles show the time of fitted temperature minima. The phase angle between temperature minimum and midsleep showed a delay of 158 minutes as a result of bright light exposure.

TABLE 11–1

Comparison of EEG sleep measures between baseline and posttreatment condition for the active (bright light) and control (dim light) groups

	Active		Control		
	Baseline	Post-Light	Baseline	Post-Light	P Value
Bedtime	11:14 P.M. (0.58 h)	11:43 P.M. (0.73 h)	00:27 A.M. (1.1 h)	11:58 P.M. (0.93 h)	<0.01
Wakeup	7:06 A.M. (0.61 h)	7:24 A.M. (0.86 h)	8:04 A.M. (0.84 h)	7:53 A.M. (0.96 h)	NS
Time in bed	472.6 min (38.0)	461.4 min (32.2)	457.1 min (47)	474.8 min (45)	NS
Total sleep time	352.7 min (19.9)	398.3 min (40.9)	326.0 min (33)	347.0 min (57)	NS
Sleep latency	13.5 min (8.1)	12.8 min (5.9)	21.1 min (16.4)	24.5 min (19.5)	NS
REMS latency	45.2 min (18.6)	69.5 min (22.1)	54.1 min (18.9)	53.7 min (18.4)	<0.02
Sleep efficiency	77.5% (3.2)	90.1% (5.1)	79.2% (5.5)	80.5% (7.7)	<0.001
Wake after sleep onset (WASO)	102.8 min (21.4)	43.2 min (21.6)	89.4 (26.5)	83.1 (36.7)	<0.001
Stage 1%	11.6 (4.1)	7.1 (2.1)	10.4 (4.2)	10.5 (3.4)	<0.01
Stage 2%	42.1 (8.2)	52.2 (6.6)	42.5 (7.6)	42.5 (7.8)	<0.01
Stage 3%	6.2 (1.6)	7.4 (2.8)	7.7 (4.0)	7.2 (4.0)	NS
Stage 4%	4.0 (2.0)	5.4 (3.8)	3.7 (5.5)	4.2 (3.9)	NS
SWS % (3 + 4)	10.2 (2.1)	12.8 (4.6)	11.4 (7.5)	11.4 (7.1)	NS
REMS %	14.3 (2.3)	17.9 (3.9)	14.8 (2.7)	16.1 (5.3)	NS
Stage changes	169.6 (26.2)	117.8 (19.4)	150.6 (34.0)	160.1 (34.1)	<0.01

Note. Means and (standard deviations) are shown. P values are for group $\times$ treatment interaction. Sleep efficiency = (ratio of total sleep time to time in bed − sleep-onset latency).

light versus the dim light control ($F = 35.3$, df $= 1,14$, $P < .0001$). Post-hoc analyses revealed that time awake was significantly reduced in the last two-thirds of the night. The results of those analyses are presented in Table 11–2.

The decline in wakefulness across the night occurred primarily as the result of an overall reduction in the *number,* rather than in the *duration,* of individual waking episodes. Following bright light exposure, the number of awakenings declined by 41.5%, from an average of 25.1 episodes per night at baseline to a mean of 14.7 per night following treatment ($F = 11.2$, df $= 1,14$, $P < .005$). Significant declines occurred in the number of brief arousals (<1 minute; $F = 5.3$, df $= 1,14$, $P < .04$), as well as intermediate (1–10 minutes; $F = 4.8$, df $= 1,14$, $P < .05$) and longer waking episodes (>10 minutes; $F = 12.5$, df $= 1,14$, $P < .005$). In addition to the reduction in waking within the night, bright light exposure also resulted in a 31% decline in the number of sleep-stage changes observed ($F = 12.2$, df $= 1,14$, $P < .01$).

The decline in wakefulness within sleep following bright light treatment resulted in an average increase in total sleep time (TST) of 45.6 minutes (SD $= 33.7$). Because of the substantial between-subjects variability in TST, and because the control group showed a 20-minute increase in TST following dim light exposure, the interaction was not statistically significant. However, post-hoc t tests re-

---

TABLE 11–2

Comparison of waking time by thirds of the night, at baseline and following treatment for the active (bright light) and control (dim light) groups

| | | Thirds of the night | | |
		First	Second	Third
Active group	Baseline	22.6 (2.0)	32.6 (5.2)*	48.4 (5.7)*
	Posttreatment	15.3 (6.0)	13.2 (4.2)*	14.7 (2.9)*
Control group	Baseline	22.3 (5.9)	32.0 (4.3)	35.0 (6.0)
	Posttreatment	17.6 (4.0)	29.7 (7.6)	35.7 (5.6)

Note. Means and (standard deviations) are shown in minutes.
*$P < .02$ (Wilcoxon matched pairs).

vealed a significant within-group effect on total sleep time for the active treatment ($P < .01$), but not for the control condition.

Our final analysis examined the composition of this increased sleep time, relative to the composition of sleep prior to treatment. For the active group, in addition to the reduction in wakefulness described previously, there was also a 38.7% decline in the proportion of stage 1 ($F = 8.5$, df = 1,14, $P < .01$). In contrast, there was a significant increase in the proportion of stage 2 sleep ($F = 2.7$, df = 1,14, $P < .003$), as well as nonsignificant increases in slow-wave sleep (stages 3 and 4) and REM sleep. As would be expected with a phase delay in the circadian timing system, the active group also exhibited a 24.3-minute phase delay in average REM latency following bright light exposure ($F = 6.8$, df = 1,14, $P < .03$).

Summary and Conclusions

A recent National Institutes of Health Consensus Development Conference on the Treatment of Sleep Disorders of Older People questioned the safety and efficacy of hypnotic and sedative medications in treating age-related sleep disturbance, and advocated the development of more effective treatment strategies including non-pharmacological methods (National Institutes of Health 1990). This position was echoed by the American Psychiatric Association Task Force on Benzodiazepine Dependency, which included high dosage and advanced age among the conditions most likely to lead to high risks of chronic toxicity, especially cognitive impairment, and true physiological dependency (American Psychiatric Association 1990). Clearly, then, an effective, nonpharmacological alternative could prove to be an important step in the management of age-related sleep-maintenance insomnia.

The application of light therapy to age-related sleep disturbance is quite recent, with no reports appearing in the literature prior to 1991. Thus, results are sparse, and those reports that do exist, including the one just described in detail, must be viewed as preliminary. Nevertheless, such findings demonstrate the potential effectiveness of this approach. Timed exposure to bright light, repeated for

12 consecutive evenings, reduced waking time within sleep by over 1 hour when compared with baseline values. Sleep efficiency increased by an average of 17%, attaining levels (90%) equivalent to, or greater than those achieved with pharmacological interventions (Carskadon et al. 1982; Roehrs et al. 1985) In addition, waking time was not simply replaced by light sleep or drowsiness (i.e., stage 1 sleep as measured by EEG). Rather, increased sleep time came in the form of a significant increase in stage 2 sleep and in nonsignificant, but perhaps clinically relevant, increases in REM and slow-wave sleep.

Similar findings were reported by Lack and Schumacher (1993), who used exposure to evening bright light in a group of patients with early morning awakening insomnia. Although the participants in the study had a mean age of only 48 years, the nature of their sleep disturbance was equivalent to that seen in older individuals. In that study, participants were exposed to either 4 hours of evening bright light (2,500 lux), or dim red light (200 lux), for two consecutive days (8:00 P.M. to midnight on the first night, 9:00 P.M. to 1:00 A.M. on the second). Bright light produced improvements in sleep, as measured by wrist actigraphy and subjective assessment: self-reported sleep duration increased significantly, whereas, actigraph movement time in the first 6 hours of sleep declined significantly following treatment. The same results were obtained in a subsequent study of nine patients (mean age of 53.4 years) with early morning awakening insomnia (Lack and Wright 1993). Following two consecutive days of bright light exposure (2,500 lux from 8:00 P.M. to midnight), actigraphically measured total sleep time increased by an average of 1.2 hours. As in the Campbell et al. (1993) study, improvements in sleep were accompanied by phase delays in the minimum of body core temperature. Lack and Schumacher observed a mean phase delay of 3–4 hours, and Lack and Wright reported an average delay of 1.85 hours.

Importantly, the improvements in sleep observed in these studies were not accomplished at the expense of time in bed. To the contrary, as a consequence of reduced wakefulness in the Campbell et al. (1993) study, total sleep time was increased by more than three-quarters of an hour following treatment, without significantly altering the time spent in bed. This is in marked contrast to most behavioral treatments, which employ various sleep restriction procedures to boost sleep efficiency (Friedman et al. 1991; Moran et al. 1988; Morin and Azrin 1988). In one such study, sleep duration was increased by more than 1 hour, but never exceeded 6 hours per night (Morin and Azrin 1988). The authors postulated that "it may be unrealistic for older adults to expect more than 6 hours of sleep" (p. 752). The current data refute that position and indicate that substantially longer sleep lengths can be obtained, and are, without sacrificing sleep efficiency, if time in bed is not artificially truncated.

The demonstrated improvements in nighttime sleep quality notwithstanding, it should be pointed out that even at 90% sleep efficiency, subjects continued to spend an average of 43 minutes each night awake. The question arises as to whether it might be possible to boost sleep efficiency still further with bright light exposure. Certainly, light exposure timed to coincide more closely with the minimum of body core temperature would produce a greater circadian phase delay (Czeisler et al. 1989; Minors et al. 1991). Whether this, in turn, would result in further sleep improvement remains a question. There is ample evidence to suggest that noncircadian factors may play an important additional role as well, in age-related sleep disturbance. A widely accepted model of human sleep regulation posits the existence of a circadian component (process C) and a sleep-wake-dependent component (process S) that interact to determine sleep tendency, duration, and composition (Achermann et al. 1993; Borbely 1982; Daan et al. 1984). Process S is thought of as a homeostatic process that rises with increasing durations of wakefulness and is reversed by increasing durations of sleep. Its level and time course are thought to be reflected in slow-wave EEG activity.

There is a large body of literature describing significant, age-related alterations in slow-wave sleep. For example, shifts in both the amplitude and frequency characteristics of slow-wave activity have been observed in middle-aged and older individuals, and it has been suggested that such alterations can change, fundamentally, the physiological and qualitative nature of sleep (see, for example, Chase and Roth 1990). It is reasonable to assume that at least a portion of the sleep disturbance observed in older individuals is the consequence of this disturbance, or fundamental change, in mechanisms governing the homeostatic component of sleep. Although there is limited evidence for a chronobiological contribution to the occurrence of slow-wave sleep (Campbell and Zulley 1989; Hume and Mills 1977; Webb and Agnew 1971), this component of the sleep process may be less responsive to circadian manipulations and, therefore, may require alternative treatment.

Elderly Nursing Home Residents With and Without Dementia

In addition to treatment of sleep disturbance per se, light therapy has been employed in nursing homes, primarily for patients with dementia, in an effort to manage behavioral disorders such as night wandering and "sundowning" (a syndrome of recurring confusion and agitation in the late afternoon or early evening). Because of the methodological and logistical difficulties inherent in obtaining polysomnographic data from patients with dementia and from other nursing home patients, no studies of light therapy in this population have been reported. Instead, behavioral observations and objective rest/activity measures have been employed to assess efficacy of bright light treatment in patients with dementia.

Okawa and co-workers (Okawa et al. 1991) examined the efficacy of morning bright light exposure (3,000 lux 9:00 A.M. to 11:00 A.M.) administered daily for 1–2 months, in a group of 24 patients (mean age: 76.6 years) with moderate or severe dementia. The patients were selected specifically because they exhibited irregularity of sleep-wake patterns and behavioral disorders. Using hourly nurses' observations to assess sleep-wake state and other behaviors, the investigators reported improvement in 12 of the 24 patients studied. Subsequently, these patients were assigned to a placebo condition (patients sat in front of lights that were not turned on), and their sleep-wake and behavioral disorders reappeared, suggesting that light exposure, rather than the behavioral structuring that accompanied such a protocol, was the important factor in treatment.

In a subsequent study (Mishima et al. 1994), again using observational data, this group reported significant improvements in nighttime sleep, and a marked reduction in behavioral disorders and daytime sleep, in a group of patients with dementia (mean age 75 years), following 4 weeks of morning (9:00 A.M. to 11:00 A.M.) bright light exposure (3,000–5,000 lux). The effects on nighttime sleep and behavioral disturbance were present 2 weeks following the end of light treatment.

In a preliminary study of 25 nursing home residents (mean age 87.1 years), Ancoli-Israel et al. (1991) compared effects on sleep of evening bright light (5:00 P.M. to 7:00 P.M.), morning bright light (9:30 A.M. to 11:30 A.M.), dim light (5:00 P.M. to 7:00 P.M.), and increased daytime activity (no time specified). A nonsignificant trend toward improved sleep (inferred from actigraphic data) was found in the group receiving evening bright light, but not in the other groups.

Satlin and co-workers (Satlin et al. 1992) employed both observational and rest/activity data to assess the effects of evening bright light (≈2,000 lux 7:00 P.M. to 9:00 P.M.) administered daily for 1 week, in a group of 10 inpatients with Alzheimer's disease (mean age 70.1 years). As in the Okawa study, patients who exhibited sundowning behavior and sleep pattern disturbance were specifically selected for participation in the study. Based on nurses' observations, 8 of the 10 patients exhibited improvements in sleep/wakefulness ratings during the week of treatment and during the subsequent week. This result was supported by data obtained from activity monitors worn by each patient. Percent of nighttime activity declined significantly from the baseline week to the light treatment week in 9 of the 10 patients. As a result, the amplitude of the cosine-fitted activity data showed a significant increase during the treatment week in 7 of the 10 patients. Interestingly, there was a significant positive correlation ($r = 0.65$) between the severity of sundowning symptoms at baseline and the degree of improvement with light treatment.

In conclusion, it should be pointed out that no study has assessed the long-term efficacy of light therapy in either healthy or pathological aging. This issue is of critical importance if light therapy is to be useful as a strategy to manage what is typically a chronic problem. In this regard, it should be emphasized that a daily, 2-hour treatment regimen is time consuming and sometimes inconvenient. Therefore, certain individuals who are likely to benefit from the program may choose alternative approaches (i.e., hypnotic medications) that require less commitment of time. Further refinements of the treatment schedule, however, may go far to ameliorate this potential drawback. We are currently conducting studies to examine the efficacy of a maintenance schedule whereby treatment is reduced to twice-weekly exposure, after an acceptable phase relationship between body temperature and sleep has been established. This, in turn, would greatly facilitate the acceptance of, and compliance with, this promising nondrug intervention.

References

Achermann P, Dijk DJ, Brunner DP, et al: A model of human sleep homeostasis based on EEG slow-wave activity: quantitative comparison of data and simulations. Brain Res Bull 31:97–113, 1993

American Psychiatric Association: American Psychiatric Association Task Force Report on Benzodiazepine Dependence, Toxicity and Abuse. Washington, DC, American Psychiatric Association, 1990

Ancoli-Israel S, Kripke D, Jones D, et al: Light exposure and sleep in nursing home patients (abstract), in SLTBR: Abstracts of the Annual Meeting of the Society for Light Treatment and Biological Rhythms, Vol. 3. Wilsonville, OR, Society for Light Treatment and Biological Rhythms, 1991

Borbely A: A two process model of sleep regulation. Hum Neurobiol 1:195–204, 1982

Campbell SS, Dawson D: Aging young sleep: a test of the phase advance hypothesis of sleep disturbance in the elderly. J Sleep Res 1:205–210, 1992

Campbell SS, Zulley J: Evidence for circadian influence on human slow wave sleep during daytime sleep episodes. Psychophysiology 26:580–585, 1989

Campbell SS, Gillin JC, Kripke DF, et al: Gender differences in the circadian temperature rhythms of healthy elderly subjects: relationships to sleep quality. Sleep 12:529–536, 1989

Campbell SS, Dawson D, Anderson MW: Alleviation of sleep maintenance insomnia with timed exposure to bright light. J Am Geriatr Soc 41:829–836, 1993

Carskadon MA, Seidel WF, Greenblatt DJ, et al: Daytime carryover of triazolam and flurazepam in elderly insomniacs. Sleep 5:361–371, 1982

Chase MH, Roth T (eds): Slow Wave Sleep: Its Measurement and Functional Significance. Los Angeles, UCLA Brain Information Service/ Brain Research Institute, 1990

Czeisler CA, Allan JS, Strogatz SH, et al: Bright light resets the human circadian pacemaker independent of the timing of the sleep-wake cycle. Science 233:667–671, 1986

Czeisler CA, Kronauer RE, Allan JS, et al: Bright light induction of strong (type 0) resetting of the human circadian pacemaker. Science 244: 1328–1333, 1989

Czeisler CA, Dumont M, Duffy JF, et al: Association of sleep-wake habits in older people with changes in output of circadian pacemaker. Lancet 340:933–936, 1992

Daan S, Beersma DG, Borbely AA: Timing of human sleep: recovery process gated by a circadian pacemaker. Am J Physiol 2:R161–R183, 1984

Dawson D, Campbell SS: Bright light treatment: are we keeping our subjects in the dark? Sleep 13:267–271, 1990

Dawson D, Campbell SS: Timed exposure to bright light improves sleep and alertness during simulated night shifts. Sleep 14:511–516, 1991

Dijk DJ, Beersma DG, Daan S, et al: Bright morning light advances the human circadian system without affecting NREM sleep homeostasis. Am J Physiol 256:R106–R111, 1989

Eastman C: Bright light improves the entrainment of the circadian rhythm of body temperature to a 26-hr sleep-wake schedule in humans. Sleep Res 15:271, 1986

Eastman CI: Squashing versus nudging circadian rhythms with artificial bright light: solutions for shift work? Perspect Biol Med 34:181–195, 1991

Eastman CI: High-intensity light for circadian adaptation to a 12-h shift of the sleep schedule. Am J Physiol 263:R428–R436, 1992

Friedman L, Bliwise DL, Yesavage JA, et al: A preliminary study comparing sleep restriction and relaxation treatments for insomnia in older adults. J Gerontol 46:1–8, 1991

Hume KI, Mills JN: Rhythms of REM and slow-wave sleep in subjects living on abnormal time schedules. Waking Sleeping 3:291–296, 1977

Lack L, Schumacher K: Evening light treatment of early morning insomnia. Sleep Res 22:225, 1993

Lack L, Wright H: The effect of evening bright light in delaying the circadian rhythms and lengthening the sleep of early morning awakening insomniacs. Sleep 16:436–443, 1993

Minors DS, Waterhouse JM, Wirz JA: A human phase-response curve to light. Neurosci Lett 133:36–40, 1991

Mishima K, Okawa M, Hishikawa Y, et al: Morning bright light therapy for sleep and behavior disorders in elderly patients with dementia. Acta Psychiatr Scand 89:1–7, 1994

Moe KE, Prinz PN, Vitiello MV, et al: Healthy elderly women and men have different entrained circadian temperature rhythms. J Am Geriatr Soc 39:383–387, 1991

Moran MG, Thompson T, Nies AS: Sleep disorders in the elderly. Am J Psychiatry 145:1369–1378, 1988

Morin CM, Azrin NH: Behavioral and cognitive treatments of geriatric insomnia. J Consult Clin Psychol 56:748–753, 1988

National Institutes of Health: NIH Consensus Development Conference Consensus Statement. Treatment of sleep disorders of older people. March 26–28, 1990

Okawa M, Hishikawa Y, Hozumi S, et al: Sleep-wake rhythm disorder and phototherapy in elderly patients with dementia, in Biological Psychiatry. Edited by Racagni G et al. New York, Elsevier, 1991, pp 837–840

Rechtschaffen A, Kales A: A Manual of Standardized Terminology, Techniques and Scoring System for Sleep Stages of Human Subjects, Vol. 204. Washington, DC, National Institutes of Health, 1968

Roehrs T, Zorick F, Wittig R, et al: Efficacy of a reduced triazolam dose in elderly insomniacs. Neurobiol Aging 6:293–296, 1985

Satlin A, Volicer L, Ross V, et al: Bright light treatment of behavioral and sleep disturbances in patients with Alzheimer's disease. Am J Psychiatry 149:1028–1032, 1992

Webb WB, Agnew HW Jr: Stage 4 sleep: influence of time course variables. Science 174:1354–1356, 1971

Weitzman ED, Moline ML, Czeisler CA, et al: Chronobiology of aging: temperature, sleep-wake rhythms and entrainment. Neurobiol Aging 3:299–309, 1982

Zepelin H, McDonald C: Age differences in autonomic variables during sleep. J Gerontol 42:142–146, 1987

TWELVE

Seasonal Affective Disorder and Beyond: A Commentary

Raymond W. Lam, M.D.

The preceding chapters illustrate how the application of light therapy has expanded from its initial use, over a decade ago, in seasonal affective disorder (SAD) and nonseasonal depression, to potential applications in other seasonal disorders, circadian rhythm disorders, and sleep disorders. In this chapter, I discuss several clinical issues concerning light therapy that are raised by the chapter authors.

Light Therapy for Seasonal and Nonseasonal Depression

The chapters on seasonal affective disorder convey the richness of the research in the past decade. This research, while adding to the understanding of SAD, also raises many new questions. The hope that SAD would be a very homogenous subtype of depression, with an easily identified etiology related to photoperiodism, has not been realized. Even the existence of SAD remains controversial to some, although, as others have pointed out, the evidence for clinical validity of SAD remains greater than for other subtypes of depression, including melancholia and atypical depression (Bauer and Dunner

305

1993; Lam and Stewart 1996; Spitzer and Williams 1989). One critique of SAD as a diagnosis is that the seasonal pattern may not remain consistent in all patients. Since the diagnosis is made by retrospective identification of a seasonal pattern, the reliability of patients to recall episode onset and offset times may be questioned. For example, several longer-term follow-up studies suggest that only a third of patients identified with SAD (or its DSM-IV [American Psychiatric Association 1994] equivalent) continue to show a regular, distinctive seasonal pattern (Sakamoto et al. 1995; Schwartz et al. 1996; Thompson et al. 1995; Wicki et al. 1992). Some patients are treated with antidepressant medications year round and may therefore have their seasonal patterns masked by maintenance treatment. Still others have occasional nonseasonal episodes, or revert to nonseasonal patterns, or go into sustained natural remission. This variability in course has prompted some investigators to suggest that the diagnosis of SAD be made only with prospective verification of seasonal patterns, or with collateral information from a knowledgeable informant (Wicki et al. 1992). Other sources criticize the validity of a diagnosis with this degree of variability, but the clinical reality is that many of the same limitations hold true for most subtypes of mood disorders, including the DSM-IV specifiers of melancholic or atypical features, rapid-cycling pattern, and even major diagnoses such as dysthymia and double depression (Holzer III et al. 1996). Instead of dwelling on the variable course, we should recognize that SAD may be more heterogeneous than initially believed. In the search for an underlying etiology (or etiologies) for SAD and the mechanism(s) of the antidepressant effect of light, this diagnostic heterogeneity must be taken into consideration.

Virginia Wesson and Anthony Levitt (this volume) have compiled a comprehensive summary of light therapy studies for SAD. As Michael Terman also points out in his chapter (this volume), the placebo issue continues to be a controversial factor in definitively establishing the efficacy of light therapy. The placebo issue is also entangled with other methodological limitations of light therapy studies, including sample size, expectation effects, and length of trial (Brown 1990). A statistically significant effect size (the difference between an active treatment and a placebo treatment) in a study depends on the magnitude of the active treatment response, the magnitude of the placebo treatment response, and the sample size. The smaller the sample size, the larger the effect size must be to demonstrate statistical significance. For any given sample size, crossover studies have greater statistical power than do parallel design studies to detect a significant effect size. Therefore, although the head-mounted unit (HMU) studies had relatively larger sample sizes than preceding light box studies, the parallel designs of the HMU studies means that they are able to detect only the same effect size as crossover studies, with about half the number of subjects. More importantly, although the effect sizes of the HMU studies were too small to be statistically significant, this was not because the active light conditions provided such poor results, but because the "placebo" dim light conditions provided such good results.

That the putative placebo conditions in these studies were so effective is not entirely unexpected, given what is known about placebo response. Factors implicated in higher pill placebo response include shorter duration of the depressive episode, outpatient participants and less severely ill patients, nonchronic illness, and shorter-duration treatment studies (Bialik et al. 1995; Brown et al. 1988, 1992). All of these factors may complicate studies of SAD and light therapy. Similar factors, however, are also found in many antidepressant drug studies. The relatively small effect sizes in antidepressant studies usually require large sample sizes (often several hundred patients) to demonstrate a significant effect of active drugs over placebo. Antidepressant clinical trials with sample sizes comparable to the HMU studies (less than 50 patients per condition or dose) often have high placebo response rates with no differentiation between active drug and placebo (e.g., Rickels et al. 1995; Shrivastava et al. 1992).

An example of antidepressant drug studies in SAD may be informative about the effect size–sample size issue. We reported a multi-center clinical trial of fluoxetine versus placebo in SAD (Lam et al. 1995). In this 5-week study involving 68 patients with depression, randomized to two groups, one of which received 20 mg fluoxetine, and the other placebo, we were unable to demonstrate a significant difference between active drug and placebo in the modified Hamilton Rating Scale for Depression (HAM-D) scores (M. Hamilton

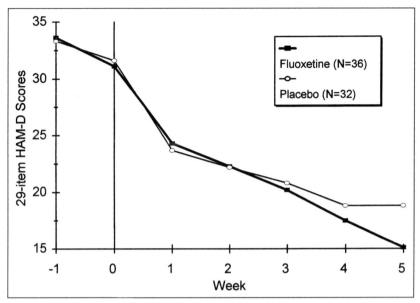

FIGURE 12-1. Mean depression scores versus week of treatment in 68 patients with SAD, randomized to 5 weeks of treatment with fluoxetine (20 mg/day) or placebo drug.
Source. From Lam et al. 1995.

1967; Williams et al. 1988); both groups significantly improved compared to baseline (Figure 12–1). However, when we examined the clinical response rates (defined as greater than 50% reduction of posttreatment scores compared with baseline scores), we found that the fluoxetine response rate (about 60%) was significantly higher than the placebo response rate (about 35%, $P < .05$). The placebo response rate was similar in magnitude to that in most outpatient studies of nonseasonal depression, thereby suggesting that patients with SAD do not have higher pill placebo responses than patients with nonseasonal depression. We also found that the greatest differences between the placebo and active drug were found in those patients with the highest baseline depression scores. That is, the more markedly depressed patients had the largest effect sizes.

In an 8-week study of sertraline versus placebo in SAD, the investigators found an effect size almost identical to that found in our fluoxetine study, with a difference between active drug and placebo of about 4 points on the HAM-D scale at study termination (Moscovitch et al. 1995). However, in this study the difference in HAM-D scores between sertraline and placebo was statistically significant ($P < .001$). The clinical response rates were also very similar to those in our study (59% response for sertraline versus 44% for placebo, $P < .05$). The major difference between the two studies was that Moscovitch and colleagues randomized 190 patients in their study, compared with the 68 patients in our study. Although the effect sizes were almost identical, the larger sample size allowed the results to be statistically significant.

These results raise the question of whether the effect sizes in the SAD antidepressant studies are smaller than those in studies of nonseasonal depression. The evidence does not support this hypothesis. A recent meta-analysis of clinical trials found a very similar effect size in most reported studies of antidepressant drugs in nonseasonal depression, with a mean difference between active drug and placebo of about 4 points on the HAM-D scale (Greenberg et al. 1992). What this illustrates is that a large placebo response is often found in outpatient depression studies, regardless of whether the depression is seasonal (Brown 1994; Lapierre 1995).

Recent studies may, however, provide more evidence to bolster the case for efficacy of light therapy. Lee (T. M. C, Lee, personal communication, November 1996) conducted a meta-analysis of light therapy studies to examine the intensity-response issue. Meta-analysis is a statistical technique that overcomes sample size limitations by comparing standardized effect sizes for each study, in contrast to the grouped analysis (which groups all patients in smaller studies as if they were in one large study) conducted by Terman et al. (1989). Rigorous and accepted techniques were utilized to sample, select, and examine 40 published and unpublished studies in the field. The results of this meta-analysis (which include the HMU studies) showed a clear dose-response relationship, as shown in Table 12–1. Medium intensity light (1,700–3,500 lux) showed a significantly greater treatment effect size (defined as the standardized difference between baseline depression scores and scores after treatment) than dim light (<600 lux), whereas strong light (greater than 6,000 lux) had the largest effect size of all. The 95% confidence intervals for

TABLE **12–1**

Effect of morning light therapy of different intensities on Hamilton Rating
Scale for Depression

Light intensity (lux)	Number of studies	Number of patients	Mean weighted effect size[1]	95% CI[2] for effect size
Dim (<600)	4	94	1.11	0.80–1.42
Medium (1,700–3500)	22	315	1.74	1.56–1.93
Strong (6,000–10.000)	3	40	2.94	2.30–3.58

[1] Effect size calculated from baseline to posttreatment, strong > medium > dim (ANOVA procedures following a fixed effect model, overall χ^2 value = 23.70, df = 2, $P < .05$).
[2] 95% confidence intervals (CI).
Source. From meta-analysis by Lee 1995.

each condition do not overlap, suggesting that this is a robust and clinically important finding.

Reports of two other recent studies also support the efficacy of light therapy. Terman and Terman (1996) and Eastman et al. (1996) conducted rigorous, well-designed, multiyear, placebo-controlled studies of light therapy in SAD. Interestingly, both used a similar placebo: negative ion generators. In Eastman and colleague's 4-week treatment, double-blind, parallel-design study, morning or evening light exposure (6,000-lux cool-white fluorescent light box for 1.5 hours/day) was compared to an equivalent time spent near a negative ion generator that was, unknown to the patient, turned off. A total of 96 patients were randomly assigned to one of the four conditions (morning light, evening light, morning placebo, evening placebo) over the 6-year study period. Clinical response was defined as greater than 50% reduction in HAM-D scores from baseline to a termination score of 8 or less. The morning light response rate was significantly greater than both the morning placebo and evening light response rates (54.5%, 16.1%, and 28.1%, respectively, $P < .05$) (Eastman et al. 1996).

The Termans compared morning or evening exposure from a 10,000-lux full-spectrum fluorescent light box for 30 minutes/day, with the same schedule of exposure to low- or high-density negative ions. Their study was a double-blind, crossover design, with each group receiving either a sequence of two 10-day treatment periods with light, or a 20-day treatment period with ions. Over 7 years, 144 patients were randomized to six groups: morning-morning light (i.e., 20 days of morning light), morning-evening light, evening-morning light, evening-evening light, low-density negative ions, and high-density negative ions. The main findings were that 1) light therapy produced greater clinical response than did low-density negative ions (the putative placebo condition), 2) morning light exposure was superior to evening light, and 3) the high-density negative ion condition was superior to the low-density negative ions (Terman and Terman 1996).

What these studies show is that when effect sizes are considered (e.g., in a meta-analysis), light therapy is significantly more effective than placebo light conditions. There is also a dose-response effect in that higher-intensity light produces more marked clinical response. With sufficient sample sizes, well-designed prospective studies have clinical response rates that show clear superiority of light therapy over credible placebo conditions.

An important question raised by clinicians concerns the longer-term outcome in SAD. After all, SAD is defined as a recurrent illness, and for other recurrent depressions there is evidence that patients do best on continuous therapy such as maintenance antidepressants. Yet in SAD, the usual clinical recommendation is to discontinue treatment in the spring and summer, and resume treatment in the fall. Should patients with SAD be on maintenance light therapy all year round? Is intermittent (winter only) light therapy as effective as maintenance medication treatment? Can prophylactic use of light prevent episodes of depression? These questions require further study. At this point, treatment recommendations are based on risk assessment with the individual patient. Intermittent, seasonal light therapy can be considered for patients who are knowledgeable about their illness, have slow onset of symptoms, are able to recognize early signs of depression and begin treatment, and do not become severely depressed. The follow-up studies show that many patients with SAD do well with winter-only light therapy (Gallin et al. 1995; Schwartz et al. 1996; Thompson et al. 1995). This also recognizes, however, that some patients may do better on year-round medication or light maintenance. For some of these patients, an insidious onset of depression means that by the time they become aware that they are depressed, they lack the motivation to seek help or begin light treatment.

Nonseasonal depression is one area in which light may play an important future role. Daniel Kripke (this volume) makes a persuasive argument for greater use of light therapy in nonseasonal depression. Two of the three controlled studies with a larger sample size showed positive results after only 1 or 2 weeks of light treatment. Situations that may suggest the clinical use of light therapy include patient preference for a nonpharmacologic treatment, as augmentation for patients who respond partially or not at all to antidepressants (especially if there is winter worsening of symptoms), or if patients have difficulty tolerating side effects of medications. Again, the converging evidence that Edwin Tam and colleagues summarize in this volume, that bright light exposure may have direct serotonergic effects, makes the adjunctive use of light therapy attractive for some patients on serotonergic medications. This is certainly an area that will be fruitful for further study.

Light Therapy for Bulimia Nervosa and Premenstrual Depression

The chapters on seasonality of subsyndromal SAD and bulimia nervosa may be thematically linked by the concept of seasonality as a dimension rather than a categorical diagnosis. Behavioral genetics studies suggest that seasonality, as a dimensional behavior, may be inherited. Madden et al. (1996) demonstrated in a study of Australian twins that 29%–45% of the variability in seasonality scores from the Seasonal Pattern Assessment Questionnaire (SPAQ) (Rosenthal et al. 1987) could be explained by a genetic factor, accounting for about 40% of the phenotypic variance in symptoms. We recently replicated those findings in a Canadian twin cohort in which the phenotypic expression of seasonality was more apparent (Jang et al. 1997). We also found that the genetic heritability for seasonality was greater in males than in females, despite the fact that females seem to have greater seasonal variation of mood (Kasper et al. 1989). We have speculated that the male genetic factor may be protective for seasonality, whereas the female factor is a vulnerability factor.

In the chapter on bulimia nervosa, Elliot Goldner and I suggest that seasonality in bulimia nervosa may be linked to SAD via a common pathophysiology such as serotonergic dysfunction (Lam and Goldner, this volume). Thus, serotonergic dysregulation may make someone susceptible to both seasonality and a particular mood or eating disorder. Interestingly, serotonergic disturbances are also implicated in premenstrual dysphoric disorder (PMDD) (Ashby et al. 1988; Bancroft et al. 1991; Yatham 1993), for which serotonergic medications are effective treatments (e.g., Brzezinski et al. 1990; Steiner et al. 1995). Do women with PMDD also demonstrate seasonal patterns? Our group recently used a modified version of the SPAQ to study seasonal symptoms patterns in women with late luteal phase dysphoric disorder (LLPDD), the DSM-III-R (American Psychiatric Association 1987) equivalent to PMDD, ($N = 100$) and nonclinical control subjects ($N = 50$). The results showed a high rate of seasonal problems, seasonal depression, and seasonal (winter) patterns in premenstrual symptoms (Maskall et al. 1997). The SPAQ-derived Global Seasonality scores (see discussion in Lam and Goldner, this volume) of the LLPDD patients were significantly higher than those of the women who were not clinically affected (mean scores ±SD: 10.9 ± 4.6 versus 7.0 ± 4.5, $P < .001$). These results show that women with LLPDD have greater seasonal changes in mood, energy, appetite, weight, sleep, and social activity. Thirty-eight percent of the LLPDD group met SPAQ criteria (Kasper et al. 1989) for SAD, compared with 7% of the nonclinically affected comparison group ($P < .001$). Similar findings emerged with regard to the seasonality of the premenstrual symptoms. Twenty-seven percent of the women with LLPDD reported "marked" or "extremely marked" seasonal changes in their premenstrual symptoms, and 30% felt that their seasonal symptoms were "marked" or "severe" problems.

It appears that, similarly to the women with bulimia nervosa, one-third or more of women with LLPDD complain of marked to severe winter worsening of mood and premenstrual symptoms, to the extent that the symptoms are described as significant problems. There may also be a high comorbidity of LLPDD with SAD. Given this high rate of seasonality (and perhaps seasonal depression), perhaps light therapy during the winter season may be most useful as a sole or adjunctive biological treatment in managing winter exacerbation of LLPDD symptoms. Barbara Parry's preliminary studies on light treatment for LLPDD were promising, although (because the studies were conducted in San Diego) there were not likely many seasonally affected patients in her study samples. Unfortunately, her extended study did not demonstrate significant differences between the results of bright and dim light conditions (Parry, this volume). Note, however, that both the bright light and the dim light conditions led to significant improvement in symptoms. As discussed, a Type II error caused by the small sample size may result in missing a difference between the conditions, especially if there is a large placebo response. Placebo response rates in the premenstrual syndrome literature are noted to be unusually high, with pill-placebo response rates of 19% to 88% reported (J. A. Hamilton et al. 1984).

One important limiting factor in Parry's studies may be that treatment was given during only a single menstrual cycle. Such a brief treatment period is more likely to lead to higher placebo responses because a patient need improve for only a short time to be considered a responder. We recently completed a small-sample ($N = 14$), controlled light therapy study of women with LLPDD, using two menstrual cycles of treatment (Lam et al. 1997). We compared two cycles of prospective baseline monitoring and no treatment, with two cycles each of an active bright light condition and a dim, placebo light condition in a randomized, crossover study design. The active light treatment consisted of daily 30-minute exposure to a 10,000-lux cool-white fluorescent light box in the early evening between 7:00 P.M. and 8:00 P.M., during the 2-week luteal phase. The control condition consisted of the same box with a red filter that was rated at 500 lux. As in our bulimia study (Lam et al. 1994), we used deception about study objectives to balance expectations between the two light conditions by telling patients we were investigating different wavelengths of light therapy. Outcome measures included the 29-item HAM-D and the Premenstrual Tension Scale (PMTS) (Steiner et al. 1980). For data analysis, the scores obtained during the follicular phase were subtracted from the scores obtained during the luteal phase; the difference score was then summed across both cycles of each condition (baseline, dim red light, bright white light).

Results are shown in Figures 12–2 and 12–3. There were significant improvements in the HAM-D and PMTS during the two cycles of bright white light compared to baseline (Friedman's two-way

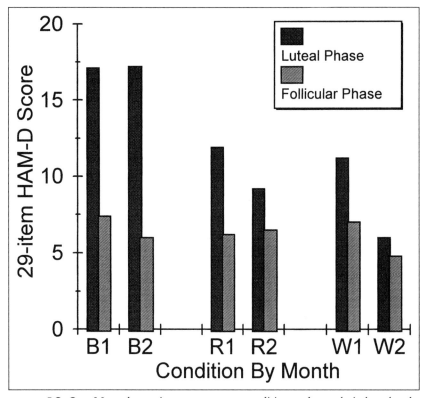

FIGURE 12–2. Mean depression scores versus condition and month, in luteal and follicular phases, in 14 patients with late luteal phase dysphoric disorder (LLPDD). Note that B1 = baseline, month 1; B2 = baseline, month 2; R1 = dim red light, month 1; R2 = dim red light, month 2; W1 = bright white light, month 1; W2 = bright white light, month 2.

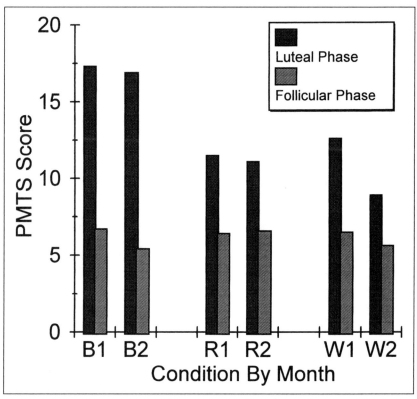

FIGURE 12–3. Mean scores on the Premenstrual Tension Scale (PMTS) versus condition and month, in luteal and follicular phases, in 14 patients with late luteal phase dysphoric disorder (LLPDD). Note that B1 = baseline, month 1; B2 = baseline, month 2; R1 = dim red light, month 1; R2 = dim red light, month 2; W1 = bright white light, month 1; W2 = bright white light, month 2.

ANOVA, $P < .05$), but no significant differences during the two cycles of dim red light. However, the figures also show that in first cycle, differences between the light conditions could not be distinguished. It was only during the second cycle that significant differences emerged, and that bright light was superior to dim light. These results hold for both mood and physical symptoms of premenstrual depression. Thus, a longer treatment duration over several menstrual cycles may be a key methodologic factor to ensure against Type II errors.

Light Therapy for Sleep and Circadian Disorders

Finally, the chapters by Rod Hughes and Alfred Lewy (this volume), and Ziad Boulos (this volume) illustrate the importance of light as a *zeitgeber* (synchronizer) of circadian rhythms. Regardless of the mechanism of action of light in seasonal disorders, the circadian phase-shifting effects of light will become increasingly important for treating circadian phase sleep disorders and disorders involving jet lag and shift work. Melatonin has recently received much public attention (some warranted, some not); although taking melatonin may be more convenient than light treatment, the phase-shifting effects of melatonin may not be as great as for bright light exposure. Indeed, in these circadian disorders, the phase-shifting effects of drugs such as melatonin may be for naught if the counteracting effects of bright light are not taken into account. Perhaps the use of combination therapy will be most effective for rapid phase shifting. Several popular books on jet lag (e.g., Oren et al. 1995) are now available to help the traveler schedule appropriate bright light and also, importantly, to know when to avoid bright light exposure, to optimize entrainment of circadian rhythms. These books are user-friendly and, with the caveats raised by Boulos (this volume), they take the complexity out of analyzing circadian phase position and shifts by providing simple charts based on the time zone at beginning of the journey, the time zone at destination, and the time taken for the journey itself.

The work of Scott Campbell (this volume) suggests that light therapy may also be a nonpharmacologic treatment for the insomnia found in the elderly, and for behavioral disturbances in dementia. Because of the wide prevalence of these disorders, and the vulnerability of the elderly to side effects of hypnotic medications, further development of a nonpharmacologic insomnia treatment is important. One of the limiting factors for light therapy has been subject compliance; it is very difficult for people (elderly or not) to sit in front of a light box for more than an hour a day. Thus, higher intensity light (e.g., 10,000 lux) should be studied to determine whether a similar intensity-duration relationship holds true for the sleep-consolidating effects as it appears to do in SAD. When using higher intensity light, as Daniel Kripke cautions (this volume), close attention should be made to retinal changes, especially in the elderly. Older people are more vulnerable to macular degeneration in the retina, which may be an asymptomatic condition in the elderly. Although there is no known direct effect of bright light on macular degeneration, it would be prudent to conduct baseline ophthalmologic assessments in older people before extended bright light exposure.

The Future

From seasonal depression to eating disorders to jet lag—a decade ago there was only speculation that light therapy would be effective for these conditions. Now, the therapeutic range of light treatment indeed seems broad, though much important research is still ahead of us. Clinical studies of light therapy are not well funded relative to antidepressant drug studies, so replication of smaller studies will be important to establish efficacy (as it is in other nonpharmacologic treatments such as psychotherapy) and encourage greater use of light therapy. Barriers that prevent wider clinical use of light therapy for SAD and other disorders include clinician inexperience with light treatment, or lack of knowledge of how to obtain a light box for clinical use. The impetus that drives the increasing clinical use of light may come more from patients as they strive to obtain the latest and most effective treatments. In this age of information, consumers may learn more about light therapy and circadian rhythms from the Internet than from their own doctors. For example, the Society for Light Treatment and Biological Rhythms (SLTBR) has a World Wide Web site (http://www.websciences.org/sltbr/) with links to a number of other Internet sites dealing with light therapy, SAD, and biological rhythms.

To buttress this enthusiasm for light therapy, however, there must be solid scientific evidence that supports the clinical application of light. The widespread use of light for any new clinical indication must be preceded by rigorous studies to demonstrate efficacy and optimal treatment parameters. The scientific studies of light therapy will need to consider the potential heterogeneity in diagnoses, and in the neural effects of light exposure. The mechanism of action of light and the psychobiology of many of the disorders under study are still not well understood. However, current evidence for therapeutic effects of light is substantial, the potential for future medical applications of light is enormous, and the increased research and clinical interest in light therapy appears well justified. The next decade in light research will no doubt provide more insights into basic mechanisms of light, as light becomes a standard treatment in our therapeutic armamentarium.

References

American Psychiatric Association: Diagnostic and Statistical Manual of Mental Disorders, 3rd Edition. Washington, DC, American Psychiatric Association, 1987

American Psychiatric Association: Diagnostic and Statistical Manual of Mental Disorders, 4th Edition. Washington, DC, American Psychiatric Association, 1994

Ashby CR Jr, Carr LA, Cook CL, et al: Alteration of platelet serotonergic mechanisms and monoamine oxidase activity in premenstrual syndrome. Biol Psychiatry 24:225–233, 1988

Bancroft J, Cook A, Davidson D, et al: Blunting of neuroendocrine responses to infusion of L-tryptophan in women with perimenstrual mood change. Psychol Med 21:305–312, 1991

Bauer MS, Dunner DL: Validity of seasonal pattern as a modifier for recurrent mood disorders for DSM-IV. Compr Psychiatry 34:159–170, 1993

Bialik RJ, Ravindran AV, Bakish D, et al: A comparison of placebo responders and nonresponders in subgroups of depressive disorder. J Psychiatry Neurosci 20:265–270, 1995

Brown WA: Is light therapy a placebo? Psychopharmacol Bull 26:527–530, 1990

Brown WA: Placebo as a treatment for depression. Neuropsychopharmacology 10:265–269, 1994

Brown WA, Dornseif BE, Wernicke JF: Placebo response in depression: a search for predictors. Psychiatry Res 26:259–264, 1988

Brown WA, Johnson MF, Chen MG: Clinical features of depressed patients who do and do not improve with placebo. Psychiatry Res 41:203–214, 1992

Brzezinski AA, Wurtman JJ, Wurtman RJ, et al: D-Fenfluramine suppresses the caloric intake and carbohydrate intakes and improves the mood of women with premenstrual depression. Obstet Gynecol 76:296–301, 1990

Eastman CI, Young MA, Fogg LF, et al: Light therapy for winter depression is more than a placebo, in SLTBR: Abstracts of the Annual Meeting of the Society for Light Treatment and Biological Rhythms, Vol. 8. Wheat Ridge, CO, Society for Llight Treatment and Biological Rhythms, 1996, p 5

Gallin PF, Terman M, Reme CE, et al: Ophthalmologic examination of patients with seasonal affective disorder, before and after bright light therapy. Am J Ophthalmology 119:202–10, 1995

Greenberg RP, Bornstein RF, Greenberg MD, et al: A meta-analysis of antidepressant outcome under "blinder" conditions. J Consult Clin Psychol 60:664–669, 1992

Hamilton JA, Parry BL, Alagna S, et al: Premenstrual mood changes: a guide to evaluation and treatment. Psychiatr Ann 14:426–435, 1984

Hamilton M: Development of a rating scale for primary depressive illness. Br J Soc Clin Psychol 6:278–296, 1967

Holzer CE III, Nguyen HT, Hirschfeld RMA: Reliability of diagnosis in mood disorders. Psychiatr Clin N Am 19:73–84, 1996

Jang KL, Lam RW, Livesley WJ, et al: Gender differences in the heritability of seasonal mood change. Psychiatry Res 70:145–154, 1997

Kasper S, Wehr TA, Bartko JJ, et al: Epidemiological findings of seasonal changes in mood and behavior. A telephone survey of Montgomery County, Maryland. Arch Gen Psychiatry 46: 823–833, 1989

Lam RW, Stewart JN: Validity of atypical depression in the DSM-IV. Compr Psychiatry 37:375–383, 1996

Lam RW, Goldner EM, Solyom L, et al: A controlled study of light therapy for bulimia nervosa. Am J Psychiatry 151:744–750, 1994

Lam RW, Gorman C, Michalon M, et al: A multicentre, placebo-controlled study of fluoxetine in seasonal affective disorder. Am J Psychiatry 152: 1765–1770, 1995

Lam RW, Carter D, Misri S, et al: A controlled study of light therapy in premenstrual dysphoric disorder (abstract), in American Psychiatric Association New Research Abstracts of the 150th Annual Meeting. Washington, DC, American Psychiatric Association, 1997, p 189

Lapierre YD: Placebo: a potent but misunderstood psychotrope. J Psychiatr Neurosci 20:173–174, 1995

Madden PA, Heath AC, Rosenthal NE, et al: Seasonal changes in mood and behavior. The role of genetic factors. Arch Gen Psychiatry 53: 47–55, 1996

Maskall DD, Lam RW, Misri S, et al: Seasonality of symptoms in women with late luteal phase dysphoric disorder. Am J Psychiatry 154: 1436–1441, 1997

Moscovitch A, Blashko C, Wiseman R, et al: A double-blind, placebo-controlled study of sertraline in patients with seasonal affective disorder (abstract), in American Psychiatric Association: New Research Abstracts of the 148th Annual Meeting. Washington, DC, American Psychiatric Association, 1995, p 146

Oren DA, Reich W, Rosenthal NE, et al: How to Beat Jet Lag: A Practical Guide for Air Travelers. New York, Henry Holt, 1995

Rickels K, Robinson DS, Schweizer E, et al: Nefazodone: aspects of efficacy. J Clin Psychiatry 56(suppl 6):43–46, 1995

Rosenthal NE, Bradt GH, Wehr TA: Seasonal Pattern Assessment Questionnaire. Bethesda, MD, National Institute of Mental Health, 1987

Sakamoto K, Nakadaira S, Kamo K, et al: A longitudinal follow-up study of seasonal affective disorder. Am J Psychiatry 152, 862–868, 1995

Schwartz PJ, Brown C, Wehr TA, et al: Winter seasonal affective disorder: a follow-up study of the first 59 patients of the National Institute of Mental Health Seasonal Studies Program. Am J Psychiatry 153:1028–1036, 1996

Shrivastava RK, Shrivastava SH, Overweg N, et al: A double-blind comparison of paroxetine, imipramine, and placebo in major depression. J Clin Psychiatry 53(suppl):48–51, 1992

Spitzer RL, Williams JBW: The validity of seasonal affective disorder, in Seasonal Affective Disorders and Phototherapy. Edited by Rosenthal NE, Blehar MC, New York, Guilford, 1989, pp 79–86

Steiner M, Haskett RF, Carroll BJ: Premenstrual tension syndrome: the development of research diagnostic criteria and new rating scales. Acta Psychiatr Scand 62:177–190, 1980

Steiner M, Steinberg S, Stewart D, et al: Fluoxetine in the treatment of premenstrual dysphoria. (Canadian Fluoxetine/Premenstrual Dysphoria Collaborative Study Group) N Engl J Med 332:1529–1534, 1995

Terman M, Terman JS, Quitkin FM, et al: Light therapy for seasonal affective disorder: a review of efficacy. Neuropsychopharmacology 2: 1–22, 1989

Terman M, Terman J: A multi-year controlled trial of bright light and negative ions, in SLTBR: Abstracts of the Annual Meeting of the Society for Light Treatment and Biological Rhythms, Vol. 8. Wheat Ridge, CO, Society for Light Treatment and Biological Rhythms, 1996, p 1

Thompson C, Rahija SK, King EA: A follow-up study of seasonal affective disorder. Br J Psychiatry 167:380–384, 1995

Wicki W, Angst J, Merikangas KR: The Zurich Study, XIV: epidemiology of seasonal depression. Eur Arch Psychiatry Clin Neurosci 241:301–6, 1992

Williams JBW, Link MJ, Rosenthal NE, et al: Structured Interview Guide for the Hamilton Depression Rating Scale—Seasonal Affective Disorders Version. New York, New York Psychiatric Unit, 1988

Yatham LN: Is 5HT-1A receptor subsensitivity a trait marker for late luteal phase dysphoric disorder? A pilot study. Can J Psychiatry 38:662–664, 1993

INDEX